D0162707

JOHNSON'S SURGERY OF THE CHEST
FIFTH EDITION

Johnson's
Surgery of the Chest

Fifth Edition

JOHN A. WALDHAUSEN, M.D.
John W. Oswald Professor of Surgery
Chairman, Department of Surgery
College of Medicine
The Pennsylvania State University
The Milton S. Hershey Medical Center
Hershey, Pennsylvania

WILLIAM S. PIERCE, M.D.
Professor of Surgery
Chief, Division of Artificial Organs
Division of Cardiothoracic Surgery
College of Medicine
The Pennsylvania State University
The Milton S. Hershey Medical Center
Hershey, Pennsylvania

Illustrated by
EDNA HILL
and
DAN BEISEL

YEAR BOOK MEDICAL PUBLISHERS, INC.
CHICAGO

Copyright © 1952, 1958, 1964, 1970, and 1985 by Year
Book Medical Publishers, Inc. All rights reserved. No
part of this publication may be reproduced, stored in a
retrieval system, or transmitted, in any form or by any
means, electronic, mechanical, photocopying, recording,
or otherwise, without prior written permission from the
publisher. Printed in the United States of America.

0 9 8 7 6 5 4 3 2 1

Library of Congress Cataloging in Publication Data
Johnson, Julian, 1906–
    Johnson's surgery of the chest.
    Rev. ed. of: Surgery of the chest / by Julian Johnson,
Horace MacVaugh, III, and John A. Waldhausen. 4th ed.
1970.
    Includes index.
    1. Chest—Surgery. I. Johnson, Julian, 1906–
Surgery of the chest. II. Waldhausen, John A., 1929–
III. Pierce, William S., 1937–   . IV. Title.
RD536.J59 1985   617′.54059   84-25766
ISBN 0-8151-9076-X

Sponsoring editor: Daniel J. Doody
Editing supervisor: Frances M. Perveiler
Production project manager: Sharon W. Pepping
Proofroom supervisor: Shirley E. Taylor

Contributors

Thomas V. N. Ballantine, M.D., Associate Professor of Surgery; Chief, Division of Pediatric Surgery, College of Medicine, The Pennsylvania State University, The Milton S. Hershey Medical Center, Hershey, Pennsylvania

David B. Campbell, M.D., Assistant Professor of Surgery, Division of Cardiothoracic Surgery, College of Medicine, The Pennsylvania State University, The Milton S. Hershey Medical Center, Hershey, Pennsylvania

William E. DeMuth, M.D., Emeritus Professor of Surgery, College of Medicine, The Pennsylvania State University, The Milton S. Hershey Medical Center, Hershey, Pennsylvania

Martin J. O'Neill, M.D., Assistant Professor of Surgery, Division of Cardiothoracic Surgery, College of Medicine, The Pennsylvania State University, The Milton S. Hershey Medical Center, Hershey, Pennsylvania

John L. Pennock, M.D., Associate Professor of Surgery, Division of Cardiothoracic Surgery; College of Medicine, The Pennsylvania State University, The Milton S. Hershey Medical Center, Hershey, Pennsylvania

William S. Pierce, M.D., Professor of Surgery, Division of Cardiothoracic Surgery; Chief, Division of Artificial Organs, College of Medicine, The Pennsylvania State University, The Milton S. Hershey Medical Center, Hershey, Pennsylvania

John A. Waldhausen, M.D., John W. Oswald Professor of Surgery, Chairman, Department of Surgery, College of Medicine, The Pennsylvania State University, The Milton S. Hershey Medical Center, Hershey, Pennsylvania

Foreword

It gives me great pleasure to introduce the Fifth Edition of this text and to have it bear the title *Johnson's Surgery of the Chest*. I am particularly pleased that John A. Waldhausen, my former associate, and William S. Pierce, my former resident, have edited this beautiful new edition and have maintained the fine tradition that the book has always enjoyed. The book has been extensively updated but still fulfills its fundamental purpose as a practical guide to chest and cardiac surgery. I am sure that it will be of great value to residents and practicing surgeons.

Julian Johnson, M.D.
Gladwyne, Pennsylvania

Preface to the First Edition

THIS BOOK is primarily an atlas of thoracic surgical operations. Our objective, both in the text and in the illustrations, has been to present the step by step details of operative technic in as clear a manner as possible. Nearly all operations of established value are included. The operative methods portrayed are those which we have found to be reliable. We believe that these methods, except for variations in minor technical details, are representative of those utilized by leaders in thoracic surgery throughout the world.

In addition to describing and illustrating operative technic, we have discussed the physiologic mechanisms which must be thoroughly understood by those who undertake thoracic surgical procedures and have stressed the abnormalities in function produced by many lesions. The features of preoperative, operative and postoperative care which are so important in assuring a successful outcome of many major intrathoracic procedures have been considered in some detail. Diagnostic technics of special value in thoracic surgery have been described in Chapter 1, but it has not been possible to include a discussion of the differential diagnosis, etiology, life history or pathology of most lesions for which the operations are performed.

In the selection and presentation of the material in this volume, we have tried to provide all the information needed by those with a background in general surgery who wish to learn the technic of thoracic surgical procedures. It has also been our desire to present the material clearly and simply enough so that students of thoracic surgery at any level of training may understand how the various operations are performed.

A bibliography has been purposely omitted and eponyms have been used in the titles of only a few operations. Progress in thoracic surgery has resulted from the efforts of a great many individuals. We believe that there is little to be gained by recording our own impressions concerning priority, and that great injustice might result from inadvertently omitting mention of important contributors. We hope it is clearly understood that only a few of the concepts and methods presented originated with us.

We wish to thank Year Book Medical Publishers for their splendid cooperation.

JULIAN JOHNSON, M.D.
CHARLES K. KIRBY, M.D.

Preface to the Fifth Edition

JULIAN JOHNSON and the late Charles Kirby originally published their short manual *Surgery of the Chest* in 1952. It soon became a classic in that students and residents dealing with surgery of the chest carried it around as their bible and would brush up on procedures late at night, before going to the operating room the next morning well prepared for the intricacies of the case at hand. Most senior thoracic surgeons in this country and abroad still own, somewhere, a tattered copy: testimony to the book's intense and practical use.

It has been 15 years since the last edition appeared. In the interim much that is new in thoracic and cardiac surgery has occurred. This edition addresses these advances and changes without altering the basic concept of the book. It is still written for the student, resident, and thoracic surgeon as a basic guide in the operating room. It is still the view of only one group of surgeons working in one cardiothoracic surgical clinic. In general, only how they practice cardiothoracic surgery is described. Rarely is an alternative approach presented. All diagnostic studies have been omitted, as have most aspects of preoperative and postoperative care, since they are complex enough to form separate subjects. As in the original text, no references are included because they add little to the information needed prior to an operation. Thus, the book truly focuses on "how to."

The general thoracic portion (Part I) has been extensively revised. However, we have kept most of the original and superb illustrations by Edna Hill. The cardiac portion (Parts II, III, and IV) has been completely redone in both text and illustrations. Dan Beisel has contributed almost all of the new drawings. His work is in the detailed and magnificent tradition of the late Edna Hill's as well as in that of his teachers in the Department of Medical Illustrations of the Johns Hopkins University School of Medicine.

We thank the Culpepper Foundation for its generous support in underwriting a large portion of the cost of redoing the book and in making the volumes more accessible to students and residents. We also thank Daniel J. Doody of the Year Book Medical Publishers, Inc., for his assistance and sage advice. It has been a great pleasure working with him.

We thank Marian T. Waldhausen, who made helpful suggestions in changing and correcting the sometimes unintelligible text; she was most patient, especially, with the senior editor. Kathleen Corbin typed and retyped the text, and we are most grateful to her for the many hours she worked on the manuscript.

This book is dedicated, with esteem and respect, to Julian Johnson, a pioneer thoracic surgeon: "A surgeon and something more."[*]

JOHN A. WALDHAUSEN, M.D.
WILLIAM S. PIERCE, M.D.

---

[*] Julian Johnson: A Surgeon and Something More; Presidential Address to the American Association for Thoracic Surgery. *J. Thorac. Cardiovasc. Surg.* 46:141–149, 1963.

Contents

Part I

Thoracic Surgery

CHAPTER 1

The Physiology and Management of Chest Injuries

SURGICAL PHYSIOLOGY OF THE THORAX

An understanding of the basic mechanics of respiration and of cardiorespiratory physiology is essential for success in thoracic surgery and the management of chest injuries. Abnormal function cannot be accurately interpreted unless normal physiologic processes are understood.

Normally, intrapleural pressure is slightly below atmospheric pressure. It is the presence of this negative pressure within the thorax that maintains the lungs in their constantly expanded state. When the thoracic cage enlarges on inspiration, as a result of the action of the respiratory muscles, and the diaphragms pull downward, the subatmospheric pressure is further decreased. The elastic lungs follow the chest wall outward, and air is sucked in through the tracheobronchial tree. On expiration, when the respiratory muscles and diaphragms relax, the thoracic cage returns toward a resting position, and air is expelled from the lungs. The normal intrapleural pressure varies from about −9 to −12 cm of water on inspiration and from about −3 to −6 cm of water on expiration.

Figs 1–1, A and B.—The mechanics of normal respiration are illustrated diagrammatically.

OPEN PNEUMOTHORAX

When there is a large opening in the chest wall, such as a thoracotomy incision or a shell fragment wound, an open pneumothorax exists. This is commonly called a "sucking wound" of the chest because of the harsh, sucking noise which is frequently heard on inspiration, when the wound edges are not widely separated.

C and D.—The abnormalities in open pneumothorax are shown. Air from the outside rushes into the pleural cavity, since it is at a lower pressure. The lung, which in its noninflated state is smaller than the chest cavity, now collapses. On inspiration, more air enters the pleural cavity through the chest wall opening than through the smaller glottic aperture. The intrapleural air competes for space with the effective ventilatory air within the lungs. As the intact chest wall on the opposite side expands on inspiration, the mediastinum is pulled over by the increased negative pressure, and the contralateral lung cannot expand completely. On expiration, more air passes out through the opening in the chest wall than through the glottis, and the mediastinum swings back to the midline or beyond it. This to-and-fro motion of the mediastinum is called mediastinal flutter. The mediastinum moves paradoxically with respect to the intact chest wall; as a result, there is a useless interchange of poorly oxygenated air between the two lungs. There are also pathologic alterations in circulatory dynamics in open pneumothorax. The efficiency of the pumping action of the thorax in returning venous blood to the right heart is impaired. The great vessels, particularly the venae cavae, may be kinked by mediastinal flutter.

These abnormalities must be corrected in treating open wounds of the thorax and must be counteracted during intrathoracic operations. An open chest wound should be converted to a closed pneumothorax as soon as possible. During intrathoracic operations, the effects of open pneumothorax are counteracted by intermittently raising the intrapulmonary pressure above that of the atmosphere. This maintains expansion of the lungs and provides a pressure differential which produces adequate ventilation.

NORMAL RESPIRATION

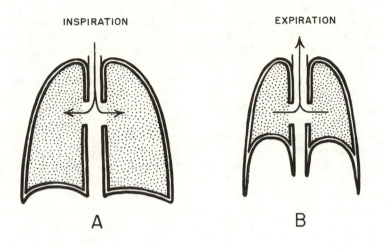

INSPIRATION

A

EXPIRATION

B

OPEN PNEUMOTHORAX

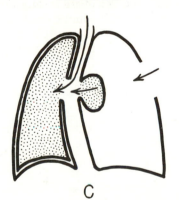

INSPIRATION

C

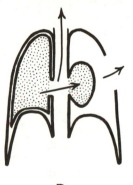

EXPIRATION

D

TENSION PNEUMOTHORAX

Injury or spontaneous rupture of the pulmonary parenchyma may cause an air leak with a valvelike mechanism. Air enters the pleural cavity as bronchi dilate on inspiration but cannot leave the pleural cavity as bronchi contract on expiration. The intrapleural pressure rises steadily; ill effects result from positive pressure within the closed hemithorax. Positive pressure is further increased when more air is forced into the pleural cavity during coughing. The ipsilateral lung is compressed, the mediastinum is pushed to the opposite side, and the contralateral lung is finally compressed. When the positive pressure rises to about 15–20 cm of water, venous return to the heart is markedly impeded.

Fig 1–2, A.—The effects of tension pneumothorax are illustrated diagrammatically. The distribution of air which may result is shown by the arrows. *Arrow 1* is the leak from the wound of the lung into the pleural cavity. *Arrows 2 and 3* represent the passage of air into the tissues of the chest wall and mediastinum through openings in the parietal and mediastinal pleurae. *Arrow 4* indicates air that has dissected proximally in the peribronchial tissues and entered the mediastinum without first entering the pleural cavity. *Arrow 5* represents leakage of air into the mediastinum through a wound of the trachea. Coughing and straining force large amounts of air into the mediastinum when there is a tracheal wound. A tracheostomy may relieve the problem by preventing the development of high intratracheal pressure. The patient may gently massage his eyelids laterally, displacing the air so that he can see. However, the air may return until the pressure forcing the air into the tissue planes is relieved.

B.—Large amounts of air may be forced into the tissue planes by tension pneumothorax. The tremendous inflation of facial tissues, shown here, resulted from a wound of the trachea. In this instance, air dissected down the arms to the fingers and down through the abdominal wall and retroperitoneal tissues to the groin.

A

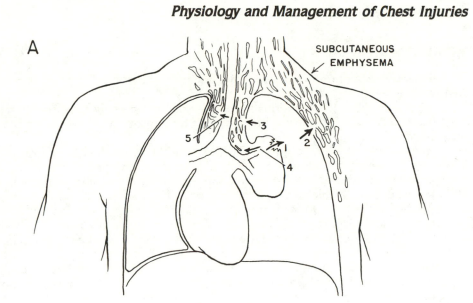

SUBCUTANEOUS
EMPHYSEMA

B

PARADOXICAL MOTION

Paradoxical motion occurs when the integrity of any portion of the thoracic bellows is lost.

Figs 1–3, A and B.—Normally, on inspiration, all portions of the thoracic cage move outward while the diaphragms move downward. Motion is in the opposite direction on expiration.

C and D.—When a portion of the chest wall becomes flexible as a result of losing its bony support, motion of the flexible area is controlled by the changing intrapleural pressures and is in a direction opposite to that of the normal portions of the chest wall. The flexible area is pulled inward on inspiration and pushed outward on expiration. This "paradoxical" motion occurs following thoracoplasty, multiple rib fractures, and diaphragmatic paralysis. Ventilatory efficiency is obviously decreased by the abnormal motion of a portion of the thoracic bellows. In addition, there is a useless exchange of stagnant air within the lungs. On inspiration, air is "inhaled" from the portion of the lung underlying the area of paradoxical motion into expanding portions of both lungs; on expiration, part of the expiratory air is "exhaled" into the portion of the lung that balloons out the flexible portion of the chest wall. On inspiration the mediastinum is pulled toward the opposite side, and on expiration it swings back to the midline or beyond it. If the area of paradoxical motion is large and there is a wide swing of the mediastinum, circulatory dynamics may be seriously altered. The venous pressure rises, filling of the right side of the heart is inadequate, and the arterial pressure eventually falls. Paradoxical motion may be increased by atelectasis.

NORMAL RESPIRATION

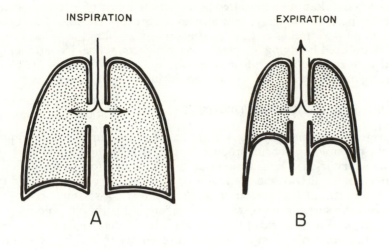

INSPIRATION   EXPIRATION

A   B

PARADOXICAL MOTION

INSPIRATION   EXPIRATION

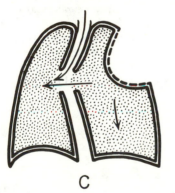   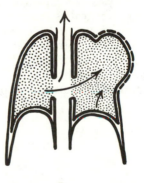

C   D

PENETRATING AND BLUNT CHEST INJURY

Injury to the chest may be caused by any of the forms of external violence that damage other parts of the body. Injuries may be broadly classified into two types: those caused by penetrating and by nonpenetrating, or blunt, assaults. Penetrating wounds are inflicted by flying missiles or sharp objects, while deceleration injuries, associated with automobile accidents and falls, account for most of the blunt injuries. Blast injuries, prevalent in warfare, are included in the latter group.

EMERGENCY EVALUATION AND TREATMENT

Management of chest injuries must be based on recognition and prompt treatment of the physiologic deficits produced rather than on specific therapy directed toward the injury itself. Oxygenation can be interrupted for only minutes, so the establishment of an airway and the return of effective alveolar ventilation must be provided before complete examination is possible. Initial assessment can be made in seconds when the surgeon understands the underlying pathophysiology.

An open, sucking wound of the thorax is immediately apparent on inspection. The open pneumothorax must be converted promptly to a closed pneumothorax (Fig 1–4).

If dyspnea is present, the cause can usually be determined by auscultation of the chest. The chief possibilities to be considered are compression of the pulmonary parenchyma by blood or air within the pleural space and obstruction of the airway by blood or tracheobronchial secretions. With compression of pulmonary parenchyma, breath sounds are diminished or absent, and the mediastinum is shifted to the opposite side. Tube thoracostomy enables removal of sufficient air or blood to relieve dyspnea. Partial obstruction of the airway produces rales and rhonchi. There may be hemoptysis. If the patient cannot clear the trachea and bronchi by spontaneous coughing, tracheal aspiration and bronchoscopy may be necessary. Intubation affords access for tracheal aspiration and ensures the vital airway. Occasionally, cricothyroidotomy or tracheostomy is required if tracheal intubation cannot be achieved, e.g., in the presence of severe facial injuries.

Shock is usually the result of blood loss. In the absence of a large hemothorax, intraperitoneal injury is usually responsible when external blood loss is not apparent.

The appropriate crystalloid solution and blood should be given without delay. Hypoxia may cause or aggravate circulatory failure; abnormalities in cardiorespiratory function resulting from injury may cause hypoxia, thus setting up a vicious cycle. Care should be taken not to overtransfuse on the assumption that blood loss is the sole cause of shock.

In the presence of a massive hemothorax, it is wise to move rapidly to the operating room for resuscitation. A thoracotomy may be required, and, if the tamponading effect of the hemothorax is providing hemostasis to major vessel injury, release of the tamponade may lead to exsanguination. However, this is not common, since most major injuries to the heart and great vessels are either immediately fatal or self-limiting and resolve without immediate operative intervention; fewer than 10% of patients require a thoracotomy. When operation is indicated, the control of hemorrhage should not be thwarted by inadequate exposure of the chest cavity.

Tension pneumothorax occurs when a large amount of air under pressure enters the pleural cavity. Subcutaneous emphysema is often an associated finding. Tube drainage of the air should be instituted immediately to prevent the development of high intrapleural pressure. If the leak is large and the lung does not reexpand with tube suction, rupture of the trachea or bronchus must be considered. When bronchoscopy confirms the presence of a rupture, a thoracotomy should be performed and the rent sutured.

Paradoxical motion is caused by severe injuries which produce multiple rib fractures. Care should be taken to inspect the posterior as well as the anterior thorax. Major paradox, associated with a flail chest, is best treated with mechanical ventilation using a volume-cycled ventilator. Respiratory support may be required for many days or weeks until the stability of the chest wall is restored by healing. Prolonged tracheal intubation raises the specter of tracheal pressure necrosis and stricture, best avoided by using a low-pressure tube cuff.

After the emergency has been controlled and adequate respiratory mechanics have been reestablished, certain problems require continued attention (see Fig 1–4).

An open chest wound is a serious emergency, the ill effects of which have been previously discussed. The open pneumothorax must be converted to a closed pneumothorax as soon as possible.

Fig 1–4, A.—An open wound caused by a shell fragment is illustrated diagrammatically.

B.—The wound is occluded with a gauze dressing so that the mechanics of respiration are those of a closed, rather than open, pneumothorax. Under field conditions, the gauze dressing may be released on expiration during several respiratory cycles in order to expel a large amount of the intrapleural air. Thoracentesis is done if a needle and syringe are available. Tight adhesive strapping is then applied over the dressing. The possibility of a subsequent tension pneumothorax must be kept in mind. Whenever possible, the insertion of a chest catheter, either next to the packing or in another location, is desirable. Air may be aspirated or the tube may be placed on waterseal drainage.

C.—After shock is controlled and the patient's condition is stabilized, the wound is debrided. Foreign material as well as necrotic and severely damaged tissue is removed. The intrathoracic injuries are cautiously inspected. If repair of an intrathoracic injury or the removal of an intrathoracic foreign body is required, access may be gained by either extending the initial wound or making a separate thoracostomy incision. The retention of radiolucent objects (shotgun or shell wads, wood, clothing fragments, etc.) should be considered.

D.—An airtight closure of the debrided wound is performed and a chest tube is inserted. When an air leak is suspected, a second chest tube is placed in the apex of the chest.

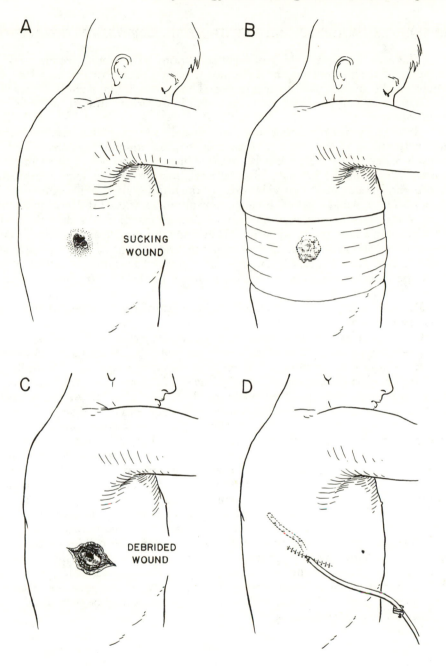

TENSION PNEUMOTHORAX AND SUBCUTANEOUS EMPHYSEMA: TREATMENT

The pathologic physiology of these conditions is illustrated (see Fig 1–2). The diagnosis of tension pneumothorax is not usually difficult to make and depends largely on the suspicion of its occurrence. The mediastinum is shifted toward the contralateral side of the chest, and breath sounds are either diminished or absent on the involved side.

Emergency treatment consists of lowering the intrapleural pressure by permitting air to escape to the outside. When thoracentesis equipment is unavailable, the largest obtainable needle should be inserted into the second or third interspace anteriorly. If a needle is unavailable, a small incision, made with any available instrument, is held open to provide egress of the trapped air. The insertion of a chest tube provides reliable relief of the pneumothorax and affords the best opportunity for uncomplicated expansion of the lung. Although insertion of a chest tube with a stylet has been advocated by some, we believe that this is generally to be condemned in view of the significant risk of puncturing the lungs, the heart, or the great vessels.

Fig 1–5, A.—A local anesthetic is infiltrated and a small skin incision is made where the chest tube is to be inserted, usually in the midaxillary line at about the fourth or fifth interspace.

B.—It is safest to thrust the finger into the pleural cavity to be certain about its position prior to tube insertion.

C.—The tube is inserted with the aid of a Kelly clamp.

D.—The tube is held in place by a skin suture to prevent its withdrawal.

E.—Negative pressure (−10 to −15 cm of water) is applied. Chest tube suction is best performed as shown. A bottle serves as a *drainage trap*. Any fluid accumulating can be measured. A second bottle, partly filled with saline solution or water, serves as an underwater seal, or *water trap,* to prevent entrance of air into the chest should suction be interrupted or absent. The negative intrapleural pressure will raise the fluid in the tube, partially under water, to a level proportionate to the negative pressure in the intrapleural space. The final bottle determines the amount of suction applied—the greater the height through which the air must be bubbled, the greater the amount of suction. The three bottles have been incorporated in their function in a commercially made disposable plastic unit. The suction usually removes air more rapidly than it enters the pleural cavity and allows increased expansion of the lung. Stronger suction to permit more rapid air removal is occasionally necessary.

Tracheal intubation tends to prevent the development of high intrabronchial pressures associated with coughing and straining against the closed glottis and, therefore, may aid in stopping the air leak more quickly. In addition, tracheal intubation ensures an adequate airway. Occasionally, in the presence of extreme subcutaneous emphysema, a suprasternal space incision may be helpful in permitting the escape of mediastinal air.

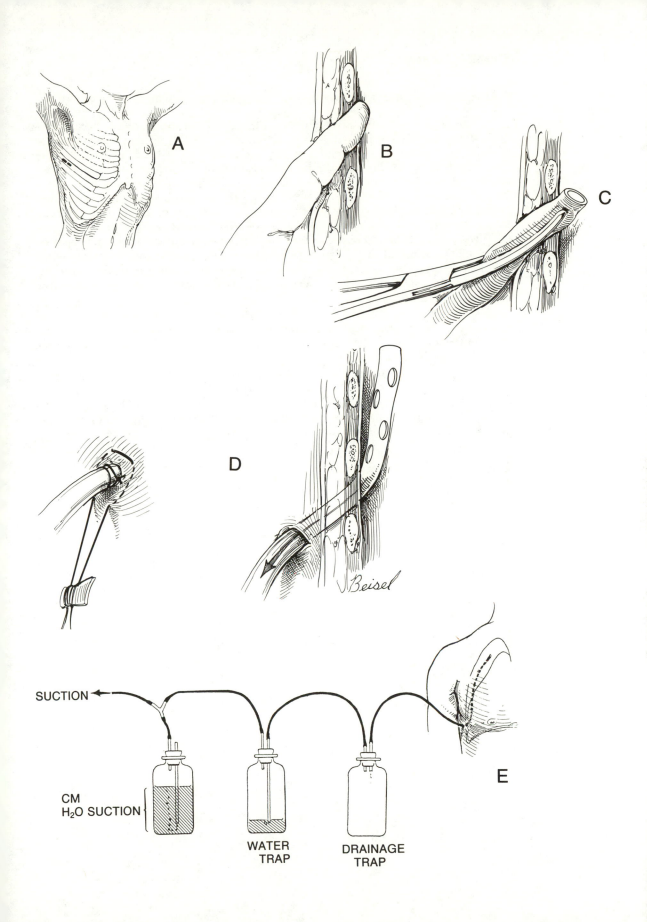

A

B

C

D

Beisel

E

SUCTION

CM
H₂O SUCTION

WATER
TRAP

DRAINAGE
TRAP

FLAIL CHEST: TREATMENT

The mechanism and adverse effects of paradoxical motion have been previously described (see Fig 1–3). This phenomenon is caused by injuries which produce multiple rib fractures.

Fig 1–6, A.—There are double fractures of the fifth through the ninth ribs. Motion of this large flail segment of the chest wall is controlled by the changing intrapleural pressure. The flail area moves inward on inspiration and outward on expiration. The method of treatment depends on the degree of impairment of ventilation as manifested by clinical status and by serial blood gas determinations.

B.—When little interference with ventilation is manifest, large gauze pads or other suitable material may be pressed into the flexible area, forming a stent. Firm adhesive strapping is applied, and a sandbag may be added for further support. Circumferential strapping impairs ventilation and may result in atelectasis and pneumonia. It should be avoided.

C.—Significant pulmonary function impairment is best treated by mechanical ventilation. This is provided by tracheal intubation and intermittent positive-pressure ventilation using a volume-cycled ventilator. Ventilatory support may be required for many days or weeks.

D.—The inspiratory phase of respiration produces a positive airway pressure which splints the flail segment and eliminates the paradoxical motion. As a result of the positive airway pressure, any lung leaks will be enhanced, with the attendant risk of tension pneumothorax. A preexisting pneumothorax should be managed by the insertion of a chest tube prior to instituting mechanical ventilation.

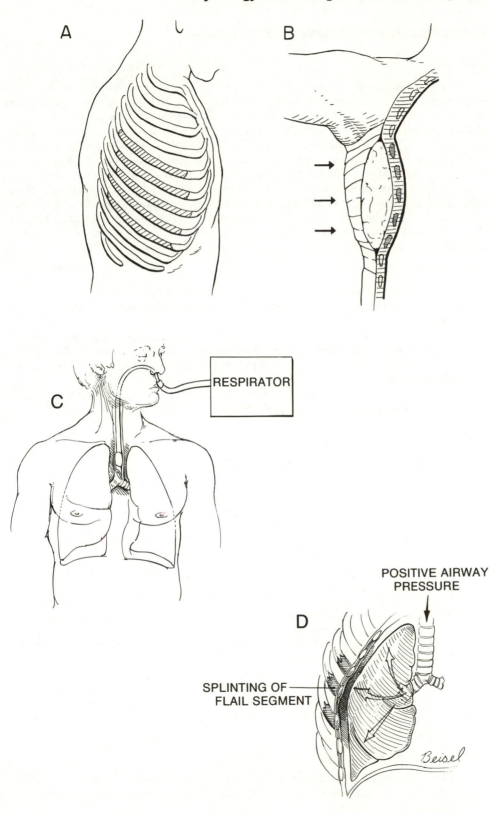

A

B

C

RESPIRATOR

D

POSITIVE AIRWAY
PRESSURE

SPLINTING OF
FLAIL SEGMENT

Beisel

PROBLEMS COMMON TO MANY CHEST INJURIES

Wet Lung

Tracheobronchial secretions ("wet lung") are a problem of as great importance in chest injuries as they are in many other phases of thoracic surgery. Causative factors are: (1) bleeding into the bronchi caused by laceration or contusion of the pulmonary parenchyma; (2) increased mucopurulent secretions caused by parenchymal injury; (3) hypoventilation and ineffective coughing due to pain. To these factors must be added the ventilatory impairment of the adult respiratory distress syndrome (ARDS), commonly associated with major trauma and sepsis.

Atelectasis is a constant threat and is easier to prevent than to treat. Relief of pain, humidification of inspired air, deep breathing, tracheal aspiration, and bronchoscopy are all useful in preventing atelectasis. The early institution of mechanical ventilation and positive end–expiratory pressure (PEEP), where required, is of enormous value in management.

Hemothorax

Collection of blood in the pleural cavity accompanes a high percentage of chest injuries. Proper management is important in shortening convalescence and preventing disability.

Patients with massive hemothorax should be moved to an operating room, where immediate thoracotomy can be performed should the insertion of chest tubes result in life-threatening bleeding owing to loss of tamponade. Autotransfusion may be of considerable value in the management of these patients.

Lesser degrees of hemothorax can be managed by chest tube insertion. Blood that is allowed to remain in the pleural cavity may require many weeks to absorb.

Clotted Hemothorax

Even when the policy of early evacuation of hemothorax is followed, clotting may occur before any or all of the intrapleural blood is removed. Why clotting occurs in some patients and not in others is probably related to the rapidity of bleeding. Defibrination with respiration will be less effective with rapid blood accumulation. Clotted blood can no longer be removed by thoracentesis or tube drainage. If the clotted blood is allowed to remain in the pleural cavity, pulmonary function may be permanently impaired. A layer of fibrin forms over the visceral and parietal pleura and prevents complete expansion of the lung. The clot is invaded by fibroblasts, and a fibrothorax develops, which limits the motion of the diaphragm and the thoracic cage on the involved side.

To prevent this series of events, the clotted blood must be removed. Fibrolytic enzymes have been useful in some patients. Under favorable circumstances, the blood clot is liquefied by these enzymes, and the blood may then be removed by thoracentesis. If use of the enzymes is unsuccessful, the patient should be operated on and a decortication of the lung performed.

Whether decortication should be performed depends on the amount of clotted blood within the pleural cavity. If a large amount is present and permanent impairment of pulmonary function seems likely, decortication is clearly indicated. If a small amount is present, the operation is not justifiable. Good judgment is required in borderline cases.

Infected Clotted Hemothorax

When infection is present in a clotted hemothorax, the blood clot must be removed and the lung promptly reexpanded. When there is a large amount of infected clot, decortication should be done. If the collection is small, it may be treated by open drainage with removal of blood clots.

Simple Rib Fractures

Simple fractures of one or more ribs at only one place is the most common chest injury in civilian life. Complications are uncommon but must be carefully excluded. Pain may be relieved by adhesive strapping, administration of analgesics, or intercostal nerve block.

Costochondral and Costosternal Separation

Dislocation of the articulations of the ribs from their costal cartilages, or of the cartilages from the sternum, usually requires no treatment other than relief of pain, unless it appears important to prevent the mild deformity which may result. A small incision is made and anatomic realignment is established by manipulation of the displaced fragment with a towel clip. An uncommon and painful sequela of costochondral separation is "slipping rib," which is the intermittent rubbing together of the articular surfaces. Excision of a short segment of rib adjacent to the cartilage may be required if the pain is severe.

Crushing Injuries

Violent injury of the chest wall by a blunt object or sudden, forceful squeezing of the chest between blunt objects results in the serious and characteristic syndrome known as a "crushing injury." Several ribs are fractured at two or more places, and the chest wall in the involved area is "flail." Paradoxical motion is prominent, and a major pulmonary contusion may lie beneath the flail segment. Shock, hemothorax, and atelectasis are almost invariably present, and tension pneumothorax, sometimes bilateral, may develop. Mechanical ventilation and other measures appropriate for the separate features of the injury are the mainstays of treatment.

Penetrating and Perforating Wounds

Penetrating wounds have only a site of entry, whereas perforating wounds have both a site of entry and a site of exit. Once an airway and ventilation are ensured, the next consideration is whether exsanguinating bleeding is imminent.

Most wounds of this type may be treated without operation except debridement of the chest wall. Blood loss and hemothorax are the principal problems. All the other problems discussed previously must be suspected and, if present, treated. After the immediate emergency period is past, it must be kept in mind that the aims of treatment are early reexpansion of the lung and the full restoration of pulmonary function.

Thoracoabdominal Wounds

Gunshot wounds and stab wounds which enter the body above or below the diaphragm may traverse both the pleural and abdominal cavities. The abdominal viscera most prone to massive blood loss when injured lies in that portion of the peritoneal cavity within the thoracic cage. The nipple line marks the level of the diaphragm in most patients. The extent of the chest injury is evaluated in the usual way and presents no unusual diagnostic problems. Peritoneal lavage is a helpful adjunct in determining the need for laparotomy. When laparotomy is indicated, a thoracoabdominal incision may be employed if circumstances suggest that the injury is confined to the upper abdominal viscera. There should be no hesitation to employ a long midline abdominal incision to give adequate exposure for the repair of intra-abdominal structures.

Blast Injury

Detonation of high-energy explosives creates an intense positive pressure followed by a relatively negative pressure in the immediate vicinity of the explosion. The blast range of nuclear weapons detonations is considerably greater. Blast pressure raises intravascular and intrapulmonary pressure, causing rupture of blood vessels and in some instances rupture of alveoli. The contusive effect on the unprotected chest wall is additive. Cerebral hemorrhage is common. Pulmonary edema and hemorrhage into the tracheobronchial tree lead to hypoxemia. Hemothorax is uncommon. Tracheobronchial aspiration, administration of oxygen, and mechanical ventilation with PEEP are helpful.

RELIEF OF PAIN FOLLOWING CHEST INJURIES

The procedures which are helpful in relieving posttraumatic chest pain, in addition to the administration of analgesics, are adhesive strapping and intercostal nerve block. Circumferential strapping should be avoided because it tends to restrict ventilation. Alternatively, application of an elastic rib belt is helpful and not as restrictive.

Fig 1–7, A.—Elastic Velcro-fastener belt.

B.—The classic type of strapping is illustrated. The hair is shaved and tincture of benzoin is applied to protect the skin. Tape sensitivity and excessive skin traction lead to skin blistering.

C.—Intercostal nerve blocks are often helpful in relieving pain. The best results are obtained when two or three nerves above and below the level of injury are blocked. Using a local anesthetic, skin wheals are raised with a hypodermic syringe over the lower rib borders, just lateral to the transverse processes.

D.—A larger needle is used for infiltrating the chest wall with the anesthetic solution. The technique recommended is to touch the rib lightly with the needle tip and then move the needle downward, far enough to clear the inferior rib border. There is such wide variation in the thickness of the chest wall that the depth of the nerve cannot be determined accurately without using the rib as a landmark. No attempt is made to inject into the nerve directly. When the needle tip is just below the rib border, the plunger of the syringe is pulled outward to make certain a vessel has not been entered. Approximately 5 ml of 0.25% to 0.75% bupivacaine hydrochloride and epinephrine injection (1 : 200,000) is injected around each intercostal nerve. This long-acting drug usually gives substantial relief for several hours and indeed may break the cycle of repeated episodes of pain related to muscle spasm. Repeat injections may be required. The serious complications of this procedure are intravascular injection and puncture of the lung, with pneumothorax. These complications are due to errors in technique and with care can be avoided.

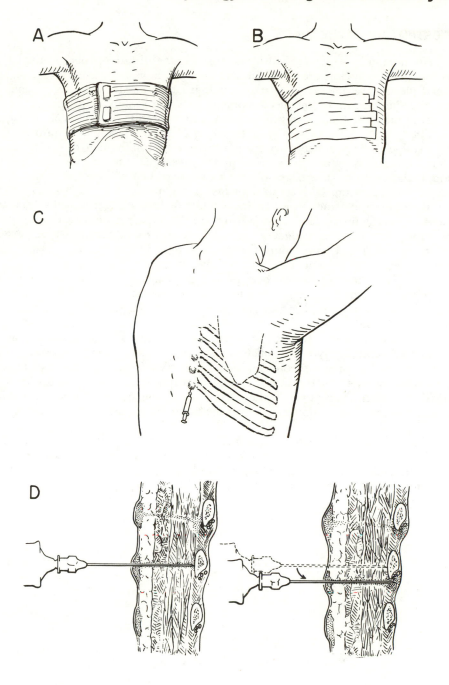

DECORTICATION OF THE LUNG

An incision is made in the fifth intercostal space with the patient in the lateral position. All blood clots are removed, and any adhesions between the parietal and visceral pleurae are divided. The anesthesiologist then inflates the lung to demonstrate the site and the extent of entrapment by the fibrinous membrane over the visceral pleura. The lung is slightly deflated, and separation of the "peel" is begun.

Fig 1–8, A.—An incision is cautiously made, transversely or longitudinally, with a scalpel. The peel may vary from a fraction of a millimeter to several centimeters in thickness. When the visceral pleura is reached, the lung begins to bulge through the incision. The edges of the incision are gently elevated with a plain forceps, and separation with a gauze pledget is begun.

B.—After the plane of cleavage is well established, a fingertip is inserted, and separation usually proceeds rapidly. When relatively adherent areas are encountered, separation with a gauze pledget is resumed. A surprising feature to those who observe or perform the procedure for the first time is that the visceral pleura is almost as shiny and glistening as in its normal state.

C.—When hemothorax has been present for many weeks or months, or when decortication is done for chronic empyema, the membrane may be adherent to the visceral pleura, and sharp dissection is required. Superficial parenchymal injuries are often unavoidable.

After the entire visceral membrane is removed and it is demonstrated that the lung expands completely when inflated, the parietal membrane is removed. This step is omitted by some surgeons but seems important to us, in some instances, to ensure full motion of the thoracic cage and the diaphragm. Usually, it can be done more quickly than the removal of the visceral membrane because the more cautious dissection required in avoiding injury to the pulmonary parenchyma is not necessary.

Maintaining a completely expanded lung during the postoperative period is essential to prevent recurrence. Two or three drainage tubes are inserted, and constant suction of −10 to −15 cm of water is applied. Air leaks may persist for several days when multiple injuries to the superficial alveoli are present.

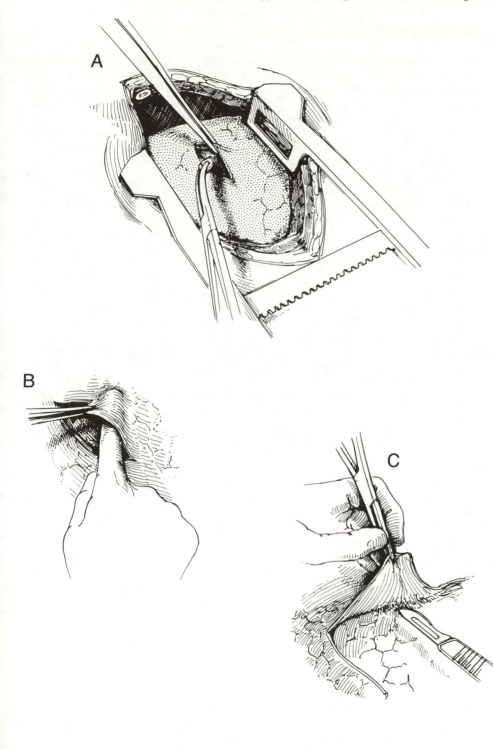

TRAUMATIC RUPTURE OF THE DIAPHRAGM

Ruptured diaphragms result from either blunt or sharp trauma. The tendency for abdominal organs to herniate through a torn diaphragm is due to an intra-abdominal pressure greater than the intrapleural pressure. The intraperitoneal pressure varies from +2 cm to +10 cm of water during quiet breathing in the supine position, while the intrapleural pressure varies from −5 cm during expiration to −10 cm during inspiration. This gradient of 7 cm to 20 cm can exceed 100 cm of water with maximum respiratory efforts. It is most likely that in crush injuries to the trunk, the momentary excessive pleuroperitoneal pressure gradient is responsible for diaphragmatic tear. Diaphragmatic injuries are far less common on the right than the left side because of the presence of the liver. The tear usually parallels the force of the impact.

The acute phase of injury is often obscured by signs and symptoms related to other multiple injuries. Diaphragm rupture due to blunt trauma to the chest or abdomen is more readily recognized, while lacerations due to stab or gunshot wounds are more easily overlooked. While inspecting wounds, it must be kept in mind that the dome of the diaphragm rises on moderate expiration, to the fifth intercostal space.

The interim phase is characterized by either absence of symptoms or only vague chronic complaints. The final phase of bowel obstruction or strangulation may occur within days after the injury, but more often occurs months or years later.

Diagnosis is based on the presence of abdominal organs in the chest, primarily using roentgenography. Gas-containing viscera are seen on chest films. A barium swallow roentgenogram will show the displaced stomach while a barium enema may show a herniated left colon.

Acute diaphragm tears should be repaired immediately after the patient's condition has been stabilized. Although the diaphragmatic injury can be managed through a thoracic incision, we now prefer an abdominal incision, which allows a better abdominal exploration for associated visceral injuries. However, in old diaphragmatic tears a thoracic approach is preferred for better lysis of intrathoracic adhesions.

The chest is entered through the lateral sixth intercostal space and the lungs are retracted superiorly and anteriorly.

Fig 1–9, A.—The diaphragmatic tear, which is often radial, is evident. Herniated viscera are replaced below the diaphragm after lysis of any adhesions.

B and C.—The diaphragm is repaired in two layers: first approximating the edges with interrupted figure-of-eight nonabsorbable sutures followed by a continuous suture of 3–0 Prolene. The chest is closed in a routine manner with chest tube drainage. Chronic herniation results in large defects that may require insertion of Marlex mesh in order to prevent undue tension in the suture lines.

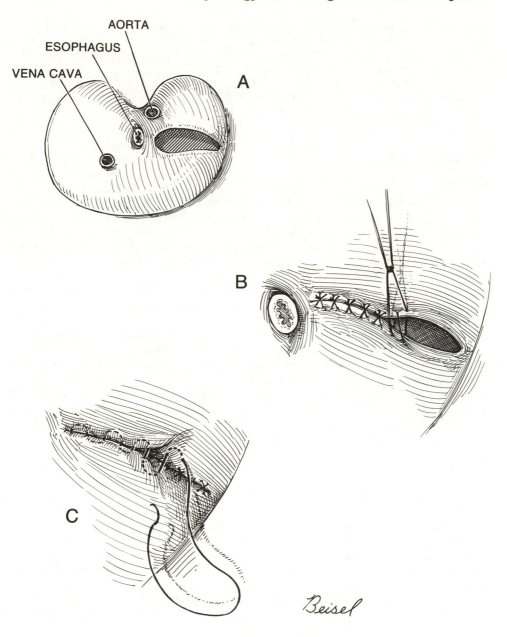

VENA CAVA

ESOPHAGUS

AORTA

A

B

C

Beisel

Fig 1–10, A.—The chest is opened through the sixth intercostal space. The herniated abdominal viscera are replaced into the abdomen. This may require lysis of adhesions. The diaphragmatic defect is quite large, and approximation of the edges would result in marked tension on the suture line.

B.—The diaphragmatic defect is closed with a double layer of Marlex mesh, the diaphragmatic edge interposed between the sheets. The mesh and intervening diaphragmatic tissue are approximated with 3–0 Prolene interrupted mattress sutures. The chest is closed in a routine manner with chest tube drainage.

WOUNDS OF THE HEART

Contusion

Steering wheel impact caused by automobile accidents causes most heart contusions, but less obvious injury may cause ECG changes suggestive of myocardial damage. Occasionally, ECG signs of the onset of cardiac injury may be delayed. The 12-lead ECG is the most reliable means of diagnosis. The treatment of myocardial contusion is similar to that of myocardial infarction. In most instances, the ECG reverts to normal within days or weeks. On rare occasions, heart failure may occur, and mechanical assistance with the intra-aortic balloon pump may be required.

Penetrating Wounds

Stab and bullet wounds produce most of the penetrating wounds of the heart. In warfare, high-velocity shell or bomb fragments frequently cause such wounds. The signs and symptoms produced may not be characteristic, and high suspicion that a cardiac wound might be present is important in making the diagnosis.

Exsanguination is the most common cause of death from penetrating heart wounds. The distress of most survivors is due primarily to cardiac tamponade, although there may be extensive blood loss due to egress of blood through the pericardial defect and associated wounds. The patient is often in an obviously desperate condition when first seen but sometimes appears deceptively well soon after the injury.

Compression of the heart by blood in the pericardial sac causes decreased cardiac filling and progressive impedance of blood flow on the venous side of the circulation. The arterial pressure gradually falls, and the pulse pressure becomes narrow. Neck and arm veins may not appear distended, but elevation of the venous pressure is nearly always demonstrable on direct measurement. A notable exception to this rule may result from significant associated blood loss and its ensuing hypovolemia. In such a case, blood volume may be so low that the central venous pressure may be normal or low.

In late stages, the pulse is weak or imperceptible, and heart sounds are very faint. The most valuable diagnostic measure is the ultrasound examination, which is quick and noninvasive, but in urgent situations treatment should not be withheld to obtain confirming evidence.

Treatment

The former practice of treating most patients with pericardial tamponade by pericardiocentesis has given way to immediate thoracotomy in most centers where a large number of these patients are seen. This change in treatment has been due in part to changes in the mechanism of injury. Ice-pick wounds are now outnumbered by knife and bullet wounds, which produce larger myocardial defects that are less likely to be self-sealing. Pericardiocentesis may provide emergency relief until operation can be undertaken. The techniques of pericardiocentesis and suture of the heart wound are illustrated in Figure 1–11.

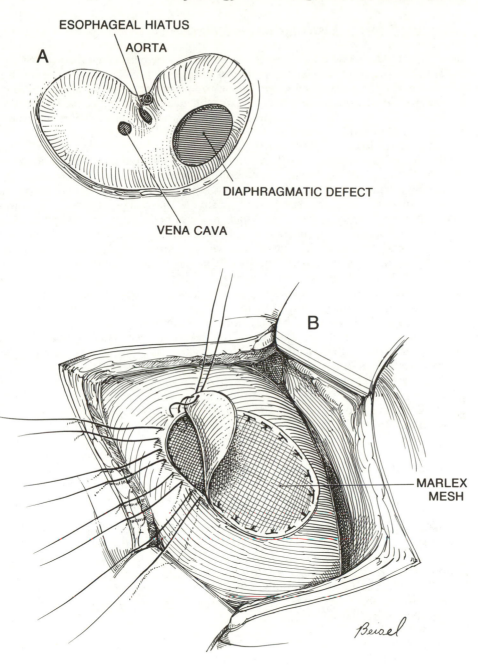

ESOPHAGEAL HIATUS

AORTA

A

DIAPHRAGMATIC DEFECT

VENA CAVA

B

MARLEX
MESH

Beisel

PERICARDIOCENTESIS: SUTURE OF HEART WOUND

Figs 1–11, A and B.—Pericardiocentesis may be performed through either of the approaches illustrated. Advancement of the needle is stopped when either intrapericardial blood appears or motion of the myocardium is felt by the fingers. It is helpful to have an ECG lead attached to the needle as the pericardiocentesis is performed. If the needle touches the myocardium, a significant change in the ECG tracing is immediately apparent.

C.—For closure of a penetrating heart wound, the operative incision is made on the side of entry, which usually is on the left. A fifth intercostal space incision is made with the patient in the supine position, and the fifth and fourth costal cartilages are divided. This incision can be made very rapidly if necessary. When the pericardium is opened and the blood clots are removed, there may be very brisk hemorrhage. Not infrequently, bleeding which has stopped temporarily is restarted by opening the pericardium or dislodging the clots. Rapid blood replacement by multiple routes may be necessary. The myocardial wound is quickly located and is covered with a finger, as illustrated. This usually controls the bleeding, so that time may then be taken for hemostasis and replacing the blood loss. The fingertip should not be thrust into the myocardial wound, because it may enlarge the size of the opening.

Atrial wounds may not lend themselves to clamping, and finger pressure may not afford adequate control. The insertion of a Foley catheter into the atrial lumen and inflation of the balloon, with slight traction, may very effectively occlude the opening. Suturing is then carried up to the catheter exit, the balloon is deflated, and the catheter is withdrawn as the last suture is tied.

D.—Deep sutures are placed in the myocardium on either side of the finger which is controlling bleeding. Crossing these sutures usually closes the wound effectively enough to permit both the removal of the finger and suture of the wound edges under direct vision. The most suitable sutures are 4–0 polypropylene. Deep interrupted sutures are placed and tied firmly, but not tightly. Pledgets of Teflon felt may be used to buttress the sutures used for the myocardial closure. Cardiac muscle is friable and tears easily. If the wound is adjacent to one of the coronary arteries, mattress sutures should be passed beneath the artery to avoid constricting it. Lacerations of coronary arteries are controlled by application of hemostatic sponges (Surgicel, Gelfoam, Avitene) whenever possible. Ligation may be required. Ideally, the repair of major coronary artery injury is performed with extracorporeal circulatory assistance. A saphenous vein bypass graft may be desirable if a major artery, such as the left anterior descending coronary artery, is involved. Otherwise, the patient may suffer a myocardial infarction with loss of a significant amount of myocardium.

After the myocardial wound is sutured, the traction sutures are removed. The pericardium is left open from top to bottom to prevent reaccumulation of fluid within the pericardial sac.

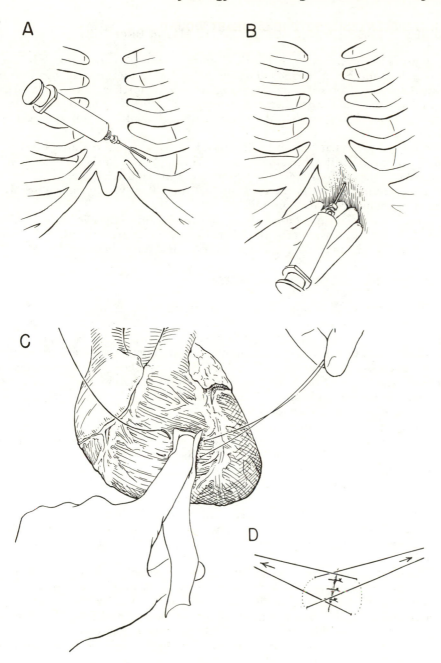

INJURIES OF THE THORACIC AORTA AND ITS MAJOR BRANCHES

Injuries to the arteries which arise from the aortic arch are commonly associated with stab and bullet wounds. The basic principle in their management is rapid proximal and distal control to avoid exsanguinating hemorrhage. No single incision affords access to all of the great vessels; consequently, the surgeon must estimate the location of injury based on clinical or roentgenographic information to obtain optimal exposure.

For rapid proximal control of the ascending aorta and aortic arch branches, a median sternotomy is the incision of choice. The upper end of the incision then can be angled to either side of the neck if exposure is inadequate.

The sternum is split in the conventional way. Rarely, clavicular resection is required to obtain adequate exposure.

The left subclavian artery is best approached through a left thoracotomy. However, since this incision provides limited access to the great vessels, the surgeon must know that the injury is limited to the proximal left subclavian artery.

TRAUMATIC TRANSECTION OF THE AORTA

When a deceleration injury causes an aortic rupture, disruption almost always occurs in the aortic isthmus just distal to the left subclavian artery. Occasionally, the tear will be in the ascending aorta. Although in most instances these ruptures result in death at the accident's site, patients admitted to the hospital with an aortic rupture usually have associated injuries. The chest film may show superior mediastinal widening, depression of the left main bronchus, and deviation of the esophagus to the right. Mediastinal widening is an indication for immediate aortography, and if rupture is demonstrated, operation is urgent.

Since repair will require occluding the aorta, the question of shunting the blood flow around the occluded aorta should be raised. Good results have been obtained using a Gott shunt (see chapter 20), but more recent studies suggest that careful anesthetic control of proximal hypertension using nitroprusside gives equally good results without the complexities of placing a shunt. Adequate blood replacement and the use of a cell saver are essential for the management of such cases.

Fig 1–12, A.—The chest is opened through a left thoracotomy in the fifth interspace. The lungs are retracted anteriorly and inferiorly. A large subpleural hematoma is evident in the region of the isthmus of the aorta just distal to the subclavian artery.

B.—An umbilical tape is placed around the proximal aorta between the origin of the left carotid artery and the left subclavian artery. A vascular clamp is placed on the aorta and occludes the left subclavian artery as well. Distal to the hematoma, the aorta has been freed also, and an umbilical tape has been placed around it. A second clamp is placed across the distal aorta. The hematoma is then entered.

C.—Usually there is a circumferential tear, with complete separation of the aortic wall. This is best managed by insertion of an appropriate-sized, preclotted Dacron prosthesis. The proximal anastomosis is made using 3–0 or 4–0 Prolene.

D.—The distal anastomosis is completed in a similar manner. The distal clamp is then removed, and the anastomoses are checked for bleeding. Any needed additional sutures are placed to control bleeding. Only then is the proximal clamp slowly released.

E.—Rarely, the tear is not circumferential, and the aorta can be repaired using a running 4–0 Prolene suture. The chest is closed in a standard manner with chest tube drainage.

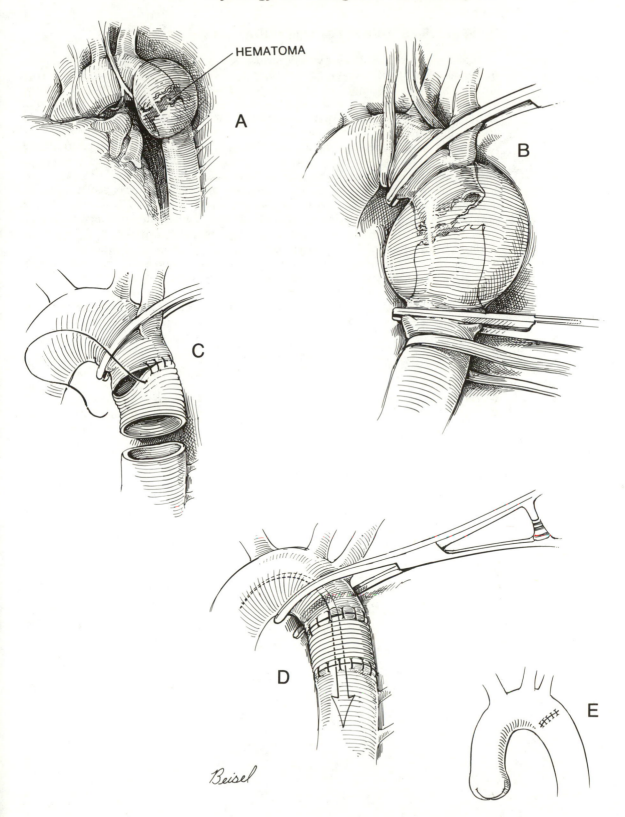

HEMATOMA

A

B

C

D

E

Beisel

CHEST INJURIES: ADDITIONAL COMMENTS

It is evident from the foregoing discussion that two separate, distinct phases are encountered in the management of chest injuries. In the first phase, which occurs immediately after the injury is received, abnormalities in the mechanics of respiration and shock are the principal problems. If the surgeon has a thorough knowledge of the physiology of the thorax, diagnosis of the type and extent of injury can usually be made by a careful physical examination. Most cases can be managed successfully without performing an immediate major intrathoracic procedure. If the basic principles are understood, surgeons who have not had prolonged training in thoracic surgery should be capable of treating most chest injuries.

In the second phase, the chief problems are infection and other sequelae which reduce pulmonary function. Early reexpansion of the lung usually prevents these problems and must be the primary aim of treatment. Clotted hemothorax has been a common cause of permanent impairment of pulmonary function, and empyema resulting from infected hemothorax has often caused prolonged disability. When these problems are managed by the methods described, and when decortication of the lung is judiciously utilized, most patients recover fully and have normal pulmonary function within a few weeks after injury.

Other problems arise in the multiply injured patient but are beyond the purview of this discussion. Shock, sepsis, and impaired immune response can lead to serious pulmonary complications that further complicate recovery.

CHAPTER 2

Surgical Diagnostic and Staging Procedures

Cᴇʀᴛᴀɪɴ ancillary procedures are of value to the thoracic surgeon for the purpose of diagnosis and staging of disease. These operations apply to certain granulomatous diseases as well as to intrathoracic malignancies. They include scalene node biopsy, mediastinoscopy, and mediastinotomy. Most often coupled with a careful bronchoscopic examination, these procedures serve to identify the patients most likely to benefit from thoracotomy in the case of malignant disease and to make a definitive diagnosis in patients with certain other diseases, such as sarcoidosis.

SCALENE NODE BIOPSY

Lung cancer spreads via the intrathoracic and mediastinal lymphatics to the supraclavicular nodes, most often in the region of the scalene fat pad. The role of scalene node biopsy or, more properly, of excision of the scalene fat pad on one side or the other, has been a controversial subject. It currently appears, however, that if a patient has probable lung malignancy and palpable nodes in the area of the scalene fat pad, the nodes should be excised before a thoracotomy is performed. The routine use of this test is not advocated in preoperative staging. These supraclavicular lymph nodes represent the last nodes in the drainage chain, and other techniques (to be discussed later) offer more sensitive diagnostic and staging information. Complications which may arise after this procedure include chylous fistula (secondary to thoracic duct injury on the left side), pneumothorax, and injury to the phrenic nerve.

Interpretation

Positive nodes, that is, the finding of metastatic malignancy, indicate that the patient is not a candidate for curative operation and that, with few exceptions, thoracotomy is ill advised.

Technique

Fig 2–1, A.—With the patient's head turned toward the opposite side, a transverse incision 5–7 cm long is made 2 cm above the clavicle, with the medial end of the incision at the posterior border of the sternocleidomastoid.

B.—The incision is carried down through the platysma, and retractors are inserted to aid in the identification of the boundaries of the fat pad. The boundaries are triangular, with a horizontal base. The lower limit is formed by the subclavian vein and transverse cervical artery, the medial limit by the internal jugular vein and sternocleidomastoid muscle, and the lateral limit by the omohyoid muscle.

C.—Removal of the scalene fat pad tissue reveals the phrenic nerve, which is covered by prevertebral fascia. The anterior scalene muscle lies behind the fat pad at its lateral aspect.

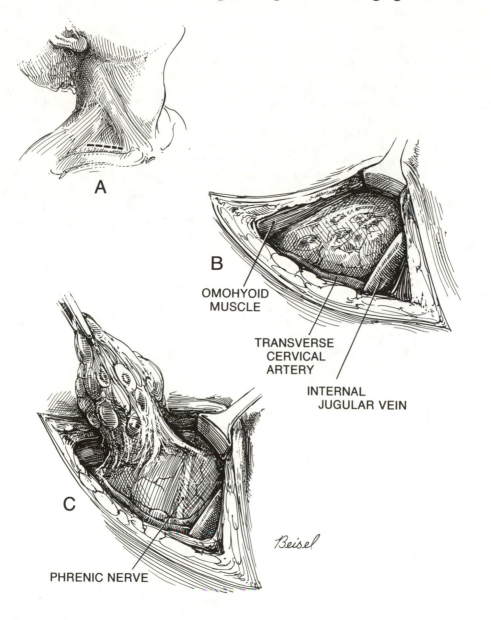

A

B

OMOHYOID
MUSCLE

TRANSVERSE
CERVICAL
ARTERY

INTERNAL
JUGULAR VEIN

C

PHRENIC NERVE

Beisel

MEDIASTINOSCOPY

This procedure has evolved as a method of clinical staging for patients with lung tumors which tend to spread via the paratracheal lymphatics. In addition, the operation is favored in making the diagnosis of sarcoidosis and is the operation of choice for establishing this diagnosis in the patient with hilar adenopathy of unknown cause. Mediastinoscopy is a safe procedure as reported in large series, which, without doubt, is due to a proper respect for the details of the procedure. One must appreciate that there are large and vital structures being manipulated through an extremely limited incision. Major vascular accidents can occur and must be recognized immediately, whereupon a median sternotomy usually offers the best opportunity to gain control. Mediastinoscopy is either denied or done with extreme caution in patients with superior vena cava syndrome, a history of neck radiation, and previous mediastinoscopy. The procedure has limited value in staging malignancies of the left upper lobe, as the nodes in the area of the aortopulmonary window are inaccessible.

Interpretation

Positive contralateral nodes and the extracapsular spread of tumor in nodes are both contraindications to thoracotomy. There appears to be a difference in resectability between epidermoid cancer and adenocarcinoma or cancers of undifferentiated type. The issue of positive low ipsilateral nodes remains unsettled, but resection appears justified in otherwise qualified patients with epidermoid cancer. Sarcoidosis is not a surgical disease, but its diagnosis by mediastinoscopy clears the way for medical management.

Technique

Fig 2–2, A.—The patient is positioned with the neck in moderate extension, and with the aid of general anesthesia, a 3-cm incision is made 1–2 cm above the suprasternal notch and carried down through the platysma. The strap muscles are either retracted laterally or divided, and the dissection is carried down to and through the pretracheal fascia onto the trachea itself. The thyroid isthmus should be immediately above this level. The pretracheal fascia is elevated and, using finger dissection, the anterior surface of the trachea is freed from the surrounding structures. These structures include the innominate artery and aortic arch anteriorly, the superior vena cava to the right, the pulmonary artery just below the carina, and the azygos vein at the lower right limit of the dissection.

B.—As the proper plane is developed and the carina is approached with the finger, the mediastinoscope is introduced, and dissection is continued. Both the dissection itself and hemostasis are achieved using an insulated suction-cautery device. The examining finger first notes any grossly palpable nodes; it is often possible to deliver these without using the mediastinoscope. The level of the nodes, that is, high or low paratracheal or subcarinal, is also noted. It is a wise practice to aspirate all structures prior to performing the biopsy. Exploration onto the right main-stem bronchus is usually of little benefit, and aggressive exploration down the left main-stem bronchus is dangerous. On completion of the procedure, meticulous hemostasis is achieved, and a few interrupted sutures are used to close the platysma and then the skin.

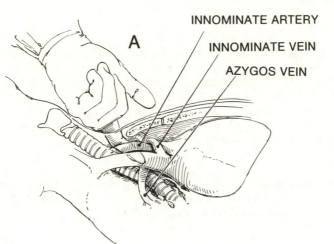

INNOMINATE ARTERY
INNOMINATE VEIN
AZYGOS VEIN

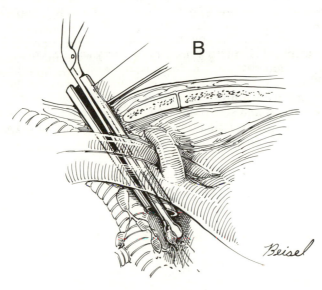

Beisel

MEDIASTINOTOMY

The pattern of lymphatic drainage from the left lung; in particular, the left upper lobe is complicated by the presence of the aortic arch. Mediastinoscopy provides limited access to the structures of the anterior mediastinum and has particular shortcomings when the area around the aortic arch on the left side must be evaluated. Anterior mediastinotomy provides a satisfactory approach to evaluate the anterior hilum and the aortopulmonary window area. Ideally, this is an extrapleural operation rather than a limited anterior thoracotomy.

Interpretation

In patients with undifferentiated tumors, especially if their pulmonary reserve is borderline, little is to be gained by a thoracotomy or an attempt at radical resection when positive nodes are found on mediastinotomy.

Technique

Fig 2–3, A.—A transverse incision is made over the second intercostal space and carried down, either within the confines of the interspace or through the bed of the second intercostal cartilage following its resection. After stripping away the perichondrium, the cartilage is popped off the sternum, and rongeurs are used for lateral division.

B.—With care, it is possible to remain outside the pleura to examine the mediastinal contents. The internal mammary artery and vein often require ligation and division. The nodes of the aortopulmonary window are embedded in adipose tissue located between the aorta and the pericardium overlying the left pulmonary artery. The phrenic nerve must not be injured. Closure consists of approximation of the chest wall muscles and soft tissue only, unless the pleura has been violated, in which case an intrathoracic drainage catheter is placed and secured. A postoperative roentgenogram of the chest is mandatory in all cases.

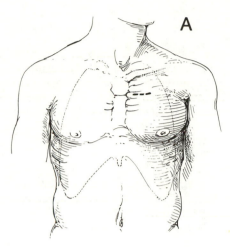

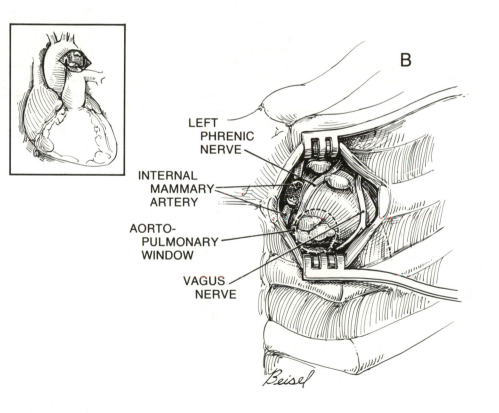

A

B

LEFT
PHRENIC
NERVE

INTERNAL
MAMMARY
ARTERY

AORTO-
PULMONARY
WINDOW

VAGUS
NERVE

Beisel

CHAPTER 3

Incisions

IN THIS CHAPTER, the methods of exposing the thoracic viscera for exploration and definitive surgical therapy are described. Small incisions, such as those used for drainage of empyema and lung abscess, are not included.

ROUTINE THORACOTOMY

Thoracotomy is the equivalent, for the thoracic cavity, of laparotomy for the abdominal cavity. The proper technique for opening and closing the thorax is important to any intrathoracic operation.

The location of the incision and the technical details of opening the pleural cavity for most intrathoracic operations depend largely on the operation to be performed. The patient is positioned on the operating table accordingly. The lateral and supine positions are most commonly used. Newer techniques of administering anesthesia and controlling ventilation have made the prone position obsolete. An oblique position is occasionally useful, e.g., for a thoracoabdominal incision (Fig 3–7).

THORACOTOMY: THE SUPINE POSITION

The patient is placed flat on his back on the operating table. The arm on the side of the incision is held away from the body to permit free access to the lateral chest wall and axilla. Excessive abduction of the arm may exert traction on the brachial plexus and, therefore, should be avoided.

Fig 3–1, A.—In females, a submammary skin incision is preferable at any age because incisions across the breast are unsightly.

B.—In males, the incision is made directly over the interspace to be entered, and the pectoral muscles are divided at the same level.

C.—The pectoralis major muscle is divided at the same level as the skin incision and is reflected upward with the skin and subcutaneous tissue to the desired interspace. The skin incision may be extended to the posterior axillary line if necessary. It is seldom necessary to extend it farther posteriorly than the midaxillary line.

The intercostal muscles are divided more closely to the rib below than to the rib above to avoid injury to the larger intercostal vessels, which course along the inferior rib margins. A small area of parietal pleura is carefully exposed, and, if no adhesions are present, the lung may be seen to move under it. The pleura is punctured with the handle, rather than the blade, of the scalpel to prevent injury to the underlying lung. The remainder of the intercostal incision is made with scissors and may be carried farther posteriorly than the skin incision to increase exposure. The lung is held away from the chest wall with the fingers of the operator's free hand as the intercostal muscles and parietal pleura are divided with the scissors.

In cases where more extensive exposure is required, such as for a pulmonary resection, the costal cartilages are divided with rib shears just lateral to the internal mammary vessels. The intercostal vessels below each divided cartilage are clamped and ligated. Should the internal mammary vessels be inadvertently injured, no harm results if they are securely ligated. A rib spreader is inserted and opened until the desired exposure is obtained. Better exposure results if the ribs, whose cartilages have been divided, are made to ride up anteriorly on top of the chest wall rather than within the pleural cavity.

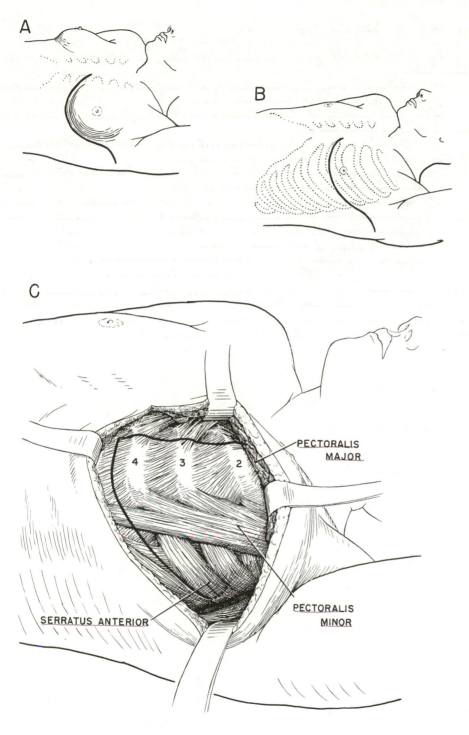

A

B

C

PECTORALIS
MAJOR

4 3 2

PECTORALIS
MINOR

SERRATUS ANTERIOR

D.—The exposure obtained on the left side through the fourth interspace is illustrated. The fourth, third, and second costal cartilages have been divided.

E.—This illustrates the exposure obtained with a similar incision on the right side.

An intercostal incision is preferable to resection of a rib in the supine position because of the wide separation of the ribs anteriorly and the relatively thin muscle layers available for closure. A secure closure may be difficult to obtain if a rib and costal cartilage are removed.

In patients with lesions of questionable operability, division of more than one costal cartilage is deferred until a preliminary exploration is made. If the lesion is inoperable, no more cartilages are divided, and the patient is spared the additional discomfort during the postoperative period.

The chief advantage of this position is that there is no interference with cardio-respiratory function owing to either restricted motion of the thoracic cage or gravitational influences. Another advantage is that the incision can be rapidly opened and closed with little blood loss and trauma. This incision has been useful in the emergency control of hemorrhage caused by penetrating heart wounds.

An important disadvantage is that exposure of some portions of the pleural cavity, particularly of the posterior aspect of the hilum, is not adequate for safe dissection. If the pleural cavity is obliterated by adhesions, the difficulty of dividing the adhesions is greatly magnified by this incision. Adhesions of the lung to the diaphragm and to the lower part of the thoracic cage are particularly difficult to reach.

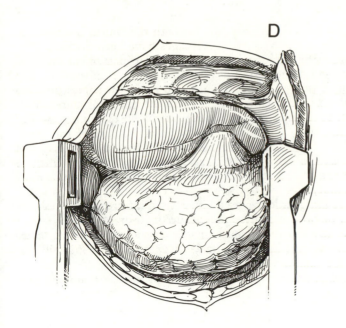

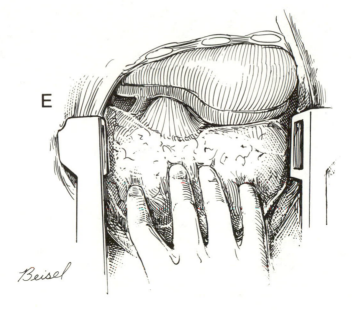

Beisel

Closure

Fig 3–2, A.—To close this incision, strong sutures are passed through the costal cartilages near their divided ends using heavy cutting-edge needles. This step is important in preventing postoperative pain. Interrupted pericostal sutures are passed around the ribs and costal cartilages adjacent to the intercostal space which was opened. The ribs are brought into close apposition with a rib approximator (not shown), and the sutures are tied. The sutures in the divided ends of the costal cartilages are not tied until after the pericostal sutures are tied, because they may pull through the cartilage if subjected to excessive strain. In large, muscular men, a single, heavy, wire suture placed around the ribs may add some protection against their separation postoperatively.

B.—The pectoralis major muscle is closed either with interrupted sutures, as shown, or with continuous sutures if more rapid closure is desirable.

C.—The superficial fascia and subcutaneous tissue are closed with great care. The pectoralis major muscle is often quite thin, and accurate closure of additional layers is required to ensure an airtight result.

Subcuticular absorbable sutures for the skin closure produce a fine scar. Any other suture ensuring accurate coaptation will suffice.

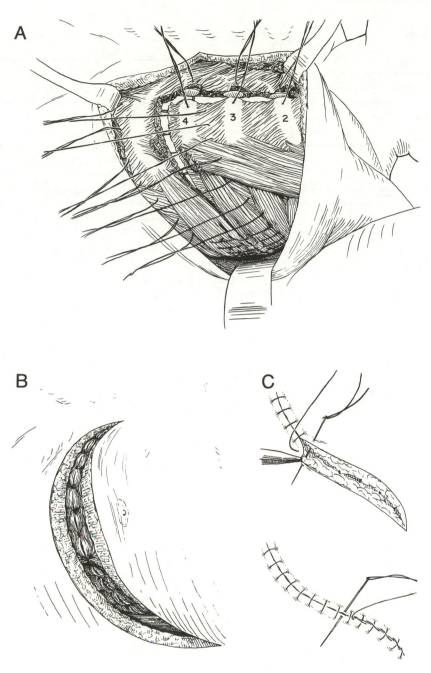

A

B

C

THORACOTOMY: THE LATERAL POSITION

Fig 3–3.—The patient is placed on his side on a standard operating table. Various devices have been developed to support the body, but adhesive strapping across the pelvic girdle and fastened to the table serves almost as well.

A.—The skin incision made in preparation for opening the chest at the fifth rib level is shown. It is deepened through the subcutaneous tissue.

B.—The trapezius, rhomboid, latissimus dorsi, and serratus anterior muscles are divided. Muscle bleeding may be controlled by finger pressure, as shown, while hemostats are applied to vessels. Electrocoagulating devices are commonly used for this maneuver.

A scapula retractor is inserted, and the chest is entered through the fourth or fifth intercostal space.

C.—A short incision is made in the intercostal muscles as shown. This exposes the parietal pleura. If no adhesions are present, the lung can be seen moving beneath the pleura. The thin membrane can be easily punctured with the scalpel handle. If adhesions are present, dissection must proceed as shown in Figure 3–5.

D.—The remainder of the interspace is opened with scissors. The index finger of the opposite hand is inserted to protect the lung.

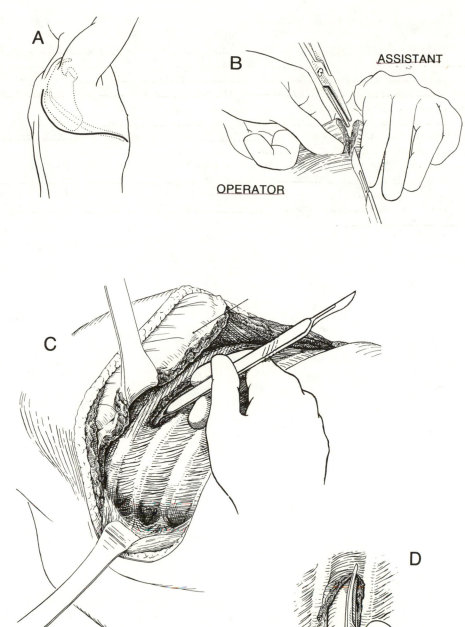

A

B

ASSISTANT

OPERATOR

C

D

E.—It is evident in the illustration that this incision provides better overall exposure than other routine thoracotomy incisions. There is greater accessibility to all portions of the pleural cavity, and the hilar structures can be approached from any direction.

The Harken modification of the Finochietto retractor (or any other retractor with one long blade) effectively holds the wound open and holds the scapula upward.

Rib resection is rarely required to obtain adequate exposure. However, division of a rib posteriorly affords wider retraction and also precludes rib fractures or dislocations as the retractor is opened.

When a seventh or eighth rib incision is made, the skin incision is placed lower than the standard fourth or fifth rib incision and need not be extended much above the tip of the scapula. In some instances, it is desirable to divide additional ribs posteriorly in the lateral position. This is done principally for the resection of high lesions of the esophagus.

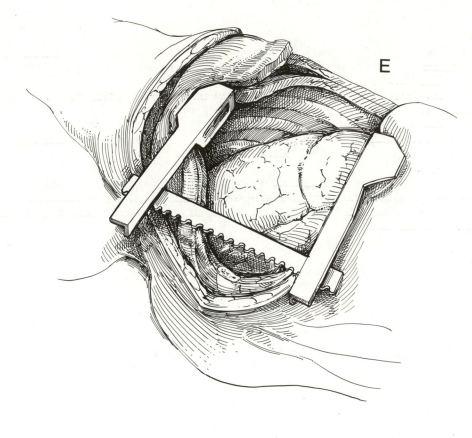

E

Closure

Fig 3–4, A.—A chest tube for aspiration is inserted through an anterior or lateral stab wound and the tip is placed near the opening for air drainage. A posterolateral tube will drain fluid adequately.

Pericostal sutures are placed around the rib above and below the intercostal space incision. The adjacent ribs are brought together with a rib approximator, and the sutures are tied. In large, muscular men, a single wire suture around the ribs may give some added security. This is especially important following a pneumonectomy when the lung is not present to seal off the incision and fluid may escape into the chest wall.

B.—The erector spinae muscle is carefully sutured to the intercostal muscles to provide an airtight closure posteriorly if the incision has extended far posteriorly.

C.—The muscles of the chest wall are closed in layers using either interrupted or continuous sutures.

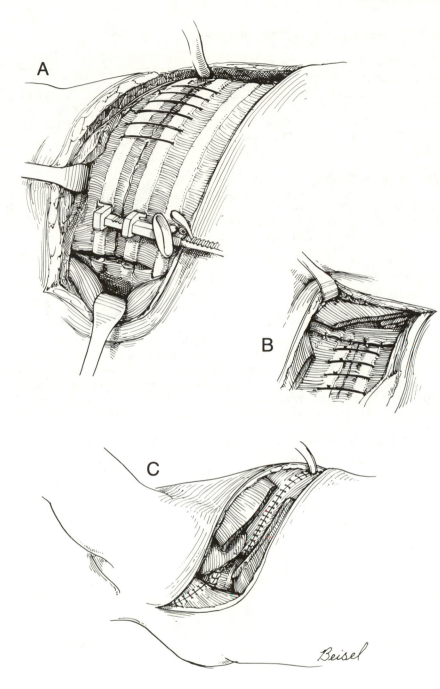

Beisel

LOCAL ANESTHETICS FOR CONTROL OF PAIN

Formerly, division of two or three intercostal nerves above and below the interspace incision was recommended in controlling pain. We now favor injection of a bupivacaine solution (0.5% with 1:200,000 epinephrine). Five or six milliliters is injected around the three intercostal nerves above and below the incision, near the spine. This is quite effective in controlling pain except in the distribution of the posterior primary division. Bupivacaine is effective for several hours, and even after the return of sensation, analgesia persists for a while longer.

PERIPHERAL ADHESIONS

Although resection of the ribs has been largely abandoned, removal of a rib is worthwhile if it is suspected that there are underlying adhesions or if an extrapleural pneumonectomy is contemplated. More room and better visibility help to avoid injury to the lung as the parietal pleura is opened or freed from the endothoracic fascia.

Fig 3–5, A.—If it cannot be seen clearly that the lung is moving, the parietal pleura should be incised slowly and cautiously with a scalpel. One edge of the parietal pleura and the internal periosteum are grasped and elevated with forceps; separation is begun gently with a gauze pledget. Pressure is applied principally against the parietal rather than the visceral pleura.

B.—In some instances, the adhesions are filmy and avascular and may be quickly separated by a sweeping motion of the index finger. In others, prolonged, tedious dissection with a pledget or with scissors is required. There may be considerable blood loss from vessels which are too small and too numerous to clamp. Such bleeding is best controlled with electrocoagulation, provided a nonexplosive gas mixture is used for anesthesia.

C.—When parietal and visceral pleurae are fused densely together, even the most meticulous dissection with a scalpel may injure the lung. If a lung abscess or tuberculous cavity is adjacent to the area of pleural adhesions, there is a real danger of penetrating the cavity. In such instances, it is safer to dissect extrapleurally. Extrapleural bleeding is best controlled by electrocoagulation. An incision is made completely around the adherent portion of parietal pleura that remains attached to the lung. Extrapleural dissection often must be done over a much wider area than is illustrated.

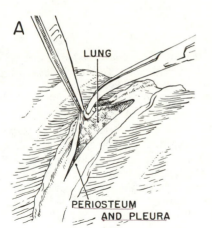

A

LUNG

PERIOSTEUM
AND PLEURA

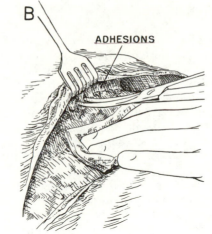

B

ADHESIONS

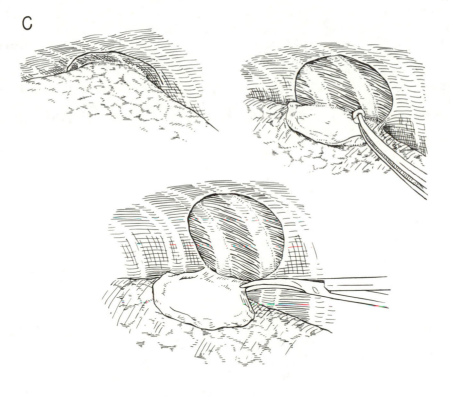

C

MEDIAN STERNOTOMY

This is probably the most widely used thoracic incision. Most cardiac procedures—pericardectomy, thymectomy, and excision of anterior mediastinal tumors—are best done by this approach. The exposure is excellent.

Fig 3–6, A.—With the patient in the supine position, a midline incision is made from 2–3 cm below the suprasternal notch to 4–5 cm below the xiphoid process. Electrocoagulation is useful in preventing excessive bleeding, especially when heparin will be administered. The oscillating power saw is advocated for division of the sternum if one is careful to keep the blunt guide against the back cortex of the sternum. Bone wax applied to the cut surface of the sternum helps to control oozing from the bone surfaces. Care must be taken if the patient has previously been operated on through the same incision. If the heart seems especially adherent to the undersurface of the sternum, it may be prudent to administer heparin, cannulate a femoral artery, and be prepared to introduce bypass support in case the cardiac cavity is entered prematurely. Shed blood can be readily reinfused.

B.—Closure of the sternal incision with heavy wire sutures is illustrated. We place the sutures around the sternum, taking care not to injure the internal mammary vessels. The suture in the region of the manubrium is often passed through the bone rather than around it because of the great width of the sternum in that area. A minimum of five wires is required for proper sternal closure. It is important that the wires be tight enough to immobilize the sternum completely.

If a tracheostomy is contemplated, it is wise to place the tracheostomy wound some distance from the sternal incision because of the likelihood of infection. Therefore, the skin incision should not extend into the suprasternal space. The prominent location of this incision makes an inconspicuous scar desirable. This is best achieved with a subcuticular skin closure.

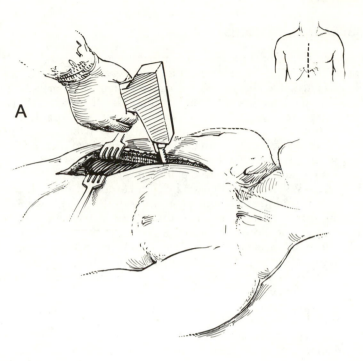

A

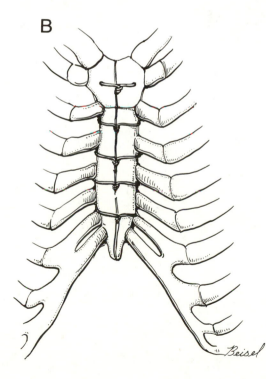

B

THORACOABDOMINAL INCISIONS

Adequate exposure of the upper abdominal viscera is often difficult to achieve through upper abdominal incisions because the overlying costal cage cannot be satisfactorily retracted. Excellent exposure can be obtained by making a low thoracotomy incision in the lateral position and opening the diaphragm. This is usually a satisfactory solution to the problem. Occasionally, it is desirable to convert an abdominal or thoracic incision into a combined thoracoabdominal incision. The exposure which results is highly satisfactory. The combined incision is not recommended for routine elective use, because considerably more time is required for opening and closing, and postoperative pain is more severe.

Fig 3–7, A.—When it is anticipated that a combined incision may be desirable, the patient is placed in an oblique position with the body at a 45° angle to the table. If a preliminary thoracic or abdominal incision is made and a combined incision is unnecessary, it should be located as shown in the *insert*. After the preliminary vertical abdominal incision is made (*dotted line*), the thoracoabdominal incision is begun at about its midpoint. The abdominal cavity is opened in the usual manner and the pleural cavity is entered through the eighth interspace. A segment of the costal arch at the anterior end of the eighth interspace is resected. This provides greater stability during closure.

The illustrated approach is satisfactory for tumors of the upper abdomen. If the contemplated surgery is to be in the retroperitoneal area, the straight lateral position is preferable. Abdominal aortic aneurysms that extend above the renal vessels may be well exposed by a long, combined incision which extends into the lower abdomen.

B.—The ribs are separated a short distance, the lung is retracted, and the incision in the diaphragm is begun. The diaphragmatic incision is usually made in the direction of the esophageal hiatus, but it may be made to point farther posteriorly for an operation on the kidney or adrenal gland.

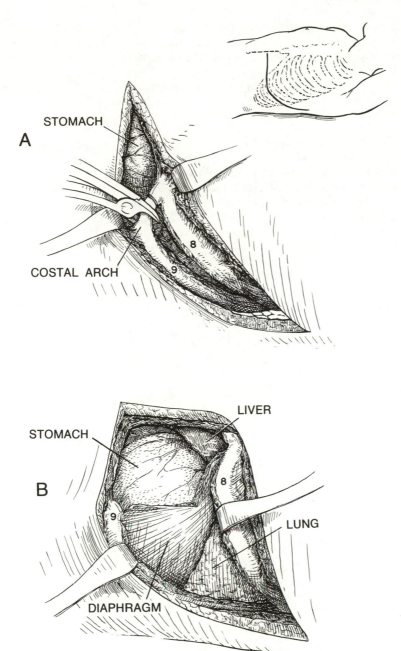

A

STOMACH

COSTAL ARCH

8

9

B

STOMACH

LIVER

8

9

LUNG

DIAPHRAGM

Fig 3–8, A.—The length of the incision in the diaphragm depends on the operation to be performed. If the distal esophagus is to be resected, the diaphragmatic incision is carried into the esophageal hiatus. When either a total gastrectomy or an infradiaphragmatic esophagojejunostomy is contemplated, the diaphragmatic incision may be somewhat shorter. An incision length of 10–20 cm usually suffices for operating on the spleen, the kidneys, and the adrenals. This figure shows the extensive exposure of the upper abdominal viscera that is obtainable with a thoracoabdominal incision.

If the contemplated operation does not require an incision in the diaphragm down to the esophageal hiatus, it may be better to cut the diaphragm in a circular manner about 2–3 cm from its attachment to the chest wall. This leaves only a small area of permanently paralyzed diaphragm.

B.—The diaphragm is closed with heavy, interrupted, nonabsorbable sutures. The abdominal wall is closed in the usual way. Paracostal sutures are passed around the ribs, and the costal arch is stabilized by passing one or two heavy sutures through the divided cartilaginous ends of the ribs with a strong cutting-edge needle. One or two steel wires around the ribs may add some security to the closure. The soft tissues of the chest wall are closed in the usual manner.

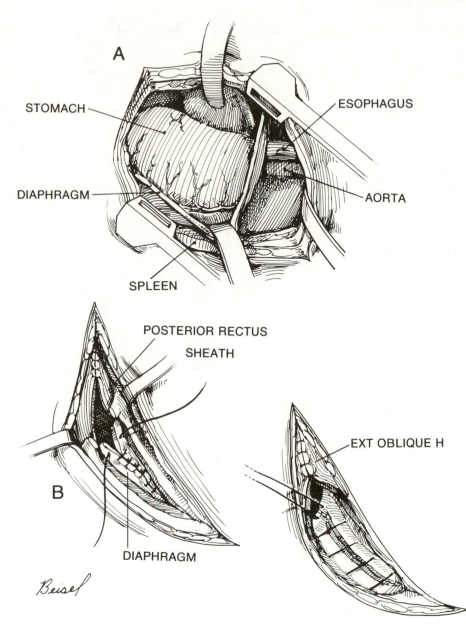

A

STOMACH

ESOPHAGUS

DIAPHRAGM

AORTA

SPLEEN

POSTERIOR RECTUS
SHEATH

EXT OBLIQUE H

B

DIAPHRAGM

Beisel

CHAPTER **4**

Surgical Anatomy of the Lungs

A THOROUGH knowledge of bronchopulmonary anatomy is essential for the thoracic surgeon to conserve healthy lung tissue and to operate safely. Anatomic variations, particularly of the pulmonary vessels, are common and will be described in this chapter. An attempt has been made to present the material from a surgical rather than an anatomic viewpoint. The structures of the primary, secondary, and tertiary hila, shown in the anatomic drawings, are those actually seen by the surgeon.

The two lungs are anatomically very similar despite the fact that there are three lobes on the right side and two on the left. The lingular segments on the left side may conveniently be regarded as the homologue of the right middle lobe, even though the lingular bronchus usually arises from the upper lobe bronchus.

Bronchopulmonary segments function as individual units, each having its own bronchus, pulmonary artery, and pulmonary vein, which are subdivisions of the lungs. The segments are held together by rather delicate connective tissue, and no bronchi or pulmonary arteries of significant size cross intersegmental planes. Disease processes may be limited to a single segment, and each segment may be excised individually without disturbing the integrity or function of adjacent segments.

The terminology proposed by Jackson and Huber for the segments and for the bronchi supplying them has been adopted throughout the world. Ten segments generally are recognized on the right side and eight on the left. The discrepancy is explained by the fact that two segmental bronchi of the left upper lobe and two of the left lower lobe originate from a common stem bronchus. These are the apical and posterior segmental bronchi of the left upper lobe and the anterior and medial segmental bronchi of the left lower lobe. The concept that there are only eight segments on the left may be useful to bronchoscopists, who are interested in the orifices they can actually visualize. From the standpoint of the thoracic surgeon, it may be well to retain the concept that there are ten segments on each side. The left apical and posterior segments may be readily resected separately, although there is no practical value in distinguishing between the left anterior and medial basal segments.

Fig 4–1.—The boundaries of the segments are shown. These boundaries cannot ordinarily be seen except when there are congenital clefts between segments, such as those not uncommonly found between the superior and basal segments of the lower lobes. The technique of demarcating the segments for accurate dissection at operation is described in chapter 8.

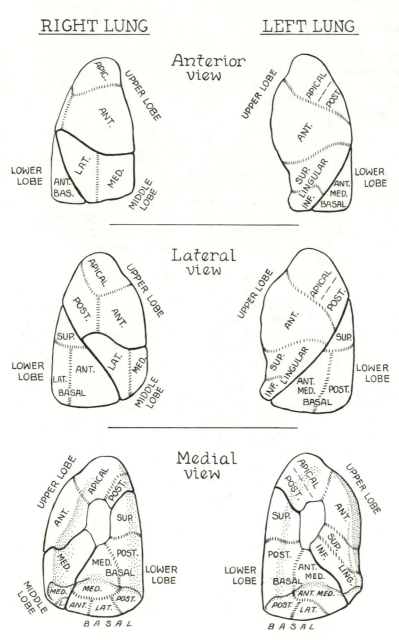

RIGHT LUNG   LEFT LUNG

Anterior view

Lateral view

Medial view

THE BRONCHIAL TREE

An understanding of hilar anatomy should be based on thorough familiarity with the anatomy of the bronchial tree (Fig 4–2). The complex relationships of the pulmonary vessels are more readily understood and remembered by regarding the bronchi as fixed points of reference. A knowledge of bronchial anatomy is essential in interpreting bronchograms.

Fig 4–2.—The left main bronchus is considerably longer than the right. The left upper lobe bronchus arises anterosuperiorly from the main bronchus and divides into two divisions, upper bronchus and lower bronchus. The upper division usually subdivides into two segmental bronchi, the apical posterior (*1, 2*) and the anterior (*3*), although the anterior bronchus may arise from either an intermediate position between the divisions or from the lower division. The lower, or lingular, division is the stem from which the superior (*4*) and inferior (*5*) lingular segmental bronchi arise. The lower lobe bronchus is very short and, after a few millimeters, gives off the superior segmental bronchus (*6*), which arises posteriorly and continues as the basal bronchus, which subdivides to form the basal segmental bronchi (*7–10*). The small medial and somewhat larger anterior basal bronchi arise from a common stem, called the anteromedial bronchus. Since the lower lobe bronchus is very short, division and suture of it, in performing lower lobectomy, may result in encroachment on the upper lobe bronchus. It is often preferable to divide and suture the superior segmental bronchus and the principal basal bronchus separately.

The right upper lobe bronchus arises posterosuperiorly, a short distance from the trachea, and divides into three segmental branches—apical (*1*), posterior (*2*), and anterior (*3*). The apical bronchus, or a supernumerary bronchus, may arise separately from the main bronchus or from the lateral wall of the trachea. The continuation of the main bronchial trunk is called the intermediate bronchus. From it arise the middle lobe trunk (*4, 5*) anteromedially and the superior segmental bronchus (*6*) posterolaterally, at about the same level. The further continuation of the main bronchial trunk is the basal bronchus, which subdivides to form the four basal segmental bronchi (*7–10*). Since the middle lobe trunk arises at the same level as or even below the superior segmental bronchus, it is usually advisable in lower lobectomy to divide and suture the superior segmental bronchus and basal bronchial trunk separately.

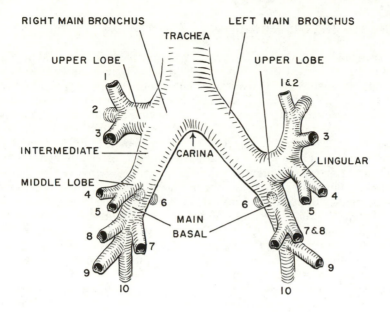

RIGHT MAIN BRONCHUS   LEFT MAIN BRONCHUS

TRACHEA

UPPER LOBE   UPPER LOBE

INTERMEDIATE   CARINA   LINGULAR

MIDDLE LOBE

MAIN
BASAL

SEGMENTAL BRONCHI

RIGHT		LEFT	
I	APICAL		
2	POSTERIOR		
3	ANTERIOR	1&2	APICAL POSTERIOR
		3	ANTERIOR
4	LATERAL	4	SUPERIOR LINGULAR
5	MEDIAL	5	INFERIOR LINGULAR
6	SUPERIOR	6	SUPERIOR
7	MEDIAL BASAL	7&8	ANTERO–MEDIAL BASAL
8	ANTERIOR BASAL	9	LATERAL BASAL
9	LATERAL BASAL	10	POSTERIOR BASAL
10	POSTERIOR BASAL		

STRUCTURES OF THE PRIMARY HILUM

The principal structures of the primary hilum, passing from the mediastinum to the lungs, are the main bronchus, the pulmonary artery, and the superior and inferior pulmonary veins. The position of the pulmonary artery is somewhat different on the two sides. On the left it lies anterior and superior to the bronchus and runs in a slightly posterior direction preparatory to curving around and behind the upper lobe bronchus. On the right it is also slightly anterior, but inferior, to the bronchus. As will be seen later, it remains anterior to the right main bronchial trunk and the upper lobe bronchus. The superior pulmonary veins are inferior and slightly anterior to the pulmonary arteries, while the inferior pulmonary veins are still further inferior and slightly posterior to the superior pulmonary veins. Below the hilum, passing from the mediastinum to the lung, is the pulmonary ligament, a pleural reflection which extends to the lowermost medial tip of the lung. Anteriorly on the right, the hilum is in close relationship to the superior vena cava, a portion of the right atrium, the phrenic nerve, and the pericardiophrenic vessels. The azygos vein is just behind the right hilum and curves up and around the right main bronchus. On the left, the pericardial sac bulges over the hilum anteriorly and is traversed by the phrenic nerve. The arch of the aorta curves around the hilum superiorly, and the descending thoracic aorta lies behind it. Anteriorly, in both hila, are the anterior pulmonary plexuses, and posteriorly are the vagus nerves and bronchial arteries.

THE PULMONARY VESSELS

A description of the pulmonary arteries and veins is given before their pictorial presentation so that the continuity of the individual vessels may be understood. A three-dimensional concept of the vessels, particularly of the pulmonary arteries, requires visualization of the entire course of each vessel.

The segmental branches of the pulmonary arteries lie closely adjacent to the segmental bronchi, usually on the superior or lateral surfaces, and have the same names as the bronchi. The arteries continue into the segments with the bronchi, branch with the subsegmental bronchi, and terminate along the borders of the intersegmental planes. It is uncommon for arteries to cross these planes.

The arrangement of the pulmonary veins is somewhat different. The venous tributaries occupy an intersegmental, rather than a central, position. Intersegmental veins drain the segment on both sides of the plane in which they lie, except on the periphery of the lobes where they are subpleural. Intersegmental veins converge at the tertiary hilum to form segmental veins. The segmental veins do not bear as close a relation to the segmental bronchi as do the segmental arteries. In general, they lie on the medial or inferior side of the bronchi and have the same names, except for the inferior vein, which drains the inferior part of the anterior segment of the right upper lobe.

Variations from the usual pattern are common. The most frequent variations should be learned so that they may be anticipated. As a general rule, the veins vary more than the arteries, and the arteries vary more than the bronchi.

The Left Pulmonary Artery

As the left pulmonary artery leaves the pericardial sac, it lies superior and slightly anterior to the left main bronchus. It then curves around behind the upper lobe bronchus and continues inferolaterally in the depths of the interlobar fissure, giving off its branches to the upper and lower lobes. The first branch, the apical posterior trunk, usually arises just as the main artery begins its posteroinferior curve and subdivides into the apical and posterior segmental arteries. It is not uncommon for the apical and posterior arteries to arise separately. The next branch is the anterior segmental artery, which arises most commonly from the anteromedial surface of the main trunk, within the fissure. Two variations of the anterior artery are frequently encountered. It may arise as the first branch of the main pulmonary artery anteriorly, in the primary hilum, or from the lingular arteries. The usual position of the lingular and superior segmental arteries is as shown in Figure 4–3, B. They may arise at exactly the same level, but the lingular trunk is usually a little lower. Both trunks soon subdivide, although the branches of either or both may arise separately from the main arterial stem. The basal segmental arteries parallel their respective segmental bronchi.

The Left Pulmonary Veins

The left superior pulmonary vein is the most anterior of the principal structures of the left primary hilum and receives all the tributaries from the left upper lobe. Its three main tributaries have the same names as the principal bronchial trunks of the upper lobe: apical posterior, anterior, and lingular. Two tributaries, which may be considered segmental, join to form the apical posterior and lingular trunks, respectively. All of these veins are superficial and may be readily exposed by dissecting laterally from the superior pulmonary vein. The most common anomaly is drainage of the inferior lingular vein into the inferior pulmonary vein.

The inferior pulmonary vein is posterior and inferior to the superior pulmonary vein and lies between the layers of reflected pleura at the top of the pulmonary ligament. It is best seen from behind (see Fig 4–3, C). It drains the entire left lower lobe, the principal tributaries being the superior segmental and the basal veins. The four tributaries which form the basal vein are roughly parallel to the segmental bronchi, in a medial or inferior position.

The Right Pulmonary Artery

As the right pulmonary artery leaves the pericardial sac, it is anterior and inferior to the right main bronchus. The main arterial trunk enters the horizontal fissure and continues inferolaterally, in a fairly straight line, remaining anterior to the upper lobe bronchus. Before entering the fissure, one large trunk arises superolaterally. From it arise the apical and anterior segmental arteries, which supply a large part, and occasionally all, of the upper lobe. The posterior segment, or part of it, is usually supplied by the posterior ascending artery, which arises deep within the fissure. Variations of upper lobe arteries are common. The apical and anterior arteries may arise separately, sometimes within the fissure, and there may be overlapping of their segmental distribution. The posterior ascending artery may arise from either the superior segmental artery or the middle lobe arteries and may supply a portion of the apical segment. The posterior artery is not found in its usual position within the fissure in 10% of patients, either being absent or arising with the apical and anterior branches.

The middle lobe segmental arteries arise anteromedially from a common stem at the junction of the horizontal and oblique fissures. They may arise separately and there may be a third, accessory, middle lobe artery. The superior segmental artery arises at the same level as the middle lobe trunk, or slightly below it. It divides into two branches, which may arise separately. The four basal segmental arteries arise just before entering, or slightly within, the pulmonary parenchyma.

The Right Pulmonary Veins

The right superior pulmonary vein lies anterior and slightly inferior to the pulmonary artery, overlapping the artery somewhat. It receives all the tributaries of the right upper and middle lobes. The areas of the upper lobe drained by the principal tributaries may overlap the bronchopulmonary segmental pattern. The terminology suggested by Boyden is used by us. From above downward, there is first the apical anterior vein which receives tributaries from the apical and anterior segments. Next is the inferior vein, which drains the inferior surface of the anterior segment. Behind it and usually entering a common trunk is the posterior vein, which emerges from the parenchyma of the posterior segment and passes just anterior to the pulmonary artery in the depths of the horizontal fissure. Its position should be noted in the fissure view (see Fig 4–3, E). The middle lobe veins drain into the inferior third of the superior pulmonary vein.

The inferior pulmonary vein lies posterior and inferior to the superior pulmonary vein and receives all the tributaries from the lower lobe. It is best seen and dissected from behind. As on the left side, there are two principal tributaries, the superior segmental and the principal basal veins, the latter receiving the basal segmental tributaries.

Fig 4–3, A.—Anterior view of the left hilum. This is a view of the anterior aspect of the left hilum as it appears to the surgeon when the patient is in the lateral position and the lung is retracted posteriorly. The surgeon is standing behind the patient. The segmental vessels which are visible were in close relation to the phrenic nerve before the hilar pleura was opened and the lung was retracted. The exposure of the hilum is slightly wider than that usually seen at operation.

The main pulmonary artery is the highest structure of the pulmonary hilum. It overlies the main bronchus slightly, just outside of the pericardium, but passes above it before curving behind the upper lobe bronchus. The apical posterior trunk is the only upper lobe artery which can be seen and dissected anteriorly, except for instances in which the anterior artery originates at about the same place. The close relation of the pulmonary artery and aorta, which makes aortopulmonary artery anastomosis possible, should be noted. The left main bronchus would be visible between the pulmonary artery and superior pulmonary vein, just lateral to the heart. More peripherally, the upper lobe bronchus and its three principal trunks—apical posterior, anterior, and lingular—can be seen. The lower lobe bronchus is usually not visible. The superior pulmonary vein is the most anterior of the hilar structures. The superficial position of the segmental veins of the upper lobe is shown.

B.—Fissure view, left. The fissure has been opened, and the interlobar portion of the left pulmonary artery is thoroughly exposed. All of the upper lobe branches and most of the lower lobe branches of the artery are seen. This view further emphasizes the point that the left pulmonary artery is the most cephalad structure of the left pulmonary hilum. The anterior segmental artery often arises proximal to the apical posterior segmental artery rather than distal to it, as shown. Anatomic variations are common, and as many as six upper lobe arteries may originate separately. It should be noted that no veins are seen in the interlobar fissure.

A

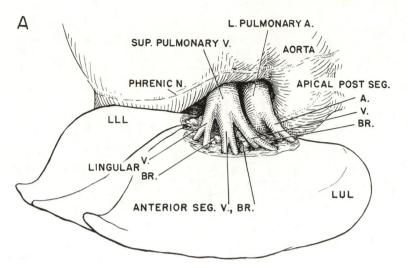

L. PULMONARY A.

SUP. PULMONARY V.

AORTA

PHRENIC N.

APICAL POST SEG.

A.

V.

BR.

LLL

LINGULAR

V.

BR.

LUL

ANTERIOR SEG. V., BR.

B

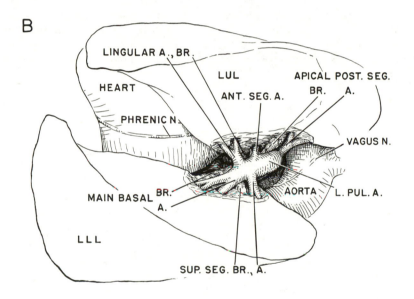

LINGULAR A., BR.

LUL

APICAL POST. SEG.

HEART

ANT. SEG. A.

BR.   A.

PHRENIC N.

VAGUS N.

MAIN BASAL   BR.

AORTA   L. PUL. A.

A.

LLL

SUP. SEG. BR., A.

C.—Posterior view of the left hilum. This is a view of the posterior aspect of the left primary hilum. The patient is in the lateral position, with the lung retracted anteriorly, and the surgeon is standing behind the patient. This view most clearly illustrates the relation of the left main pulmonary artery trunk to the left upper lobe bronchus. It is evident that the pulmonary artery is in jeopardy when the posterosuperior aspect of the hilum and the upper lobe bronchus are dissected. This view is also helpful in clarifying the statement that, in general, the segmental arteries are superior and lateral and the segmental veins are inferior and medial to the segmental bronchi. The close relation of the hilar structures to the esophagus is shown. When inflammatory adhesions are present, the esophagus may easily be injured during dissection of the main bronchus. The inferior pulmonary vein lies at the upper end of the pulmonary ligament and can be more advantageously approached when the pulmonary ligament is divided first, exposing the inferior as well as the posterior surface of the vein. The extrapericardial portion of the inferior pulmonary vein is usually quite short. In about one fifth of all patients, the left superior and inferior pulmonary veins join to form a common vein as they enter the pericardial sac.

D.—Anterior view of right hilum. A comparison of this view with Fig 4–3, A, illustrates the anatomic differences in the primary hilum on the right and left sides. The right lung is retracted posteriorly, and the surgeon is standing behind the patient. On the right, the main bronchus is the most cephalad structure. The pulmonary artery is anterior and inferior and overlies the bronchus to a greater or less extent. It is apparent that the position of the right pulmonary artery is not as favorable for performing an anastomosis to the aorta (in patients with a right aortic arch) as its position on the left side. Another important difference is that the right superior pulmonary vein receives at least one deeply placed tributary, the posterior segmental vein. Dissection must be carefully performed to avoid injury to this vein.

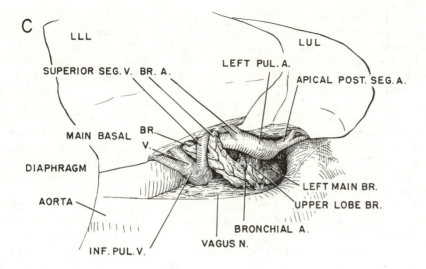

C

LLL

LUL

LEFT PUL. A.

SUPERIOR SEG. V. BR. A.

APICAL POST. SEG. A.

BR.

MAIN BASAL

V.

DIAPHRAGM

LEFT MAIN BR.

AORTA

UPPER LOBE BR.

BRONCHIAL A.

INF. PUL. V.

VAGUS N.

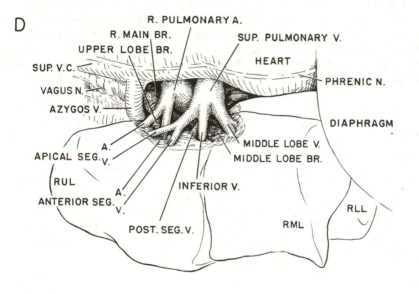

D

R. PULMONARY A.

R. MAIN BR.

SUP. PULMONARY V.

UPPER LOBE BR.

HEART

SUP. V.C.

VAGUS N.

PHRENIC N.

AZYGOS V.

DIAPHRAGM

A.

MIDDLE LOBE V.

APICAL SEG.

V.

MIDDLE LOBE BR.

RUL

A.

INFERIOR V.

ANTERIOR SEG.

V.

POST. SEG. V.

RML

RLL

E.—Fissure view, right. The major fissure of the right lung has been opened widely to expose the interlobar portion of the right pulmonary artery. The main trunk remains anterior to the upper lobe bronchus. The usual pattern and sites of origin of the segmental arteries are shown. The posterior artery is the most variable of all the segmental arteries. It may arise from any part of the intermediate trunk, from within the minor fissure or from a superior or middle lobe artery. In about 10% of patients, it is not found during interlobar dissection. There are often two or even three middle lobe arteries. The arterial supply to the middle lobe often arises somewhat more proximal to the superior segmental artery than is shown. In contrast to the left side, a segmental vein is often encountered during fissure dissection on the right. This is the posterior segmental vein, which is frequently closely related to the posterior segmental artery just adjacent to the upper lobe parenchyma. The posterior segmental vein is often somewhat larger than illustrated here.

F.—Posterior view of right hilum. The right lung is retracted anteriorly to expose the posterior aspect of the hilum. The patient is in the lateral position. It should be noted that there are no major structures posterior to the right upper lobe bronchus. The middle lobe bronchus, which cannot be seen in this view, is directly opposite the superior segmental bronchus. This must be kept in mind when performing a lower lobectomy.

The bronchial arteries originate from the systemic rather than the pulmonary circulation. They arise most commonly from the aorta just beyond the arch, but may originate from the aortic arch, from the subclavian or innominate arteries or from any of the upper intercostal arteries. There may be one to three branches for each lung. The bronchial arteries approach the main bronchus from the posterior aspect but are not in close contact with the membranous posterior wall until they reach a point slightly proximal to the upper lobe bronchus. They then branch into dorsal and ventral bronchial arteries, and these branches accompany the progressively smaller bronchi.

Bleeding from bronchial arteries is usually controlled by the bronchial sutures but, occasionally, a bronchial artery requires ligation. The bronchial arteries may be very large in the presence of either chronic pulmonary disease or certain forms of congenital heart disease. In tetralogy of Fallot, the bronchial arteries may function, in effect, as pulmonary arteries in increasing the blood flow to the alveolar capillaries. Except in such instances, ligation of the bronchial arteries has no deleterious effects.

The bronchial veins are normally small and of little anatomic or functional significance. Bronchial flow may be of great importance, however, during cardiac bypass. When large bronchial arteries have developed as a result of the patient's lesion, the return flow to the left atrium may pass through a septal defect and flood the operative field.

E

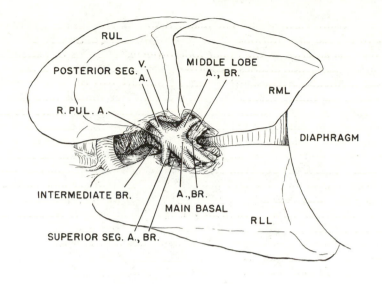

RUL

POSTERIOR SEG. V. A.

MIDDLE LOBE A., BR.

RML

R. PUL. A.

DIAPHRAGM

INTERMEDIATE BR.

A., BR. MAIN BASAL

RLL

SUPERIOR SEG. A., BR.

F

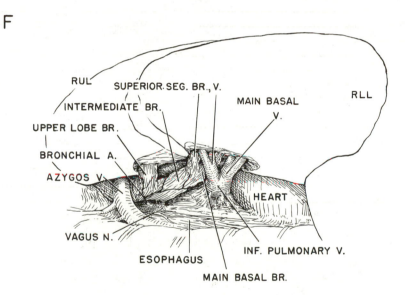

RUL

SUPERIOR. SEG. BR., V.

INTERMEDIATE BR.

MAIN BASAL V.

RLL

UPPER LOBE BR.

BRONCHIAL A.

AZYGOS V.

HEART

VAGUS N.

INF. PULMONARY V.

ESOPHAGUS

MAIN BASAL BR.

CHAPTER 5

Pulmonary Resections:
General Considerations

Two basic questions must be answered when resection is planned for patients with lung lesions. The first relates to the patient in general and to the amount of pulmonary tissue which can be removed. The second relates to the lesion itself and to the scope of the operation required for its removal. These two issues must be reconciled for each individual patient and form the basis for preoperative workup.

Extreme limitations of activity and a poor quality of life because of pulmonary insufficiency are unsatisfactory postoperative results. Information which aids in the determination of operability and resectability includes impressions from the history and physical examinations, the results of laboratory tests of other organ functions, the arterial blood gases, and pulmonary function tests. Some measure of exercise capacity, breathing characteristics, and general physical condition must be taken into consideration. The grave surgical decision is whether the patient will be offered reasonable hope of cure for lung cancer. The basic philosophical tenet is that it is better to deal with the disease by nonsurgical, perhaps noncurative, means than to embark on a resection which will likely leave the patient a pulmonary cripple.

Documentation of recent changes on plain chest films, as well as the appearance of the lesion in that study, tomography, and computer-assisted tomography all serve to assist in formulating the operative strategy. This information, combined with the results of the staging procedures discussed in an earlier chapter, allows a reasonable estimate of the scope of the operation required for definitive treatment.

Contraindications to pulmonary resection include markedly impaired arterial blood gases (resting, room-air), with either extreme hypoxia or carbon dioxide retention (P_{O_2} < 60 mm Hg; P_{CO_2} > 50 mm Hg). Pulmonary hypertension, cor pulmonale, recent myocardial infarction, and clinical and laboratory evidence of multiple system compromise also contraindicate surgery. In the case of cancer, documented metastatic disease, the superior vena cava syndrome, new onset of hoarseness secondary to vocal cord paralysis (laryngeal nerve involvement), or positive cytology in any associated pleural effusion signifies inoperability on the basis of the cancer's spread beyond the confines of standard resections. Relative contraindications to operation include paralysis of one diaphragm (phrenic nerve involvement) and contiguous chest wall involvement. For a diagnosis of small cell undifferentiated ("oat cell") carcinoma, chemotherapy would be the primary treatment.

Tests of lung function may be used to estimate the margin of safety for an operation of magnitude. Spirometry serves to reinforce clinical impressions of breathing function and capacity, and guidelines have been offered to suggest what measure of resection is safe for a patient with given test results. Most patients can function at an acceptable level if, after operation, their measured values are at least 50% of their original capacity. For a 70-kg man, a vital capacity (VC) of over 2 L, a one-second forced expiratory volume (FEV_1) of over 1 L, and a maximum voluntary ventilation (MVV) of over 50 L/min are representative of these minimal values. Preoperative findings of FEV_1 < 1,000 ml or MVV < 50% of predicted capacity would generally prohibit pneumonectomy. Greater impairment would challenge the wisdom of performing either a lobectomy or a wedge resection for a given problem. Computer-assisted radionuclide scanning, which furnishes information on ventilation and perfusion of the lung segments in question, may also help in providing an estimate of how much the diseased segments contribute to breathing and therefore extend the number of patients who would qualify for operation.

BRONCHOSCOPY

A careful bronchoscopic examination by the operating surgeon is mandatory before thoracotomy. There is no substitute for a personal examination of the bronchial anatomy. The important features to be appreciated are not subtle and can be seen readily with either a fiberoptic or rigid instrument shortly before positioning the patient for thoracotomy. A separate takeoff of a right upper lobe segment from the bronchus intermedius, for example, can be dealt with easily when its presence is known. In addition, the precise appearance and location of intrabronchial tumors must be known to plan for an adequate margin of resection when the bronchus is divided.

In patients with primary or secondary suppurative processes such as bronchiectasis or abscess distal to an obstructing tumor, bronchoscopy is done immediately following resection to aspirate spilled or residual secretions from the remaining airways and to give the patient a "head start" on postoperative pulmonary toilet work. Routine postoperative bronchoscopy also allows inspection of the bronchial closures and anastomoses as well as repeated measurements to satisfy any lingering questions regarding the adequacy of the resection.

MANAGEMENT OF THE AIRWAY

Skilled anesthesia support and improved double-lumen endotracheal tubes can reduce the difficulty of the operation by permitting routine use of the lateral position and the best possible exposure of the operative field by lung deflation. With a properly positioned tube, it is possible to ventilate the contralateral lung and to totally deflate the lung in the operative field. It is necessary to monitor arterial blood gases, however, since this maneuver can create a considerable right-to-left shunt through the nonventilated lung, causing systemic hypoxemia and difficulties secondary to CO_2 retention. Occasionally, it is necessary to control the ipsilateral pulmonary artery with a snare to eliminate this shunt.

POSITION OF THE PATIENT

The various ways to approach the intrathoracic viscera have been discussed in chapter 3. From the standpoint of the surgeon, the lateral patient position is preferable to the prone and supine positions because it offers the greatest amount of flexibility in the conduct of the operation. Exposure and access to all hilar structures is good, and therefore the operation can be done more safely than otherwise. Either the patient's disease or the capabilities of the anesthetist may, on occasion, dictate the use of one of the other positions. The principal consideration is to avoid contamination of the uninvolved lung by purulent secretions when the use of a double-lumen endotracheal tube is not possible. Such circumstances include abscess secondary to either carcinoma or another obstructive lesion, multiple lung abscess, bronchiectasis, and tuberculosis.

Fig 5–1, A.—A double-lumen endotracheal tube is shown with separate bronchial and tracheal cuffs. Inflation of the cuffs allows selective control of ventilation in each lung. Deflation of a lung is tolerated well for short periods, and many patients will remain stable throughout the procedure.

B.—Tubes are most often placed with the tip (bronchial lumen) in the right bronchus. Accurate positioning is required to avoid occlusion of the right upper lobe orifice by the bronchial cuff, and the tube is carefully secured before turning the patient for thoracotomy. It is possible, but frequently challenging because of the more acute angulation of the left bronchus at the carina, to place the tube in the left bronchus.

DISSECTION

In formal procedures for either segmental or lobar disease, particular attention must be given to the anatomy of the area. Bronchoscopy by the surgeon before the thoracotomy allows recognition of any unusual bronchial anatomy. A thorough familiarity with both normal and variant hilar anatomy is essential to a safe and efficient operation.

The approach to hilar dissection depends on which structures the surgeon wishes to address first. In cases of suppurative disease, for example, it may be prudent to gain early control of the bronchus, while in malignant disease, division of the pulmonary veins may be the most prudent first step. If the operation is being done for hemorrhage, it seems wise to address the pulmonary artery first. One great virtue of the lateral position is that any sequence is possible without difficulty. It is now unusual for the operation to require having the patient in the prone position, which was common in the era preceding effective antibiotics and double-lumen endotracheal intubation.

The initial steps involved in any thoracotomy include freeing the pleural adhesions (best done sharply) and mobilizing the lung. It is frequently advantageous to divide the inferior pulmonary ligament up to the level of the inferior pulmonary vein as one of the initial steps in dissection. This increases mobility of the lung and allows clamping of the entire hilum if massive hemorrhage should occur. Individual hilar structures are delineated using careful sharp and blunt dissection. A curved clamp holding a small gauze pledget is a safe, effective tool for gaining greater exposed length on hilar structures.

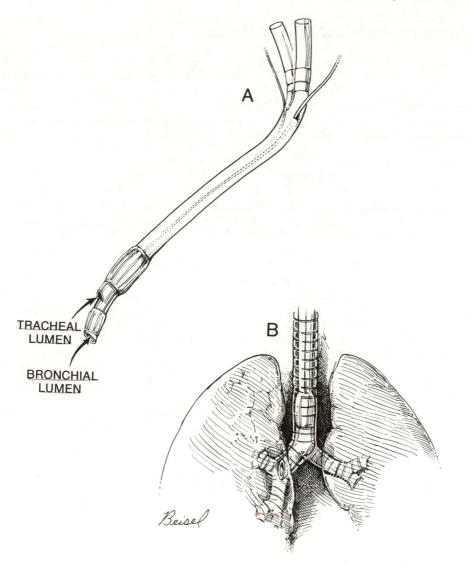

A

TRACHEAL
LUMEN

BRONCHIAL
LUMEN

B

Beisel

DIVISION AND SUTURE OF THE HILAR VESSELS

Proper technique for dealing with the hilar vessels is of the greatest importance. These vessels are so large that hemorrhage due to injury during dissection may be difficult to control. If the technique of ligation does not include the use of suture ligatures and long cuffs, as illustrated, fatal hemorrhage due to the slipping of a ligature may result.

Fig 5–2, A.—To dissect a pulmonary artery or vein, the surgeon picks up adjacent tissues with a smooth forceps, and the adventitial cleavage plane is opened by gentle spreading of the tissues with a long, curved hemostat.

B.—After a proper cleavage plane is established, the index finger is introduced to further develop it. In general, this is safer than continued dissection with instruments, particularly when working around the far side of the vessel, where direct vision is not possible. A gauze pledget is helpful in freeing adherent areas. Occasionally, the perivascular tissues are so adherent that the entire dissection must be done with instruments.

C.—The method of passing a ligature around a hilar vessel is illustrated.

D–F.—The objective of proper ligation and division is to place a snugly applied free ligature and a suture ligature on the proximal end of the vessel, and have a cuff of vessel at least 1 cm long beyond these ligatures. Free and suture ligatures are also applied distally. The application of proximal and distal ligatures is shown in this series of figures. It is a safe and reliable method of preventing back-bleeding during the rest of the procedure.

When there seems to be an inadequate length of vessel, it is usually possible to obtain additional length distally by ligating several branches, but this may not be possible in the presence of a tumor. If there is to be any compromise in this method of ligation, it should be made at the expense of the distal end. Kocher clamps may be applied to the vessels and parenchyma distally in order to leave an adequate cuff proximally. Intrapericardial ligation may be the best solution to the problem when an adequate cuff cannot be obtained in the usual way. If the available vessel is too short for this technique, dividing it between the clamps and suturing the ends, as for a patent ductus arteriosus, should be considered.

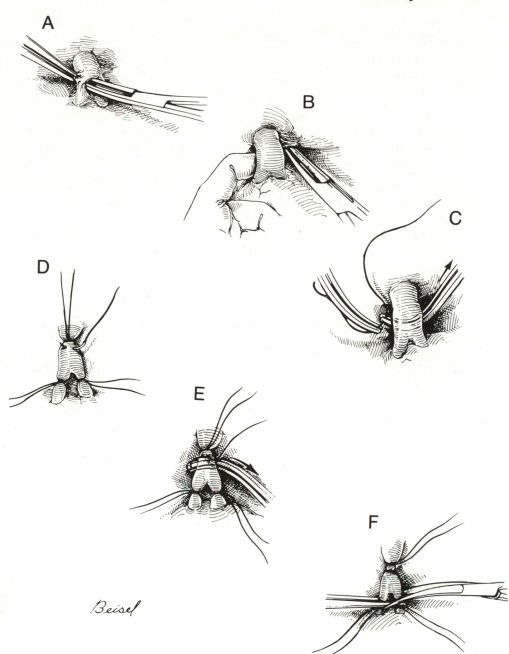

Beisel

DIVISION AND SUTURE OF THE BRONCHUS

Fig 5–3, A.—The clamps are placed 0.5–1 cm apart, and the area is walled off with sponges. The bronchus is cut with a scalpel half-way between the clamps, leaving a short cuff, which further prevents slipping. The proximal bronchus clamp is for airway control and is unnecessary if a double-lumen endotracheal tube is used.

B.—Since granuloma formation may result from the use of silk or other braided nonabsorbable suture, interrupted end sutures of either 000 monofilament, nonabsorbable material or synthetic absorbable material is used for the bronchial closure. After all of the sutures are placed, the bronchus clamp is removed, and the ends of the sutures are brought together with some tension applied to minimize the leakage of air and anesthetic gases. At this point, tension on the sutures may be relaxed so that the inside of the bronchial stump and carina can be inspected, and so that a suction tip to remove secretions can be introduced.

C.—The bronchial sutures are then quickly tied. Soiled sponges are discarded, and the bronchial stump is checked for air leaks. An additional suture or two may be required. The closure is tested by flooding the operative field with saline solution and then inflating the airway with continuous pressure of 30–40 cm H_2O. All but three or four of the sutures are cut close to the knot; the uncut sutures may be used to anchor a pleural flap.

D.—Usually, an adequate flap may be procured by elevating and advancing the pleura posterior to the hilum. If insufficient pleura is available, enough alveolar tissue can almost always be mobilized by careful dissection.

E.—The remaining bronchial sutures are passed through the pleural flap, as shown, and tied.

F.—Additional sutures may be inserted between the free edge of the pleural flap and the mediastinal tissues anterior to the bronchus. In many instances, the bronchial arteries are occluded by the proximal bronchus clamps, severed as the bronchus is cut, or caught by the bronchial sutures, and require no additional attention. If they do bleed after the bronchial sutures are tied, they must be ligated individually.

Special consideration to reinforcement of the bronchial closure is advised for patients given either steroid therapy or radiation therapy during either the preoperative or postoperative period. Coverage with a viable muscle flap affords perhaps the greatest insurance against a bronchopleural fistula. This additional step is used for any patient in whom the adequacy of wound healing is questioned and is illustrated in the following chapter.

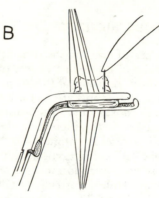

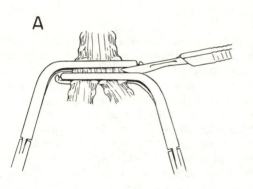

A

B

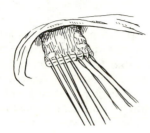

C

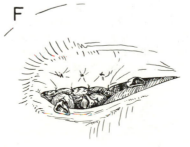

D

E

F

STAPLING INSTRUMENTS

The use of stapling instruments in pulmonary surgery has been demonstrated to be safe and effective in a variety of situations. The illustrations show their use for wedge biopsy, division of the bronchus, and division of major vascular structures. In addition, these tools are useful in the treatment of apical blebs, in cases of recurrent pneumothorax, and in the completion of (incomplete) fissures.

There are three different staples with which the surgeon must be familiar, and they vary in size and configuration. "Vascular" staples are made in only one size and have a tight "B" configuration which is hemostatic. The other two types are identical to those used in abdominal surgery and come in 3.5- and 4.8-mm sizes, both of which are available in cartridges of 30-, 55-, and 90-mm widths. The smaller staples (3.5 mm) can be used for wedge biopsies and fissure completion; the larger ones can be used for the same purposes but should be the only choice for division of the bronchi.

To minimize tearing of the lung during subsequent reexpansion, the lung parenchyma should be partially or fully inflated before these instruments are used. The same precautions apply as with suture technique regarding testing for air leaks at closure sites, hemostasis of bronchial vessels, and protection of anastomoses and closures.

Fig 5–4, A.—A 30-mm wide instrument with 4.8 mm staples is applied to a main-stem bronchus apposing the membranous trachea to the cartilage rings. The bronchus is controlled distally with a bronchus clamp before division and is cut flush with the edge of the applied stapling instrument before it is released. Bronchial vessels should be closely inspected, because hemostasis is not always ensured.

B.—A wedge excision of a peripheral pulmonary nodule, using an instrument which places parallel 5-cm lines of staples and cuts between, is shown. Several applications may be necessary for larger lesions. Routine oversewing for hemostasis and control of air leaks is unnecessary.

C.—If a stapling instrument is to be used to divide a major vascular structure such as a pulmonary artery or vein, it is recommended that the instrument be placed, fired, and removed before the vessel is divided to ensure that massive hemorrhage does not occur as a result of instrument failure. The specimen side of the vessel can be controlled with a clamp as the vessel is divided. A stapling instrument loaded with "vascular" staples is applied to a pulmonary vein.

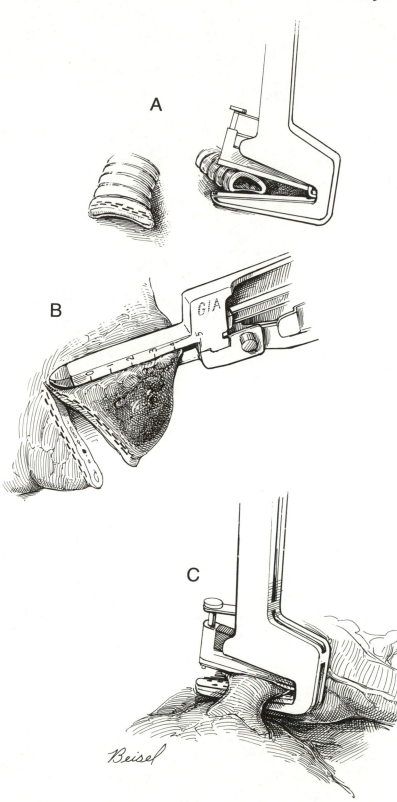

A

B

C

Beisel

CHAPTER 6

Pneumonectomy

Pneumonectomy means removal of an entire lung as opposed to lesser resections, such as lobectomy, segmental resection, and wedge resection. Other resections are often combined with pneumonectomy, such as resection of mediastinal lymph nodes, resection of portions of the chest wall or diaphragm, and removal of the parietal pleura.

INDICATIONS

The chief indication for pneumonectomy is bronchogenic carcinoma, which is currently the most frequent cause of cancer death in males, and which is overtaking breast cancer as the most common lethal cancer in females. Despite advances in the treatment of other forms of cancer by radiation therapy and chemotherapy, resection offers the only hope of cure for lung cancer at present. Surgical therapy for lung cancer has not much changed over the past 30 years, and the results of treatment have not significantly improved. This disappointing truth continues due to the aggressive nature of the disease and to delays in its diagnosis. Surgery is curative at an early stage of the disease, and the importance of clinical suspicion and aggressive workup deserve emphasis. In the surgical treatment of lung cancer, pneumonectomy remains the standard against which lesser resections are to be compared.

Bronchogenic carcinoma is protean in its manifestations and may simulate any other pulmonary lesion. All lung diseases developed during or past middle age must, therefore, be regarded with suspicion, even though the lesion at first appears to be inflammatory. Pneumonectomy is the treatment of choice for carcinoma of the lung, unless the lesion is located peripherally, in which case a lobectomy appears to give equal results. Lobectomy must sometimes be performed even for large peripheral tumors in poor-risk patients when the conservation of functioning lung tissue is an important consideration.

Less common indications for pneumonectomy include multiple lung abscesses, bronchiectasis, and extensive unilateral tuberculosis. Lobectomy and segmental resection are used more often than pneumonectomy in treating these lesions to conserve normal lung tissue. Pneumonectomy is advisable for an inflammatory disease only when the involvement is so great that it is not possible to save a significant amount of pulmonary parenchyma. Pneumonectomy is occasionally done for unusual lesions in which there is extensive parenchymal involvement, such as sarcoma, endothelioma, or metastatic disease to the lung.

POSITION OF THE PATIENT

In the past, consideration was given to the performance of this operation in varying patient positions—lateral, prone, or supine. The easiest orientation for the surgeon is the lateral position, because it offers the best overall access to the hilar structures and allows flexibility in managing the various stages of the operation. The use of a double-lumen endotracheal tube weakens the arguments made for the use of the other positions, since it nearly eliminates the possibility of spilling purulent secretions into the unaffected lung.

INCISIONS

The standard incision for pneumonectomy is a generous posterolateral thoracotomy through the fifth intercostal space. Posterior dislocation of the rib articulation, either division or resection of the rib, and extension by division of the costal cartilages, either superiorly or inferiorly, are all means by which exposure can be facilitated.

GENERAL OPERATIVE CONSIDERATIONS

The lung is mobilized by dividing any adhesions present between the parietal and visceral pleurae. The pulmonary ligament is then divided so that the surgeon may grasp and compress the hilum if hemorrhage occurs. The order in which the hilar structures are divided is subject to some variation. In general, the pulmonary artery is dealt with first, then the superior and inferior pulmonary veins, and finally the main-stem bronchus. If a double-lumen endotracheal tube is not used, and if spillage of purulent secretions is a possibility, then early control of the bronchus is advised. In addition, early division of the bronchus is sometimes helpful because the bronchus has the least flexibility. After its division, the lung may be displaced further laterally and larger segments of the great vessels become accessible for dissection, ligation, and division.

If the operation is being done as an emergency or semi-emergency because of recent intrapulmonary bleeding, it is probably not wise to ligate the pulmonary veins before the artery is ligated, because the increased pressure may restart the bleeding. Under most circumstances, however, it seems to make no difference which vessels are ligated first. When dealing with malignancy, some surgeons have suggested that the veins be ligated first, before handling the tumor, in the hope of avoiding dissemination of tumor cells through the bloodstream.

PNEUMONECTOMY: LATERAL POSITION

A right pneumonectomy in the lateral position is illustrated (Fig 6–1). The appearance of the hilar structures is that seen when the surgeon stands behind the patient. It is often advantageous for the surgeon to stand in front of the patient, particularly when the bronchus is divided first. The hilar structures then have approximately the appearance seen in the prone patient.

Fig 6–1, A.—The first step, after freeing peripheral adhesions and dividing the pulmonary ligament, is to incise the anterior hilar pleura with the lung retracted posteriorly. The pleural borders are reflected laterally and medially, and loose areolar tissue is entirely separated to expose the hilar structures. The superior pulmonary vein is the most anterior of the major hilar vessels. It overlies and partially obscures the pulmonary artery. The artery is dissected out first, while the superior pulmonary vein is displaced gently downward. The cleavage plane between the artery and vein must be developed with great care.

B.—The technique of dissecting the extrapericardial portion of the pulmonary artery is illustrated. In some instances, the main artery is long enough so that both proximal and distal ligatures can be applied to it. In general, it is better to use the method illustrated, i.e., to dissect out about 1 cm of the apical anterior and intermediate arteries. Application of the distal ligatures to the branches provides a long cuff and decreases the tendency to employ dangerous maneuvers in an attempt to mobilize excessively the main artery.

C.—The pulmonary artery is divided just distal to the bifurcation. The superior pulmonary vein is freed and ligated in the same manner as the pulmonary artery. Even greater care is necessary in dissecting out the vein because of its thinner walls and the risk of systemic air embolism if a tear occurs.

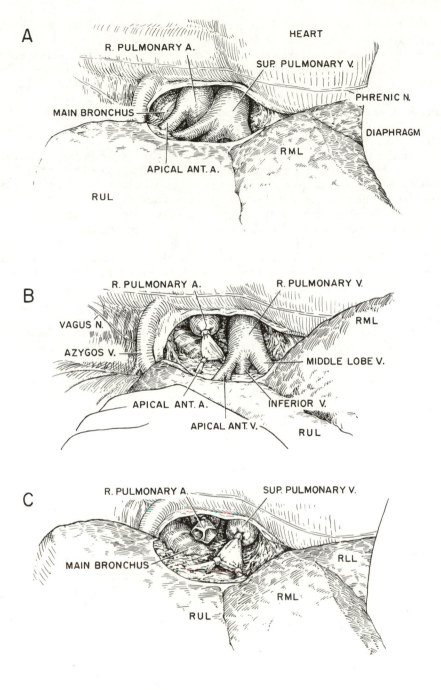

D.—The incision in the hilar pleura is extended around the superior and posterior aspects of the hilum, and the lung is retracted anteriorly. Separation of loose areolar tissue exposes the main-stem bronchus as well as the inferior pulmonary vein, which lies just above the divided pulmonary ligament. The vein is freed by blunt dissection and ligated and divided in the same manner as the other great vessels. Distally the superior segmental and main basal segmental veins are ligated separately. Usually, the extrapericardial portion of the inferior pulmonary vein is the shortest of the three great vessels, and ligation of the separate branches distally is essential in dealing with this vein.

With the three large vessels divided, the bronchus is the principal remaining structure to be severed. A certain amount of unimportant connective tissue surrounds the bronchus and spans the hilum in the areas where the vessels have been dissected out. This tissue is divided between clamps and ligated. Blunt dissection is adequate for clearing the bronchus except when there are adherent lymph nodes. The bronchus should not be denuded proximal to the point planned for division, since this may decrease the blood supply.

E.—The bronchus is divided and sutured in the usual manner. The bronchial stump should be no more than 1 cm long. A longer stump will collect secretions and can cause chronic infection and aspiration. The azygos vein is divided, and the bronchial stump is covered with a pleural flap by placing sutures in the manner illustrated.

The excellent exposure of all portions of the hilum is apparent in these figures and is the outstanding advantage of the lateral position. The incision is closed in the usual way and the intrapleural pressure is adjusted.

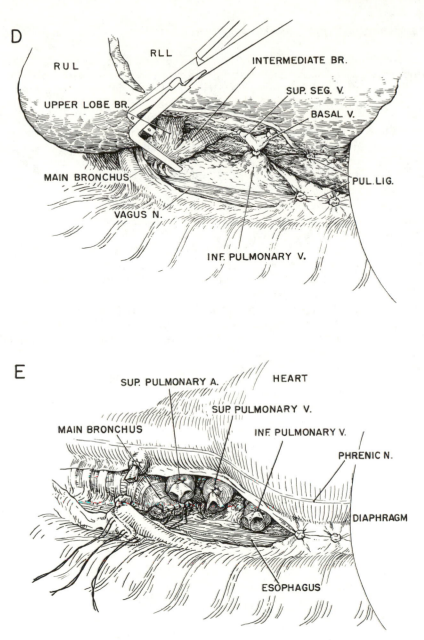

D

RUL
RLL
INTERMEDIATE BR.
SUP. SEG. V.
UPPER LOBE BR.
BASAL V.
MAIN BRONCHUS
PUL. LIG.
VAGUS N.
INF. PULMONARY V.

E

SUP. PULMONARY A.
HEART
SUP. PULMONARY V.
MAIN BRONCHUS
INF. PULMONARY V.
PHRENIC N.
DIAPHRAGM
ESOPHAGUS

LEFT PNEUMONECTOMY: SUPINE POSITION

In the supine position most, if not all, of the dissection must be done from the anterior aspect. Even if the intercostal incision is carried far posteriorly, it is not impossible to obtain an entirely satisfactory exposure of the posterior surface of the hilum by retracting the lung anteriorly. It is important to free all peripheral adhesions and to divide the pulmonary ligament before beginning the hilar dissection so that the hilum can be compressed between the thumb and fingers if hemorrhage occurs. When this operation is performed with the patient in the lateral position, the anterior hilar exposure is the same as depicted in these figures. It is easier and safer to expose and deal with both the inferior pulmonary vein and the left main-stem bronchus from the posterior aspect.

Fig 6–2, A.—The pleural reflection on the anterior and superior surfaces of the hilum is divided and the hilar structures are exposed by separating the loose areolar tissue which covers them. The *arrow* indicates that the apex of the lung is retracted downward and backward. The pulmonary artery is the most cephalad structure of the left hilum and is exposed by dissecting anterosuperiorly. The proximal ligatures are applied to the main pulmonary trunk beyond its origin.

B.—The superior pulmonary vein is dissected, ligated, and divided in the usual way. Being very superficial, it is usually most easily dealt with in this position. The segmental veins are just beneath the pleura and are readily mobilized to permit application of the distal ligature at a considerable distance from the main venous trunk.

A

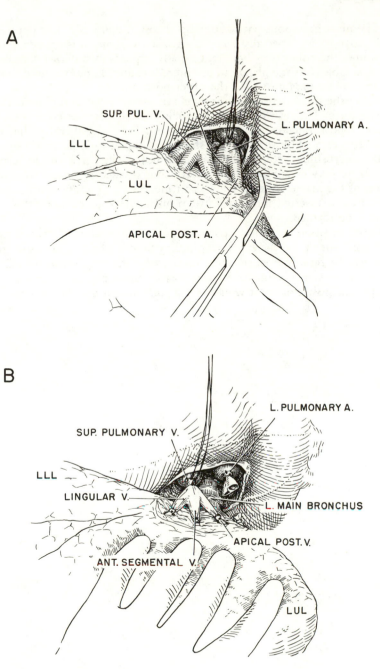

SUP. PUL. V.

LLL

L. PULMONARY A.

LUL

APICAL POST. A.

B

L. PULMONARY A.

SUP. PULMONARY V.

LLL

LINGULAR V.

L. MAIN BRONCHUS

APICAL POST. V.

ANT. SEGMENTAL V.

LUL

C.—The most hazardous part of the dissection in this position is exposing the inferior pulmonary vein, especially when the tissue overlying it is matted and indurated. Division of the pulmonary ligament usually exposes the inferior surface of the vein so that a suitable cleavage plane can be entered readily. Ligation and division are performed in the same manner as in the other positions.

D.—After the three major hilar vessels are divided, the bronchus is the only remaining structure. The relation of the bronchus to the hilar vessels is well shown in this figure. The bronchus may be divided and sutured either by the method described in chapter 5 or by the method shown in Figure 6–2, E.

E.—If noncrushing bronchus clamps are not available, a single, crushing, right-angle clamp may be applied and the bronchus divided proximal to it. Only a small portion of the bronchus is divided at a time, and, as each portion is divided, bronchial sutures are inserted and tied. Little bronchial leakage occurs if this maneuver is carefully performed.

The supine position is highly satisfactory for pneumonectomy when the hilar dissection is not difficult and the cardiorespiratory function of the patient is optimal. The incision can be rapidly opened and closed with little blood loss. Dividing the intercostal nerves posteriorly may decrease postoperative pain. However, division of adhesions to the posterior chest wall or to the diaphragm may be very difficult in this position.

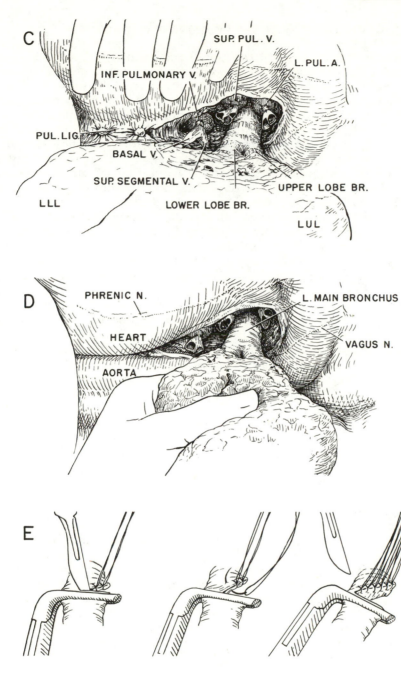

C

SUP. PUL. V.

L. PUL. A.

INF. PULMONARY V.

PUL. LIG.

BASAL V.

SUP. SEGMENTAL V.

UPPER LOBE BR.

LLL

LOWER LOBE BR.

LUL

D

PHRENIC N.

L. MAIN BRONCHUS

HEART

VAGUS N.

AORTA

E

INTRAPERICARDIAL LIGATION OF THE PULMONARY VESSELS

Ligation of one or more of the great vessels within the pericardial sac is desirable under the following circumstances: (1) when a tumor encroaches on the hilum to such an extent that complete removal is not otherwise possible; (2) when the hilar dissection is unusually difficult because of the presence of inflammatory tissue or fibrosis; and (3) when a vessel is torn close to the pericardium.

Intrapericardial ligation is not difficult if the relations between the pericardium and great vessels are understood. The great vessels can be seen intrapericardially only if they cause an invagination of the serous pericardium. The pulmonary arteries can nearly always be identified on both sides. The superior and inferior pulmonary veins protrude into the pericardial sac sufficiently to be identified in about 75% of the cases. Seldom more, and often less, than three fourths of the circumference of the vessel is covered with serous pericardium. It is almost always necessary, therefore, to puncture the pericardial sac either above or below a specific major intrapericardial vessel in order to pass a ligature around it.

Representative examples of intrapericardial anatomy are illustrated in these figures. The pericardial incision may be made either anterior or posterior to the phrenic nerve, depending on its location.

Fig 6–3, A.—On the right, the pericardial reflection usually passes obliquely across the pulmonary artery as illustrated. When the pericardial reflection is more medial, ligation of the pulmonary artery at this point is not feasible. Ligation may then be performed medial to the superior vena cava. The pericardial incision is extended, and the aorta and superior vena cava are gently separated to expose the right pulmonary artery near its origin.

B.—On the left, the pulmonary artery is a prominent intrapericardial structure. The fold of Marshall, which arches downward below it, is a fairly constant landmark and may contain a patent vessel (persistent left superior vena cava). About 75% of the superior and 30% of the inferior pulmonary vein is covered with serous pericardium in this instance.

RADICAL PNEUMONECTOMY

All hilar and closely adjacent mediastinal lymph nodes should be removed en bloc with the resected specimen. Whether a more extensive dissection of mediastinal lymph nodes should be done routinely in the absence of gross lymph node involvement is not yet settled. Many surgeons excise only those mediastinal nodes which appear enlarged, whereas others remove all that can be found, from the thoracic inlet to the diaphragm. There seems to be an increased incidence of bronchial fistula following so-called radical pneumonectomy. This is probably due to operative interference with blood supply of the remaining structures, particularly the bronchial stump. Local extension of the tumor is a relative contraindication to resection when the involvement is of the chest wall, diaphragm, or pericardium and phrenic nerve. The entire specimen should be removed en bloc, if possible, to avoid spilling tumor cells.

EXTRAPLEURAL PNEUMONECTOMY

In patients with tuberculous empyema either with or without bronchopleural fistula and extensive unilateral parenchymal inflammatory disease, removal of the lung within the investing envelope of parietal pleura may offer the best chance of disease resolution. This is called extrapleural pneumonectomy. The extrapleural plane is entered just beneath the periosteum of the resected rib, and separation from

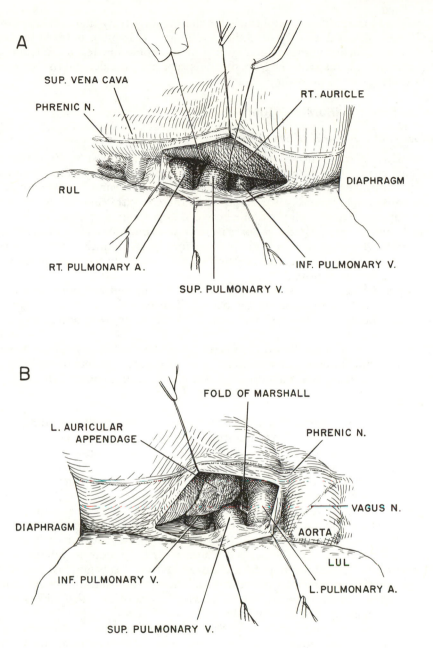

A

SUP. VENA CAVA

PHRENIC N.

RT. AURICLE

RUL

DIAPHRAGM

RT. PULMONARY A.

INF. PULMONARY V.

SUP. PULMONARY V.

B

L. AURICULAR APPENDAGE

FOLD OF MARSHALL

PHRENIC N.

VAGUS N.

DIAPHRAGM

AORTA

LUL

INF. PULMONARY V.

L. PULMONARY A.

SUP. PULMONARY V.

the chest wall is readily accomplished, for the most part, by finger dissection. The most adherent area is usually over the diaphragm. It is often possible to free the entire parietal pleura without spilling any of the contaminated intrapleural fluid. When the hilum is reached, the hilar pleura is reflected laterally and the hilar dissection is done in the usual manner.

FINAL STEPS IN PNEUMONECTOMY

Reinforcement of the Bronchial Stump

If there is any concern about the bronchial stump closure, or if there is a reasonable chance that the patient will undergo radiation therapy following operation, reinforcement of the bronchial stump is advised. A pleural flap is preferred, but a more substantial buttress is warranted when there is extra concern. An intercostal pedicle flap consisting of all the tissue between two adjacent ribs can be developed anteriorly and cleared posteriorly. Care is taken to avoid traumatizing the neurovascular bundle which runs just beneath the superior rib. (A simpler method of preserving the integrity of the neurovascular bundle is to remove the superior portion of the flap in a subperiosteal plane.)

Fig 6–4, A.—A mass of intercostal tissue is ligated anteriorly and divided from the superior margin of the rib below. The periosteum of the upper rib is incised, and the flap is developed and cleared from front to back in the subperiosteal plane.

B.—The end of the flap is then carefully tacked down around the bronchial closure with fine sutures and superficial bites of tissue. As with pleural flaps, the sutures used for closure of the bronchus also can be used to anchor this flap.

Thoracoplasty

It is generally agreed that a modified type of thoracoplasty should be performed when tuberculosis is the indication for pneumonectomy. The purposes are to prevent overdistention of the remaining lung and to obliterate dead space, thus decreasing the risk of bronchopleural fistula and tuberculous empyema. It has been customary to perform the thoracoplasty at a second operation, three to six weeks after the pneumonectomy. More recently, it has been recommended that a concomitant thoracoplasty be performed in good-risk patients, with the advantages that a second operation is avoided and that the dead space is obliterated more rapidly. A five- to six-rib thoracoplasty is adequate to accomplish these objectives. The first rib is not usually resected, but the parietal pleura is stripped from its inferior surface. Resection of the second through the sixth or seventh ribs is begun just lateral to the transverse processes, which are not removed. The second and third ribs are removed almost to their costal cartilages, but progressively less of the other ribs is resected anteriorly because of their downward slope.

Concomitant thoracoplasty heightens the risk of operation by increasing both blood loss and postoperative pain and by causing paradoxical motion, which impairs the efficiency of ventilation and coughing. The paradoxical motion may be minimized by dividing each of the second through the seventh ribs in three or four places instead of resecting them. The chest wall may then be displaced inward so that it is more rigid, making paradoxical motion less of a problem. It can be further minimized by immobilizing the external chest wall with a splint, but the maneuver may decrease ventilation on the opposite side and predispose to atelectasis. An excessive chest wall resection may prohibit early adequate ventilation, and the patient will require prolonged postoperative intubation and ventilatory support. It is recommended that thoracoplasty be deferred until a second stage unless the patient is in excellent condition.

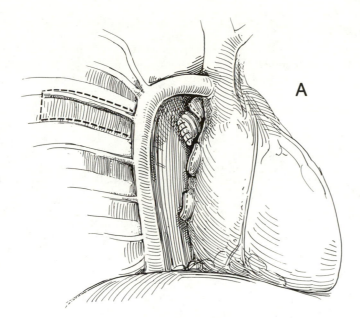

A

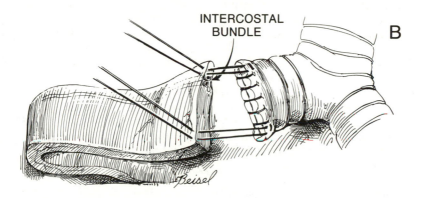

INTERCOSTAL
BUNDLE

B

Phrenic Nerve Paralysis

Routine crushing or division of the phrenic nerve at the completion of pneumonectomy is not recommended. The paralyzed diaphragm interferes significantly with ventilatory efficiency, and more perioperative complications may be expected. Later, after pneumonectomy, a fibrothorax forms and the diaphragm becomes elevated and fixed whether or not the phrenic nerve was paralyzed at the time of operation.

DRAINAGE OF THE PLEURAL CAVITY

Except under special circumstances, routine drainage of the pleural cavity is not required following pneumonectomy. The empty space formerly occupied by the resected lung is decreased as the mediastinum and diaphragm shift, and it is gradually filled with a serosanguinous effusion which eventually clots and is invaded with fibroblasts. It is not necessary or desirable, therefore, to remove the fluid which forms following a clean, uncomplicated pneumonectomy unless it accumulates too rapidly. However, if there has been heavy contamination of the pleural cavity with pathogenic organisms, which may occur when a primary or secondary lung abscess is ruptured during resection, the risk of empyema is great. This risk can be considerably reduced by copious intraoperative irrigation and subsequently by keeping the pleural cavity free of fluid, which is an excellent culture medium, for five to seven days. A large catheter (32 F) is led out from the lower portion of the pleural cavity through the eighth or ninth interspace and connected to very low (5–10-cm) H_2O suction. A small catheter (16 F) is inserted higher in the chest. At intervals, air is let in through the upper catheter as suction is applied to the lower catheter to remove all fluid from the pleural cavity. The lower catheter is then clamped, and a solution containing antibiotics is used to irrigate the hemithorax. The solutions used include penicillin-streptomycin, cephalosporins, and iodophors. Both tubes remain clamped for several hours following each injection, and the lower tube is then opened. When the tubes are removed on about the seventh postoperative day, the effusion which then forms is usually sterile and will remain so.

If there is more than the usual amount of chest wall bleeding, as may occur following an extrapleural pneumonectomy, it is probably wise to drain the pleural cavity. When a resection is done with concomitant thoracoplasty, drainage is indicated because a small volume of blood will materially affect the position of the mediastinum.

Some surgeons use drainage routinely following pneumonectomy and believe that being certain of the position of the mediastinum outweighs the possibility of introducing infection by this route. When drainage is used following a pneumonectomy, its purpose is to remove not fluid from the pleural cavity, but only the air, which is gradually replaced by blood and plasma. A small catheter may, therefore, be left and connected to a low-suction drainage. Strong suction is dangerous and should not be employed, since hemodynamic problems can be introduced by an exaggerated mediastinal shift. An underwater seal alone is also dangerous, since a cough can displace enough water to result in considerable negative pressure. The tube may be removed the day after surgery, when the chest film appears satisfactory, and danger of appreciable bleeding has passed.

ADJUSTMENT OF INTRAPLEURAL PRESSURE

The final step in pneumonectomy, if the pleural cavity is not to be drained, is adjustment of the intrapleural pressure. Early removal of the endotracheal tube is desirable in most lung resections, because air leaks and contamination are minimized when positive-pressure ventilation is avoided. For some time following resection of a lung, the mediastinum remains mobile. As fluid accumulates within the hemithorax and as fibrosis begins to occur, the mediastinal structures become fixed. In the immediate postoperative period, it is well to monitor the position of the mediastinum with follow-up roentgenogram examinations to be certain that a marked shift does not occur. An acceptable method of adjusting the intrapleural pressure on the resected side is to leave a small intercostal catheter in place at the end of the procedure and to adjust the pressure, using a manometer, to between -5 and -10 cm H_2O by aspiration of air. When chest closure is complete, the catheter is removed. This usually results in the displacement of both the trachea and the heart slightly toward the resected side. If necessary, and using sterile technique, the adjustment can be repeated with a needle and manometer.

PNEUMONECTOMY: COMPLICATIONS

The major and minor complications which may occur after any major operative procedure may follow pneumonectomy. Only those which are particularly related to pneumonectomy are discussed here. It must be reemphasized that meticulous surgical technique and aggressive postoperative management are of great importance in minimizing problems after operation. Preoperative instruction in pulmonary toilet exercises, adequate pain control, early mobilization, and measures directed at controlling and eliminating secretions all serve to better the chances of a smooth recovery.

Cardiovascular Instability

Pulmonary edema and cardiac arrhythmias are both sufficiently common following pneumonectomy to deserve special mention. Because the entire cardiac output is directed through the remaining lung, these patients are in jeopardy of fluid overload. Routine postpneumonectomy intravenous (IV) fluids should be given at lower-than-normal maintenance rates. Intraoperative and postoperative monitoring with either central venous or pulmonary artery catheters provides continuous information on the intravascular volume status. Both supraventricular and ventricular arrhythmias are common following major pulmonary resections and should receive aggressive treatment. Preoperative digitalization of all patients about to undergo pneumonectomy is favored by some surgeons; close postoperative cardiac rhythm monitoring is indicated.

Empyema

Postpneumonectomy empyema is uncommon following uncontaminated operations if antibiotic prophylaxis has been properly employed and irrigation of the pleural cavity at the time of operation has been carried out. In the presence of gross contamination, the pleural cavity is often drained for seven to ten days and treated with antibiotic irrigation as previously described. When a pleural space infection, or empyema, does develop, symptoms and signs are often masked by the antibiotics or may be delayed for several weeks. The diagnosis is made by clinical signs and symptoms of infection, regardless of how far in the past the patient underwent the pneumonectomy. Confirmation is obtained by culture of aspirated pleural fluid.

The options available for the treatment of empyema are dictated by the clinical picture of the patient and the nature and scope of the infectious process. If the infection is small, liquid, and well localized, either tube drainage or daily aspiration plus instillation of antibiotics may be successful. The classic method of treating larger, older, or loculated infected spaces is by open drainage, after which the intrathoracic volume may be reduced by thoracoplasty, if necessary.

BRONCHOPLEURAL FISTULA

A most significant problem which can follow any pulmonary resection but is somewhat more common following pneumonectomy is breakdown of the bronchial stump closure, creating a fistula between the airway and the pleural space. Whether caused by technical inadequacy, residual disease at the suture line, or surgical devascularization, this complication can be life-threatening. Bronchopleural fistula is also associated with bronchial stumps of excessive length, residual infection, and preoperative or postoperative radiation therapy. Pleural flaps and the intercostal muscle flap previously described minimize its frequency.

Fever and cough associated with large amounts of bloody, serous liquid (the old effusion) are diagnostic indicators and usually occur within two weeks of surgery. Depending on the cause, however, this problem may appear much later. The immediate threat to the patient is that of drowning, and the patient should immediately be positioned with the operated-on side down. Tube thoracostomy is urgent, and small leaks may actually heal if drainage and supportive care are continued. In severely infirm patients, maintenance of tube drainage may be accepted as definitive treatment as long as the air loss through the fistula is not great. To achieve closure of the fistula in most instances, however, direct intervention is necessary.

When diagnosis is made early, technical problems can be corrected by resuture of the bronchus. Reinforcement of the closure with an intercostal muscle flap should be performed, and irrigation and drainage of the chest is prudent because of the contamination which accompanies the fistula. The mediastinum becomes fixed, and a progressive fibrothorax develops following pneumonectomy. Late occurrence of bronchopleural fistula cannot be successfully treated by simple closure of the fistula. Considerable evidence suggests that thoracotomy, debridement, and transfer of a large, viable, predicled muscle flap offer the greatest chance for resolution. Latissimus dorsi, serratus anterior, pectoralis major, and rectus abdominis muscles have been used with success.

Closure with Muscle Flap

The following series demonstrates one technique of closure of a bronchopleural fistula which becomes manifest late after pneumonectomy. The pectoralis muscle flap has a hardy and predictable blood supply, and the technique of preparation is straightforward.

Fig 6–5, A.—An anterolateral thoracotomy provides access to the mediastinum for identification of the fistula and debridement of the tissues nearby. Vigorous irrigation of the chest with saline and antibiotic solutions is carried out next.

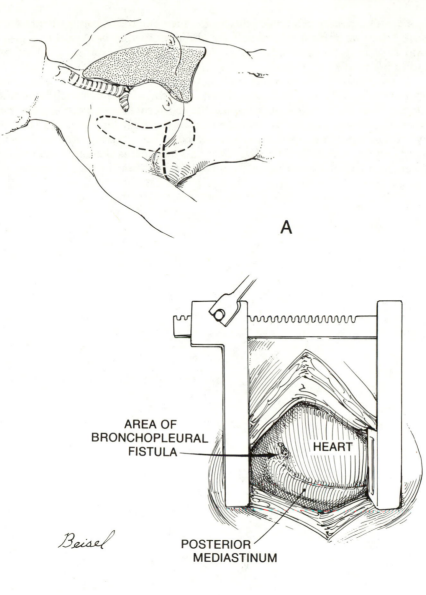

A

AREA OF
BRONCHOPLEURAL
FISTULA

HEART

Beisel

POSTERIOR
MEDIASTINUM

B.—The pectoralis major muscle is taken off the chest wall inferiorly and medially, leaving a vascular pedicle from the axillary vessels. A short section of the second rib has been removed to provide entry of the flap into the chest without tension or kinking.

C.—The debrided fistulous tract is oversewn with synthetic absorbable suture, and the muscle flap is tacked down over the area. In bronchopleural fistula following pneumonectomy, it is impossible to fill the entire pleural space with the mass of the muscle. The thoracotomy wound is therefore left open and packed twice daily with iodophor-dampened gauze until exuberant granulations are present over the flap and the interior of the chest cavity. The chest is then filled with antibiotic solution, and the thoracotomy incision is closed without further drainage.

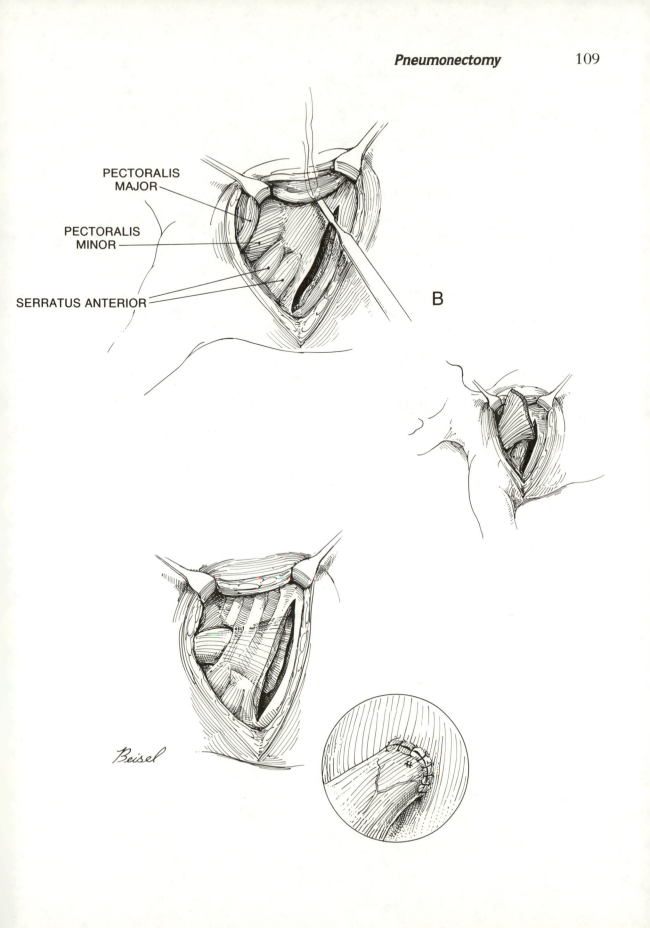

PECTORALIS MAJOR

PECTORALIS MINOR

SERRATUS ANTERIOR

B

Beisel

CHAPTER 7

Lobectomy

IN GENERAL, lobectomy is a more difficult operation to perform than pneumonectomy. Dissection of the secondary hilar structures is tedious and time-consuming, the anatomic relationships are complicated, and anomalies occur frequently. In many instances, the fissures between the lobes are incomplete and must be developed by careful dissection. Finally, peripheral adhesions can be a problem because lobectomy is often done for inflammatory rather than neoplastic lesions. On the other hand, since smaller vessels are being handled, catastrophic hemorrhage is less likely to occur.

INDICATIONS

Lobectomy is now performed frequently for bronchogenic carcinoma, since experience has shown that the results are just as good as those for pneumonectomy when the tumor is peripherally located and hilar nodes are not involved. A review of the lymphatic drainage patterns of the lobes shows why there are four basic lobectomy operations for bronchogenic cancer: left upper and lower lobectomies, right upper lobectomy, and the right middle and lower bilobectomy.

The most frequent indication for lobectomy in the past was bronchiectasis. The disease is seldom confined to one lobe, and the removal of additional segments on the same side, or of an additional lobe or segments on the opposite side, is often necessary. Lymphatic drainage patterns do not generally indicate the scope of resection for inflammatory disease. Considerations which lead to the choice of operation for lung abscess have been discussed previously. Lobectomy for pulmonary tuberculosis was once common, but now is less frequently used. The operative strategy in the treatment of tuberculosis is covered in chapter 10. Additional indications for lobectomy include giant emphysematous blebs or bullae, large or centrally located benign tumors, chronic nonspecific suppurative disease, fungus infections, and congenital anomalies.

Preoperative Preparation

A prolonged period of preparation may be necessary, particularly in patients with bronchiectasis, chronic lung abscess, or other types of chronic suppurative disease. The objectives are to clear active infection and to reduce tracheobronchial secretions to a minimum. Helpful measures are antibiotic therapy, postural drainage, and repeated bronchoscopic aspiration. Operation should be deferred, if possible, until the daily output of sputum is less than 25 ml.

POSITION OF THE PATIENT

Whenever feasible, the lateral position is used for lobectomy because it gives the surgeon the greatest maneuverability. However, the danger of spillover of purulent secretions, the skill of the anesthesiologist, and the facility of hilar dissection must also be considered. A double-lumen endotracheal tube should be used in resection for tuberculosis and suppurative disease when there is danger of spilling infected material into the other lung. If one is not available, consideration might be given to operating with the patient prone, even though the operative procedure is usually more difficult in that position. The supine position may be used for upper and middle lobe resections, especially in poor-risk patients. Knowledge of the anatomy of the secondary and tertiary hilar structures must be so thorough that orientation will be easy regardless of the position of the patient.

In the lateral position, a fourth intercostal space incision is used for the upper lobes, and a fifth or sixth interspace incision is used for the right middle lobe, lingula, and lower lobes. In unusual situations when the supine position is used, additional exposure is gained by either transection or resection of adjacent ribs or cartilages. In all of the lobectomies illustrated, the use of the lateral position is shown.

PROBLEMS COMMON TO MANY LOBECTOMIES

Before describing the technique of removing the different lobes, problems which frequently arise deserve special attention.

Peripheral Adhesions

Since many lobectomies are performed for inflammatory lesions, there are frequently adhesions between the parietal and visceral pleurae. They may be thin and avascular, so that division with scissors or even by blunt dissection with the fingers or a sponge stick is a simple matter. Often, however, a dense layer of fibrous tissue binds the parietal and visceral pleurae firmly together. Sharp dissection with scissors or a scalpel is required if the lung is to be freed intrapleurally; it is difficult to avoid cutting into the pulmonary parenchyma. Cavities may be caused by tuberculosis, lung abscess, or bronchiectasis, and the densest adhesions usually overlie these areas. Entering such cavities during the dissection of adhesions inevitably contaminates the pleural cavity with pathogenic organisms. Usually this can be avoided by dissecting extrapleurally when the parietal and visceral pleurae are densely fused. An incision is made in the parietal pleura adjacent to the adherent area, and the extrapleural fascial plane is developed by blunt dissection with the index finger or a gauze pledget. The parietal pleura overlying the densely adherent area is then excised. If this maneuver is painstakingly executed, it is nearly always possible to avoid opening into parenchymal cavities, except in instances of erosion of the cavity through the pleura. If a cavity is entered, the extent of soiling can be minimized by quickly walling off the area with sponges and removing the contents of the cavity by suction. Dissection may continue after the cavity is firmly packed with gauze sponges.

Incomplete Fissures

Interlobar fissures are often incomplete from the periphery to the interlobar hilum. Incomplete fissures are due to either inflammatory adhesions or congenital failure to develop completely. Fusion of a fissure may also be due to the extension of an inflammatory lesion or a tumor from one lobe to another.

The technique for opening an incomplete fissure is usually not difficult. Care must be used, however, to avoid complications. In the case of inflammatory adhesions, blunt dissection should be tried first, for it is usually successful. A gentle, sweeping motion with a sponge stick will suffice if the adhesions are filmy, whereas pushing with a gauze pledget is necessary if they are moderately firm. Dense adhesions must be separated by spreading with a long, curved hemostat or by cutting with scissors. Pressure with a gauze sponge can control capillary oozing, but large bleeding vessels must be clamped and ligated. The principal task is that of remaining in the true interlobar plane, thus avoiding injury to the pulmonary parenchyma on either side. The area of dissection is kept dry by constant suction and sponging, while frequent reference is made to adjacent landmarks which localize the position of the fissure. When adhesions are tough and vascular and it is difficult to stay within the interlobar plane, two other maneuvers should be considered. One is to place clamps across the adherent area, cut between them, and suture the edges with a basting stitch reinforced by an over-and-over suture. Alternatively, a stapling instrument may be used. The other maneuver is to dissect and divide the secondary hilar structures first and then to complete the separation of the adherent lobes by the retrograde technique (to be illustrated for right middle lobectomy). When the diseased lobe is thoroughly deflated and the adjacent lobe expanded, separation of the fissure may be accomplished accurately by either blunt or sharp dissection. Bleeding vessels and air leaks which persist after pressure has been applied for several minutes are clamped and ligated.

When an incomplete fissure is due to a congenital failure of development, the stapler or the clamp-and-suture method is advisable because vessels and bronchi of moderate size are often divided. The retrograde technique may be used, however, and is preferable if the area of incomplete separation is extensive, because the distortion of the remaining lobe (caused by the clamp and suture method) is avoided. Bleeding points and air leaks must be controlled with great care.

LEFT UPPER LOBECTOMY

This procedure is illustrated with the patient in the lateral position. The plan is to divide the segmental arteries first, then the veins, and finally the upper lobe bronchus. The arteries to the apical and posterior segments are on the anterosuperior surface of the primary hilum. The arteries to the anterior and lingular segments are found within the fissure between the upper and lower lobes, except for those instances in which the anterior segmental artery comes off proximal to the apical posterior artery. All of the upper lobe veins drain into the superior pulmonary vein, which is approached on the anterior surface of the hilum.

Fig 7–1, A.—With the upper lobe retracted downward and backward, the anterosuperior portion of the hilar pleura is incised and separated. The left main pulmonary artery is identified and followed distally until the first upper lobe branch is encountered. This is usually the apical posterior trunk, but the apical and posterior segmental arteries may arise separately. Often the anterior segmental artery is the most proximal branch of the left pulmonary artery. In any event, all branches which originate at the point where the main pulmonary artery trunk begins to curve around the left upper lobe bronchus on the superior aspect of the hilum are divided and ligated. The technique of ligation and division is the same as that for the primary hilar vessels, except that finer ligatures are used. The principle of ligating branches distally to obtain the longest cuff possible is important. It is not always necessary to use suture ligatures in addition to free ligatures distally, because the segmental or subsegmental arteries concerned are often small and back-bleeding, if it does occur, is not a serious problem.

B.—The fissure between the upper and lower lobes is then opened to divide the arteries into the anterior and lingular segments. Dissection of the pulmonary artery in the depths of the fissure must be sufficiently extensive to identify all upper lobe branches which originate within the fissure and to exclude anomalies. Usually only an anterior and a lingular trunk require ligation and division (*insert*), but the occurrence of three or four branches with separate origins is not uncommon. The superior segmental artery arises at about the same level as the lingular artery.

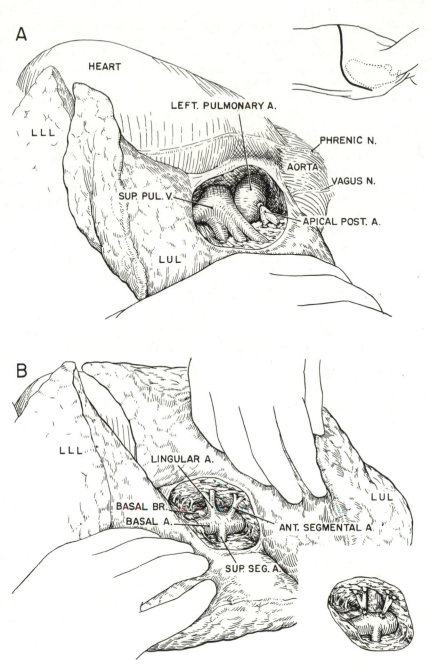

A

HEART

LEFT. PULMONARY A.

LLL

PHRENIC N.

AORTA

VAGUS N.

SUP. PUL. V.

APICAL POST. A.

LUL

B

LLL

LINGULAR A.

BASAL BR.

BASAL A.

ANT. SEGMENTAL A.

LUL

SUP. SEG. A.

C.—The lung is retracted posteriorly for dissection of the superior pulmonary vein. This step is usually deferred until all of the upper lobe arteries have been divided and may be important if the patient has had recent bleeding from the lobe. Dissection, ligation, and division of the superior pulmonary vein do not differ from the technique employed during pneumonectomy except that the region of the lingular tributaries should be exposed with greater care to exclude the possibility of anomalous drainage from the lower lobe to this area. In the *insert,* the superior pulmonary vein has been divided, and the upper lobe bronchus is clearly visible.

D.—After the upper lobe arteries and veins are divided, the upper lobe bronchus is the only important remaining structure. Considerable care must be taken in dissecting all other remaining tissues, however. The bronchus is freed by blunt dissection unless the peribronchial lymph nodes are unusually adherent. The left upper lobe bronchus is usually so short that encroachment on the remaining airway to the lower lobe may result if it is divided and sutured. The proximal bronchus clamp should be placed at least 1.5–2 cm from the main bronchial trunk, usually at the bifurcation of the upper and lower divisional bronchi, as illustrated. The divisional or segmental bronchi are sutured rather than the upper lobe bronchus. In clearing the bronchus and applying the bronchus clamps, the main trunk of the pulmonary artery should be kept in full view and protected by retracting the upper lobe anteriorly.

E.—The stump of the upper lobe bronchus, or the stumps of the branch bronchi, are closed with either fine (4–0) monofilament sutures or a stapling instrument (4.8-mm staples) and covered with a pleural flap, as illustrated.

The most common technical accident in performing left upper lobectomy is injury to the main trunk of the pulmonary artery as it curves around the upper lobe bronchus. Injury is most likely to occur during dissection of an incomplete fissure or while freeing an adherent bronchus. Since the relative position of the artery may be altered by inflammatory changes, the surgeon should be cautious in executing any maneuver in the region of the posterosuperior aspect of the hilum.

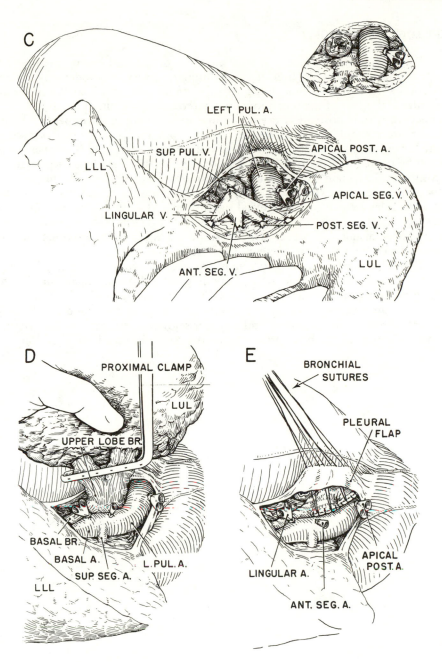

C

LEFT PUL. A.

SUP. PUL. V.

APICAL POST. A.

LLL

APICAL SEG. V.

LINGULAR V.

POST. SEG. V.

LUL

ANT. SEG. V.

D

PROXIMAL CLAMP

LUL

UPPER LOBE BR.

BASAL BR.

BASAL A.

L. PUL. A.

SUP. SEG. A.

LLL

E

BRONCHIAL SUTURES

PLEURAL FLAP

LINGULAR A.

APICAL POST. A.

ANT. SEG. A.

LEFT LOWER LOBECTOMY

Fig 7–2, A.—The first step is to open the fissure and expose the lower two thirds of the interlobar portion of the pulmonary artery. A moderately extensive dissection verifies which branches go to the upper and which to the lower lobe, minimizing the risk of ligating anomalous intercommunicating branches. Often, it is unnecessary to expose the artery to the anterior segment of the upper lobe, but the lingular artery should be exposed. The one or two branches to the superior segment of the lower lobe may originate proximal to the lingular artery to the upper lobe and should be ligated and divided first. A third, smaller branch to this segment is not uncommon. The main basal trunk is then followed downward, and the basal segmental branches are exposed. If the proximal ligature is placed just distal to the lowest lingular branch, a single distal ligature placed at the point of origin of the basal segmental branches may provide a sufficient cuff. It is often necessary to ligate the branches distally, however, and in some instances both proximal and distal ligatures must be placed on the segmental branches.

B.—The inferior pulmonary vein is exposed by retracting the lung anteriorly, opening the posterior hilar pleura, and dividing the pulmonary ligament. The technique for ligating this vessel is the same as that for all the great vessels. The proximal free and suture ligatures are placed proximal to the bifurcation, and the distal ligatures are placed on the main basal and superior segmental tributaries. The tributaries are divided distal to the bifurcation so that the cuff will be a least 1 cm long.

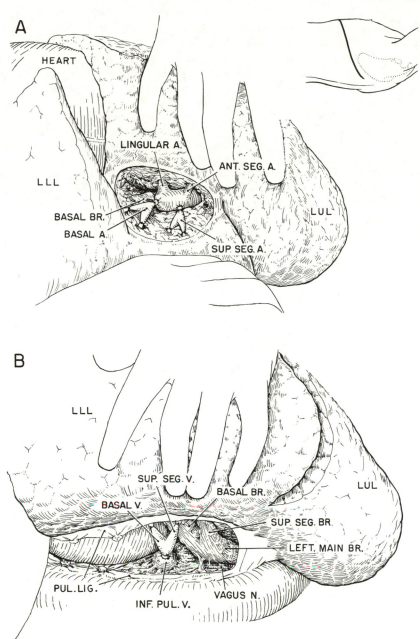

C.—After dividing the arteries and veins of the lower lobe, the bronchus is the only important remaining structure. Considerable dissection may still have to be done to separate the lobes, however. The upper and lower lobes below the bronchus are often quite adherent and must be separated. Even more often, the fissure between the superior segment of the lower lobe and the posterior segment of the upper lobe is incomplete. The retrograde technique should be used if the adherent area is broad, but if only a thin layer of tissue remains, either a stapling instrument or the clamp-and-suture technique may be used without appreciably altering the contour of the upper lobe. Freeing of the bronchus presents no special problem, except that the point of origin of the superior segmental bronchus may be only slightly distal to the point of origin of the lingular bronchus. When this is the case, division of the short lower lobe bronchus above the superior bronchus may not be possible without encroaching on the lingular bronchus. Separate division of the superior and main basal bronchi is then preferable. Unless care is taken to see the actual position of the lingular bronchus, this procedure should not be used. When the landmarks are carefully identified, it is usually possible to place a single proximal bronchus clamp just at the bifurcation of the basal and superior bronchi, as illustrated.

D.—Bronchial sutures are inserted in the usual way. It is normally simple to advance the pleura overlying the aorta to cover the bronchus.

Lingulectomy often accompanies left lower lobectomy, and the segmental technique is usually used, as illustrated in chapter 8.

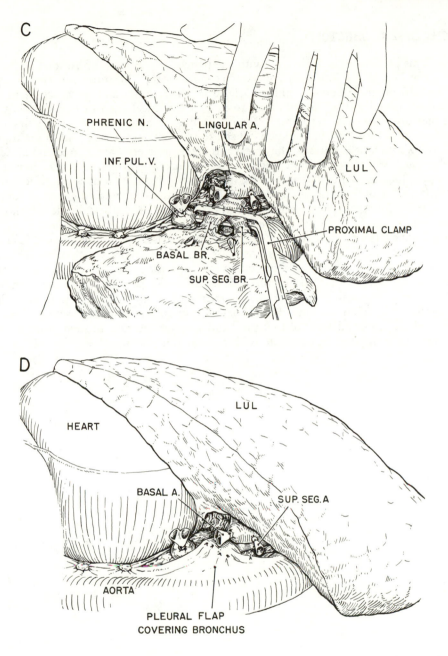

C

PHRENIC N.

LINGULAR A.

INF. PUL. V.

LUL

PROXIMAL CLAMP

BASAL BR.

SUP. SEG. BR.

D

LUL

HEART

BASAL A.

SUP. SEG. A

AORTA

PLEURAL FLAP
COVERING BRONCHUS

RIGHT UPPER LOBECTOMY

This procedure is illustrated with the patient in the lateral position.

Fig 7–3, A.—With the lung retracted posteriorly, the anterosuperior portion of the hilar pleura is opened, and the arteries to the anterior and apical segments are dissected. Usually these arteries arise from a single apical anterior trunk as shown, but they also may arise separately. When they do, the apical artery appears first and the anterior artery may be somewhat distal to it, even originating within the minor fissure. Whatever the pattern, the apical and anterior arteries are ligated and divided in the usual way. On the right side the main pulmonary artery remains anterior to the upper lobe bronchus rather than passing posterior to it, as it does on the left side.

B.—The oblique fissure is then opened to expose the remaining arterial supply to the upper lobe, and the posterior segmental artery is ligated and divided. It should be noted that on the right side the posterior segmental artery arises within the fissure, while on the left side the anterior segmental artery arises within the fissure. Usually on the right side there is a single posterior ascending artery which arises as illustrated. However, it may start from either the superior artery or one of the middle lobe arteries, and the dissection within the fissure must often be to the extent shown to exclude such possibilities. The other important variant to be kept in mind is that in about 10% of all patients the arterial supply to the posterior segment arises anteriorly, from or adjacent to the apical and anterior arteries. In such instances, no arteries to the upper lobe originate within the major fissure.

A

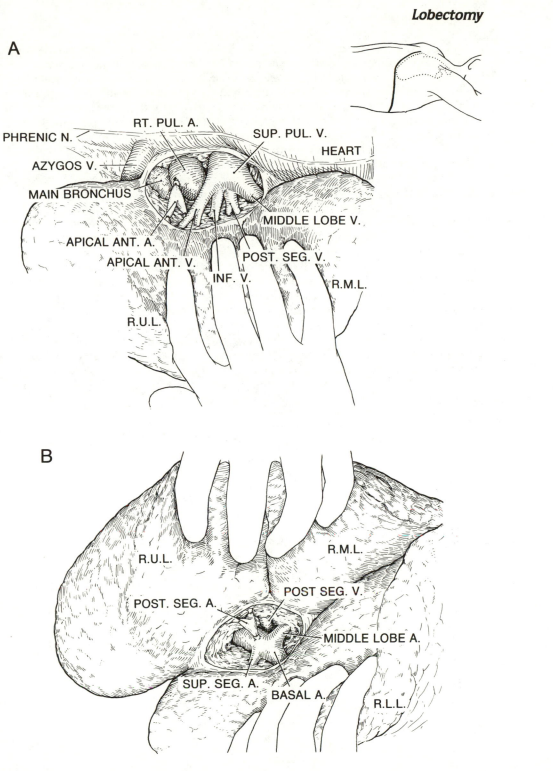

PHRENIC N.

AZYGOS V.

MAIN BRONCHUS

RT. PUL. A.

SUP. PUL. V.

HEART

APICAL ANT. A.

APICAL ANT. V.

MIDDLE LOBE V.

POST. SEG. V.

INF. V.

R.M.L.

R.U.L.

B

R.U.L.

R.M.L.

POST. SEG. A.

POST SEG. V.

MIDDLE LOBE A.

SUP. SEG. A.

BASAL A.

R.L.L.

C.—After the upper lobe arteries are divided, the lung is again retracted posteriorly, and the upper lobe veins are disposed of. The distribution and nomenclature of these veins are variable. The segmental branches usually join to form either two or three main tributaries which enter the upper two thirds of the superior pulmonary vein. The objectives are to dissect the branches sufficiently to provide adequate cuffs without causing injury and to differentiate the middle lobe vein or veins which enter the inferior portion of the superior pulmonary vein. The middle lobe vein or veins must be spared. The posterior segmental vein often arises at a sharp angle from an adherent fissure and can be easily overlooked.

It should be remembered that both the inferior vein (from the anterior segment) and the posterior vein lie deep within the minor fissure. The posterior vein is usually seen as it emerges from the parenchyma during dissection of the posterior artery. In opening an adherent minor fissure, the posterior and inferior veins are vulnerable behind the point of ligation and may cause annoying bleeding if they are injured.

D.—Freeing the upper lobe bronchus is less hazardous on the right than on the left side, because there are no major vessels immediately posterior to it. In most instances, it is advisable to carry the dissection far enough distally to place the proximal bronchus clamp just distal to the trifurcation.

E.—The three segmental bronchi rather than the upper lobe bronchus are sutured, so that encroachment on the airway to the remaining lobes is avoided. A good pleural flap to cover the bronchial stump is nearly always available. The pleura above the hilum is relatively mobile, and the anchoring sutures may be passed under the azygos vein, as illustrated. When this is done, it is advisable to ligate the vein to prevent embolization if thrombosis should occur.

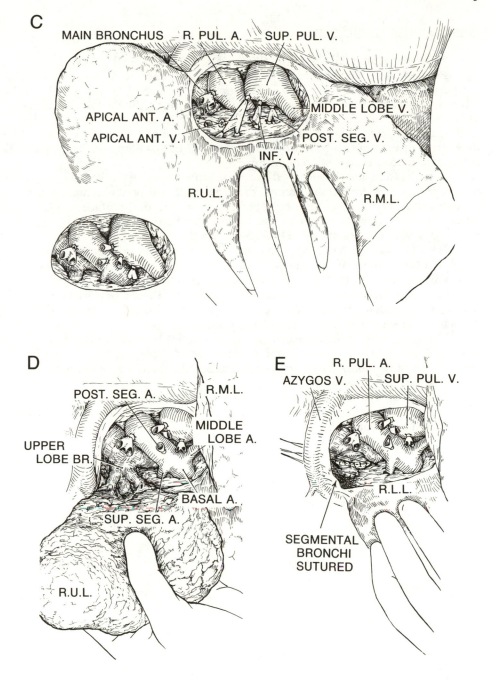

C

MAIN BRONCHUS   R. PUL. A.   SUP. PUL. V.

APICAL ANT. A.

APICAL ANT. V.

MIDDLE LOBE V.

POST. SEG. V.

INF. V.

R.U.L.

R.M.L.

D

POST. SEG. A.

R.M.L.

MIDDLE LOBE A.

UPPER LOBE BR.

BASAL A.

SUP. SEG. A.

R.U.L.

E

R. PUL. A.

AZYGOS V.

SUP. PUL. V.

R.L.L.

SEGMENTAL BRONCHI SUTURED

RIGHT MIDDLE LOBECTOMY

This procedure is illustrated with the patient in the lateral position.

Fig 7–4, A.—The first step is to open the major fissure and expose the interlobar portion of the pulmonary artery. There may be one, two, or three middle lobe arteries, all arising at about the same level as the superior segmental artery. Usually, as shown here, there is a single common trunk, and the middle lobe bronchus is easily palpable just behind it. The possibility of an anomalous branch of a middle lobe artery to the upper lobe must be kept in mind. In this figure the first ligature is being placed around the middle lobe artery.

After ligation and division of the arterial supply, it is easy to free the bronchus by deepening the dissection through the fissure. If the peribronchial tissues are adherent, it is best to retract the lung posteriorly and to deal with the middle lobe veins from the anterior aspect of the hilum. Inadvertent injury to the superior pulmonary vein can result from blind dissection through the fissure.

B.—The lung is retracted posteriorly. Normally, a single middle lobe trunk enters the lower third of the superior pulmonary vein, and ligation is as shown.

Dissection of the middle lobe bronchus presents no difficulties after the arteries and veins are ligated and divided. The bronchial sutures should be placed far enough distally so that edema will not cause encroachment on either the lumen of the main bronchial trunk or the superior segmental bronchus.

C.—The most difficult maneuver in middle lobectomy is dissection of the minor fissure, which is rarely complete. The use of sponge sticks to separate the upper and middle lobes, dissection with a gauze pledget, and dissection with a long, curved hemostat are illustrated.

The retrograde technique of removing the right middle lobe is illustrated in Figures 7–4, D–G. This includes use of the maneuvers that demarcate intersegmental planes in segmental resection.

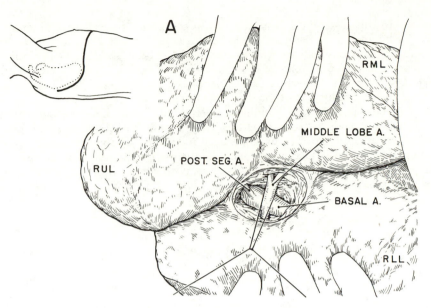

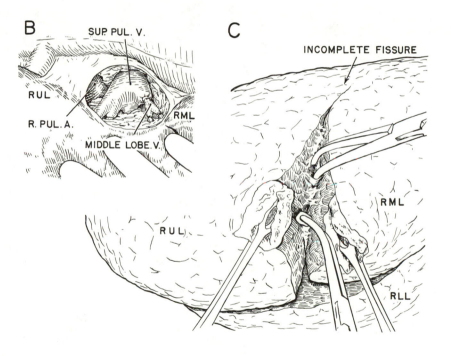

D.—In this instance, a large portion of the minor fissure is so adherent that separation by any other method would be difficult. No attempt is made to dissect the minor fissure before all the hilar structures have been divided. The middle lobe arteries and veins have been ligated and divided. The middle lobe bronchus has been dissected, and the first bronchus clamp is about to be applied. Before occluding the bronchus, the entire lung is deflated.

E.—The middle lobe bronchus has been divided, and the bronchial stump has been closed. The ends of two of the bronchial sutures have been retained to use in anchoring the pleural flap. The lung has been reinflated, but the middle lobe remains airless because the bronchus clamps were applied while the lung was deflated. This technique of differential inflation clearly shows the demarcation between the upper and middle lobes.

D

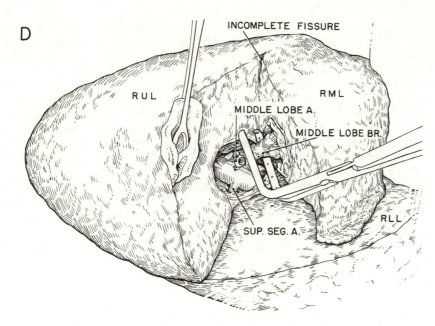

INCOMPLETE FISSURE

RUL

RML

MIDDLE LOBE A.

MIDDLE LOBE BR.

SUP. SEG. A.

RLL

E

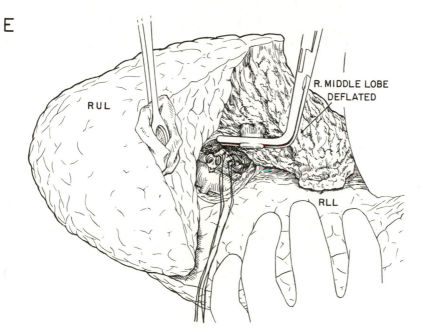

RUL

R. MIDDLE LOBE DEFLATED

RLL

F.—The visceral pleura has been divided at the line of demarcation between the inflated upper lobe and the deflated middle lobe. The surgeon is gently squeezing the tissue along this line between his right thumb and index finger. Tissue which does not yield to this maneuver is cut with the scissors. If there is doubt as to whether dissection is proceeding exactly in the interlobar plane, as there may be when extensive inflammatory adhesions are present, care is taken to dissect slightly on the middle lobe side of the plane so that the upper lobe, which is not to be removed, will not be injured. The dissection may be done with a gauze pledget or by spreading with dissecting scissors as well as by the method illustrated. Dissection should be started at the hilum and continued peripherally, since this offers the best opportunity of staying in the proper plane.

G.—Separation of the minor fissure has been completed and the lobe has been removed. The upper lobe surface is slightly irregular, but there are no significant bleeding points or air leaks. The middle lobe bronchus has been covered with a pleural flap, although it is often difficult to advance a flap to cover it. Loose areolar tissue can be used instead of pleura and is usually available in the immediate vicinity.

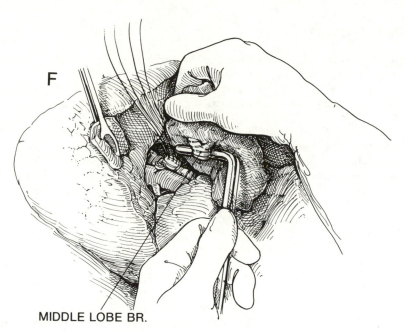

F

MIDDLE LOBE BR.

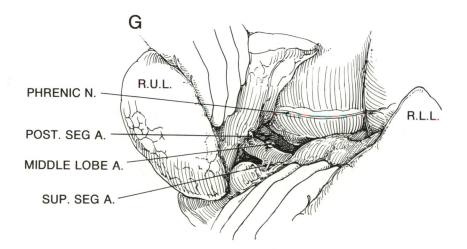

G

PHRENIC N.

R.U.L.

POST. SEG A.

R.L.L.

MIDDLE LOBE A.

SUP. SEG A.

RIGHT LOWER LOBECTOMY

The procedure is illustrated with the patient in the lateral position.

Fig 7–5, A.—The great fissure is opened. The interlobar portion of the pulmonary artery is exposed in the depths of the fissure, and the dissection is carried to approximately the extent shown in order to detect possible anomalous branches between the lobes. The one or two branches of the superior segmental artery, which arise at the same level as the middle lobe arterial supply (two branches in this instance), are ligated and divided. The basal arterial supply is ordinarily no more difficult to deal with than the arterial supply on the left side. The proximal ligatures are placed just distal to either the lowest superior segmental or middle lobe branch, and the distal ligatures are placed just beyond the bifurcation of the basal artery. The completed division of the arterial supply is shown in the insert.

It is not uncommon on the right side, however, for the four basal segmental arteries to originate separately just below the superior segmental and middle lobe arteries and to plunge immediately into the pulmonary parenchyma. All the ligatures must then be placed on the basal segmental arteries. Freeing these arteries from the lung substance sufficiently to provide an adequate cuff entails some risk of injury to them.

B.—The inferior pulmonary vein is exposed by retracting the lung anteriorly, opening the posterior hilar pleura, and ligating and dividing the pulmonary ligament. For division of this vein, the proximal ligatures are placed proximal to the bifurcation, and the distal ligatures are placed on the superior segmental and main basal tributaries. The proximal bronchus clamp should be placed just distal to the bifurcation of the basal and superior segmental bronchi, so that these bronchi are actually sutured separately even though they are caught in a single clamp. This is advisable to avoid injury to the middle lobe bronchus, which frequently lies close to the bronchus of the superior segment of the lower lobe. The problem is similar to that encountered with the lingular bronchus in a left lower lobectomy, except that the margin of safety is somewhat smaller on the right.

The clamp-and-suture method of dealing with an incompletely developed fissure is illustrated. There is congenital underdevelopment of the fissure between the superior segment of the right lower lobe and the posterior segment of the right upper lobe.

A

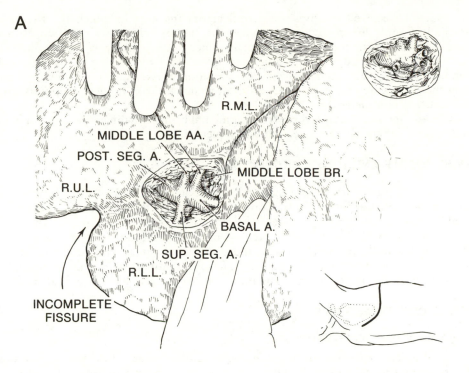

R.M.L.

MIDDLE LOBE AA.

POST. SEG. A.

MIDDLE LOBE BR.

R.U.L.

BASAL A.

SUP. SEG. A.

R.L.L.

INCOMPLETE
FISSURE

B

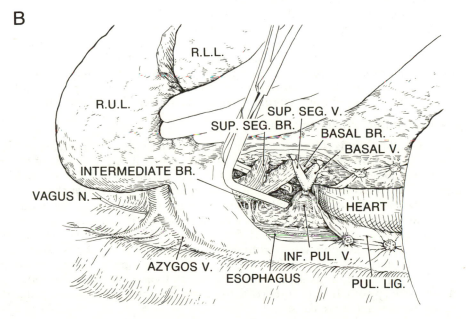

R.L.L.

R.U.L.

SUP. SEG. V.

SUP. SEG. BR.

BASAL BR.

BASAL V.

INTERMEDIATE BR.

VAGUS N.

HEART

AZYGOS V.

INF. PUL. V.

ESOPHAGUS

PUL. LIG.

C.—Three Kelly clamps are placed across the area in which the fissure is normally found. When dividing between the clamps with a scalpel, two clamps should be left on the lobe that is to remain, since a single clamp will often slip off.

D.—The cut edge of the lobe may be secured by placing a basting stitch behind the clamps and then an over-and-over suture through the crushed lung tissue after the clamps are removed. There are seldom any air leaks or bleeding points after the suture is completed.

E.—The main basal and superior segmental bronchi, which have been divided and sutured separately, are covered with a pleural flap.

RIGHT MIDDLE AND LOWER BILOBECTOMY

The lymphatic drainage of the right middle and lower lobes is to a central area around the bronchus intermedius. Complete removal of the nodes, as is prudent for lung carcinoma of the right lower lobe, therefore requires sacrifice of the right middle lobe as well. The conduct of the operation and the exposure are the same as for a right middle lobectomy, with the division of artery and bronchus at the intermediate level within the fissure. The inferior pulmonary vein is also divided. As in the case of middle lobectomy, the minor fissure is completed as a final step.

LOBECTOMY: FINAL STEPS

Drainage of the Pleural Cavity

Complete expansion of the remaining pulmonary tissue at the site of operation and obliteration of the pleural cavity are important objectives following lobectomy. The pleural cavity is always drained to remove fluid and air which would prevent apposition of the parietal and visceral pleurae. Small air leaks seal rapidly, and the removal of fluid decreases the likelihood of empyema by depriving any contaminating organisms of a culture medium in which to flourish.

As a general principle, it is wise to insert two drainage tubes following lobectomy. One is placed in a posterobasal position for the removal of fluid and the other in an apical position for the surest evacuation of air. It is helpful to anchor the tubes with a small absorbable suture to the parietal pleura to prevent migration. Chest tubes are left in place for at least 24 hours after air leaks have stopped, until fluid drainage is minimal. Antibiotic prophylaxis is maintained throughout this period.

Expansion of the Remaining Lobes

Before the chest is closed, the lung is fully inflated by the anesthesiologist while the surgeon makes sure that no atelectatic areas remain. Any remaining adhesions between the parietal and the visceral pleura should be divided so that the residual pulmonary parenchyma can expand uniformly and fill the new interior chest geometry comfortably. Finally, any tendency toward rotation on the hilar axis should be noted, and, if present, the remaining lobe or lobes should be anchored in such a way as to correct the problem. It is prudent, for example, to place a few sutures between the lower and middle lobes after right upper lobectomy to prevent possible torsion of the middle lobe. The chest roentgenogram is examined closely to confirm expansion of the remaining lung tissue after operation, and vigorous chest physiotherapy and incentive spirometry are important to ensure complete expansion during the first several postoperative days.

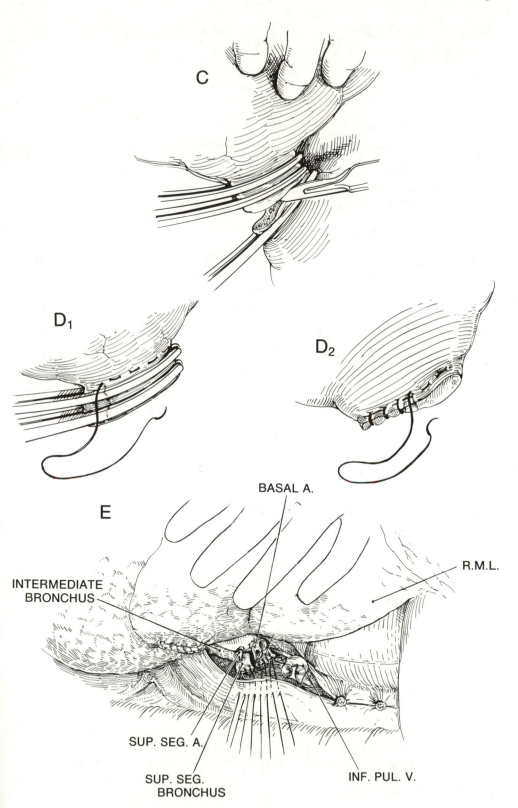

C

D₁

D₂

BASAL A.

R.M.L.

INTERMEDIATE
BRONCHUS

E

SUP. SEG. A.

SUP. SEG.
BRONCHUS

INF. PUL. V.

ANCILLARY PROCEDURES

Thoracoplasty

Although this practice has been nearly abandoned, some surgeons perform a limited thoracoplasty when a lobectomy has been done for tuberculosis. The rationale for this is that recurrent tuberculosis appears to develop more frequently in pulmonary tissue that has become overdistended as the result of a previous resection. Concomitant thoracoplasty also aids in early obliteration of the pleural cavity and may decrease the risks of empyema and bronchopleural fistula. This additional procedure adds to the risk of lobectomy in that there is increased blood loss, increased postoperative pain, and some paradoxical motion, which decreases the efficiency of ventilation and coughing. Thoracoplasty should be done as a second-stage procedure in poor-risk patients.

Decortication

Lobectomy may be done under circumstances in which expansion of the remaining pulmonary tissue is restricted by the presence of a fibrinous exudate which has formed over the visceral pleura. Examples are chronic pneumothorax due to ruptured blebs and unexpandable lung following prolonged artificial pneumothorax for tuberculosis. The "peel" over the remaining lobe or lobes must be removed.

Phrenic Nerve Paralysis

It is not advisable to crush the phrenic nerve at the end of lobectomy. The resulting paradoxical motion of the diaphragm might embarrass cardiopulmonary function to the point of compromise. Phrenic nerve crushing has been recommended when more than one lobe has been resected and when difficulty with full obliteration of the pleural space is anticipated. An attractive alternative is pneumoperitoneum, which assists in the process of decreasing the size of the pleural space, is controllable, and carries very little risk.

POSTOPERATIVE CARE

The general care of the patient following lobectomy is essentially the same as that following other major thoracic procedures. Excessive tracheobronchial secretions are more commonly serious, however, because lobectomy is often done for an inflammatory lesion. It should be stressed again that every effort must be made to prevent atelectasis. Spontaneous coughing by the patient is the most desirable method of expelling secretions but, if this is not effective, tracheal aspiration and bronchoscopy must not be neglected. Finally, tracheostomy may be advisable in some instances, particularly when secretions are unusually voluminous.

Management of Drainage Tubes

If there is an air leak, constant suction (-10 to -20 cm H_2O) is desirable. Whether it is due to an alveolopleural fistula or a bronchopleural fistula, closure of the leak is aided when the residual pulmonary tissue is maintained in a more expanded state. Both the upper and lower drainage tubes may be connected through a Y-tube to the same suction source. Constant controlled suction should be continued until the leak has sealed over and full expansion is achieved. Unless a bronchial suture line breaks down or a relatively large branch bronchus on the raw surface of a lobe is not closed, a leak usually stops within 24–48 hours. If a small air leak persists for several days, the negative pressure should be increased. This is most common in patients with emphysema, but the air leak seldom persists more than a week. A persistent large air leak or one that increases should receive prompt bronchoscopic investigation for bronchopleural fistula. Early reoperation with resuture of a failed bronchial closure is often successful, and muscle flap reinforcement is wise.

In the absence of an air leak, continuous suction is not essential except for upper lobe resections. Fluid is expelled adequately as the intrapleural pressure is increased by coughing and straining. The application of suction every two or three hours may help to dislodge fibrin clots, which tend to plug the tube, and ensure complete drainage. Any type of suction apparatus may be used to apply suction intermittently.

POSTOPERATIVE COMPLICATIONS

A discussion of the complications which may occur after any major thoracic procedure need not be given here. However, two complications which are particularly related to lobectomy deserve consideration.

Bronchopleural Fistula

In a nontuberculous patient, reopening of a bronchial stump is rare if the stump is properly sutured and covered. It occurs even less often after lobectomy than after pneumonectomy because expansion of the remaining pulmonary tissue obliterates adjacent dead space. Breakdown of an improperly sutured bronchial stump early in the postoperative period may cause tension pneumothorax, and this possibility must be kept in mind if the patient experiences sudden respiratory distress. Leaks more often than not occur late and are either caused by or followed by empyema. A chest roentgenogram shows a new cavity with an air-fluid level within. The insertion of a large tube into the cavity and the use of constant suction is sometimes a successful treatment. Suction may have to be continued for several weeks. If the fistula persists, resuture of the bronchus and decortication of the remaining lobe or lobes may be required, or a pneumonectomy may have to be done. Muscle flap transfer may aid in healing the stump and in obliteration of the persistent air space as well.

Postlobectomy Empyema

The incidence of pleural space infection, or empyema, following pulmonary resection is currently low when appropriate antibiotic prophylaxis and meticulous surgical techniques are employed. This complication was much more common in the past. Various treatment options were developed that are worthy of mention.

Empyema is most frequently associated with operative contamination. Other possible etiologies include infection secondary to a bronchopleural fistula that closed and secondary infection of fluid in the pleural space by hematogenous spread from another source.

Treatment of "early" empyema is drainage, either open or closed. Intermittent aspiration and instillation of antibiotics into the cavity every few days has been successful for small empyemas diagnosed soon after surgery. Several limitations with this form of closed drainage must be recognized. Clotting, organization, and fibrothorax eventually result, and pulmonary function is decreased. If the empyema cavity is loculated, there is little likelihood of successful resolution with this method, and if clinical and radiologic signs are not clearly favorable after seven to ten days, surgical drainage should be instituted.

Tube thoracostomy will often be adequate treatment for a localized area of infection if the contents of the cavity are liquid and if loculations are not present. The techniques of insertion of an intercostal thoracostomy tube were presented in chapter 1. Preliminary needle aspiration of the cavity confirms the diagnosis, provides a specimen for culture and sensitivity testing, and ensures correct drainage tube position. Placement of the chest tube in the most dependent part of the cavity is desirable. The catheter is then connected to high (40–100-mm Hg) suction in an effort to evacuate completely the contents and shrink the cavity. Many of the limitations of intermittent drainage apply to closed tube drainage as well, and ultimate drainage and decortication will be required for those empyema cavities which fail either of these closed drainage techniques.

When the empyema is loculated or contains thick pus with large fibrin clots, open drainage is indicated. A small thoracotomy incision is used, with resection of short segments of one or two ribs. The operation includes evacuation of inflammatory exudate and large fibrin clots. The method illustrated in Figure 7–6 is utilized to provide an airtight seal, and powerful suction is applied to reexpand the lung and obliterate the cavity.

Open drainage should be performed before the inflammatory membrane overlying the visceral pleura becomes so thick that the lung cannot be expanded by suction. Delay in performing open drainage often leads to chronic empyema, for which a much more extensive operation is required.

Fig 7–6, A.—The most dependent portion of the empyema cavity is localized as accurately as possible, and a needle is introduced to confirm the presence of pus at that point.

B.—A vertical incision about 3 in. long is made, and the muscles of the chest wall are divided. A short (2-in.) rib segment is then resected subperiosteally.

C.—An incision parallel to the long axis of the rib is made in the external periosteum, and transverse incisions are made at right angles to it. It is important not to denude the remaining rib ends of periosteum because this increases the likelihood that osteomyelitis will develop.

D.—Separation posteriorly is begun by working downward on the superior border and upward on the inferior border of the rib, so that the periosteal elevator moves in approximately the same general direction as the fibers of the intercostal muscles. This tends to force the periosteal elevator back inside the periosteum if it accidentally breaks through. If the periosteum is freed in the opposite direction, the periosteal elevator tends to follow the fibers of the intercostal muscles if it breaks through the periosteum.

E.—Separation posteriorly is completed with a Doyen rib stripper. The rib segment is resected with rib shears.

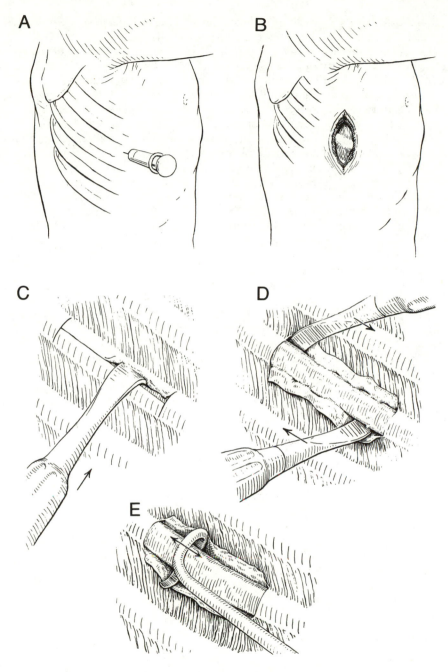

F.—An aspirating needle is introduced through the internal periosteum to make certain that the cavity will be entered by incising at that point.

G.—A small incision is made through the internal periosteum and the parietal pleura, which may be very thick. Pus is removed with the suction apparatus, and the index finger is inserted for exploration of the cavity. The relationship of the incision in the parietal pleura to the bottom of the cavity is determined. If the pleural incision is somewhat above the bottom of the cavity, the opening should be extended downward so that there will not be pocketing at the bottom of the cavity.

H.—A short segment of an additional rib is removed. The intervening intercostal muscles and underlying parietal pleura are excised (*dotted lines*), the intercostal vessels being ligated adjacent to the divided rib edges.

I.—An opening of this size is made so that as much inflammatory exudate as possible can be removed. Exudate and fibrin clots can best be removed by wiping with sponges held with a sponge stick.

A large tube is then inserted and suction is applied. If the empyema is relatively old and the lung is adherent to the chest wall, the empyema cavity may be packed with gauze and the application of suction deferred for 48–72 hours. Much of the residual exudate comes out with the packing.

Chronic Empyema

Empyema is termed chronic when the fibrinous membrane overlying the pleura becomes so thick and strong that expansion of the lung and obliteration of the cavity cannot be achieved by the methods just described. Major operative intervention will be required for resolution of the problem, and poor-risk patients may be best treated by long-term open or closed drainage.

The surgical approach used for treatment of a long-standing empyema is thoracotomy and decortication (chapter 1). Thoracoplasty (chapter 10) often is required if the empyema cavity is large.

F

G

H

I

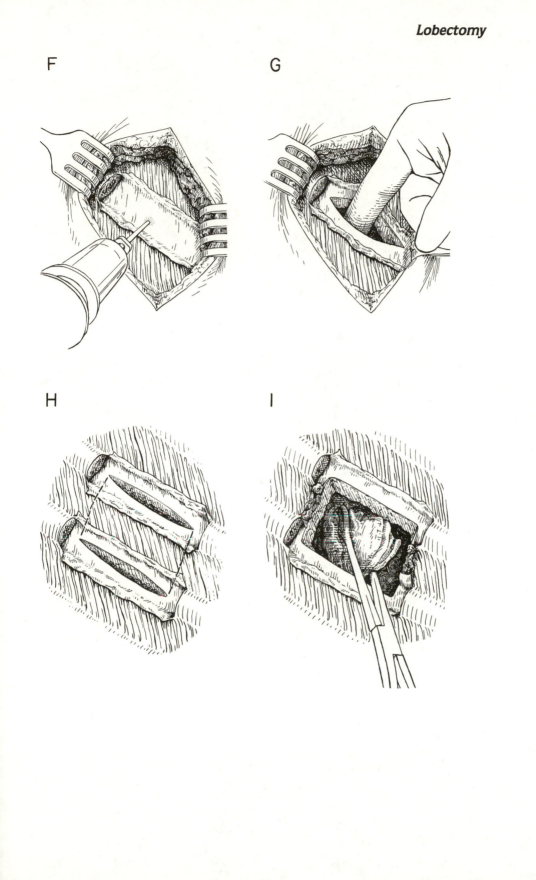

CHAPTER **8**

Segmental Resection

R ESECTION of anatomic subdivisions of the pulmonary lobes is frequently desirable when there is a localized lesion. The concept of segmental resection evolved from the demonstration that bronchopulmonary segments are sufficiently distinctive anatomic units to be removed individually and that certain lesions are often confined to such units.

The principal advantage of segmental resection is that only the segments which include diseased tissue need to be removed. Healthy, functioning pulmonary tissue is therefore conserved. If only the superior segment of the right lower lobe contains a lesion, for example, the four basal segments may be spared, whereas in lobectomy they would be sacrificed. An additional advantage over lobectomy is that there is more residual pulmonary tissue to fill the hemithorax on the side of operation, and the handicap imposed by compensatory overdistention is therefore not so great.

It must be emphasized that segmental resection is usually not an easy operation. A thorough knowledge of the anatomic relations of the tertiary hilar structures and of their frequent anomalies is essential. Accurate identification of segmental vessels requires the most careful dissection and is often time consuming. Separation of the diseased segment from adjacent segments must be done precisely if postoperative complications, such as empyema and bronchopleural fistula, are to be avoided. Even when the most careful technique is employed, the incidence of complications is somewhat higher than that following lobectomy.

INDICATIONS

Segmental resection is indicated for any benign lesion which has a segmental distribution. Whether segmental resection is preferable to lobectomy depends on the extent and distribution of the disease and the cardiorespiratory reserve of the patient. For example, if all but one segment of only a single lobe is diseased and the cardiorespiratory reserve is good, conservation of that single segment would scarcely justify the increased risk of segmental resection. However, when multiple segments in different lobes, unilaterally or bilaterally, are involved and the cardiorespiratory reserve is limited, it is obviously important to save all undiseased segments.

Bronchiectasis is the most common indication for segmental resection. Four fifths of the patients have multisegmental involvement, and one third have bilateral involvement. A subnormal cardiorespiratory reserve is common. Before the technique of segmental resection was introduced, removal of the major portion of the diseased areas without causing pulmonary invalidism was less often possible. Careful and complete bronchographic studies must be done preoperatively, because the involved segments cannot be delineated with certainty in any other way. The objective of treatment is to remove all severely diseased segments wherever possible, since the satisfactory relief of symptoms and the avoidance of subsequent complications cannot otherwise be ensured. The most badly diseased areas are removed, and the lesser involved ones are left alone. Antibiotics may then be used to control any further infection. Indeed, if bronchiectasis extensively involves both lungs, an antibiotic program may be wiser than multiple segmental resections.

Other indications for segmental resection include hamartoma, lung abscess, pulmonary cyst, metastatic tumor, and well-localized areas of tuberculosis.

Position of the Patient and Incisions

Considerations governing the choice of the position of the patient during operation are the same as those for lobectomy. The lateral position is always considered preferable unless the patient has too much residual secretion. If it seems likely that secretions or purulent exudate may be a problem, the use of a double-lumen endotracheal tube is advised. The incisions made are the same as those made for lobectomy but vary according to the segments involved.

Preoperative Preparation

Suppurative tracheobronchial secretions must be reduced to a minimum by antibiotic therapy, postural drainage, and bronchoscopy. In patients with bronchiectasis, all segments must be outlined by bronchography, since their external appearance and operative palpation can seldom be relied on to ascertain which segment is diseased.

GENERAL TECHNICAL CONSIDERATIONS

Peripheral adhesions and incomplete fissures are handled by the methods previously described. The general plan of procedure is essentially the same for all segments. The segmental artery, vein, and bronchus are divided in that order, as they are in most other pulmonary resections. Identification of the segmental artery first is of great value in verifying the segmental bronchus, which is immediately adjacent to it and easily palpable. If there is any doubt about the distribution of the veins, ligation and division of the vein should be deferred until after the bronchus is divided.

Delineation of Intersegmental Planes

Much of the success of segmental resection is dependent on differential inflation of the diseased and undiseased areas, for this demarcates intersegmental planes. The usual procedure is to deflate the lung before clamping the segmental bronchus and to inflate it after the bronchus is occluded. The diseased segment remains collapsed, and the dividing line between it and the remaining expanded portion of the lobe is usually clear-cut. In some instances the diseased segment soon begins to fill with air from adjacent segments. The reverse method of differential inflation is then used. The lung is expanded before the bronchus is occluded and deflated after the bronchus clamps are applied. The trapped air remains in the diseased segment and apparently has only little tendency to leak into adjacent, healthy segments. In addition, inflammatory changes and fibrosis often maintain the diseased segment in an expanded state.

Separation of Intersegmental Planes

The actual separation of the diseased segment from the rest of the lobe is done largely by blunt dissection. A useful maneuver is to squeeze the tissue at the line of demarcation between the thumb and index finger and, when in doubt, to apply pressure slightly to the diseased side of the intersegmental plane to avoid injury to the unresected parenchyma. Strands of tissue which do not separate readily are usually veins but may be tiny bronchi; in either case they should be ligated. Strands of fibrous tissue may also be present and should be ligated if they cannot be distinguished from veins or bronchi. Other helpful maneuvers are gentle pushing and a side-to-side sweeping motion with the tip of the index finger or a gauze pledget.

As mentioned in the section on anatomy, the principal venous tributaries of the segments occupy an intersegmental position and join at the tertiary hilum to form the segmental veins. Intersegmental veins drain both segments adjacent to the plane in which they lie, except subpleural veins, which drain only a single segment because of their peripheral position. In removing a segment from a lobe, it is important to preserve the intersegmental veins so that venous drainage from adjacent segments will not be restricted. Many of the tributaries entering the intersegmental veins are so small that they do not bleed significantly. However, some are of sufficient size to require ligation. It is better to identify such tributaries and to ligate them carefully than to resort to tearing them off the intersegmental vein.

Intersegmental veins serve as valuable guides to the intersegmental plane when separation of a segment is begun. As gentle traction is placed on the divided tertiary structures distally, and the adjacent parenchyma is gently separated, one or more veins will be seen to enter the adjacent segmental vein proximally. Veins which do not accompany bronchi are intersegmental veins, and the intersegmental vein to be followed is that which leaves the plane between inflated and deflated parenchyma. Veins which accompany bronchi are subsegmental veins, and they usually enter the adjacent segmental vein more distally. The most precise technique for segmental resection is to identify intersegmental veins at the hilum and follow them and their tributaries distally, ligating and dividing branches from within the segment as they are encountered. Dissection of the relatively filmy tissues which bind the segments together is carried slightly ahead of the dissection along the veins.

Technique for Individual Segments

The technical maneuvers just described are applicable to any bronchopulmonary segment, and resection of any one of the segments may sometimes be advisable. It is common practice, however, to excise certain segments together, such as the superior and inferior lingular segments, the lateral and medial segments of the middle lobe, and all of the basal segments of the lower lobes. The reason for combined resections is that these segments are frequently involved in the disease process as groups, and the conservation of an additional segment or two does not warrant the increased risk entailed in the difficult dissection of more peripheral segmental structures. Resection of individual segments of the right upper lobe is the most exacting, as a rule, because of the frequent presence of anomalies and an overlapping blood supply.

The techniques for four commonly performed segmental resections follow.

LINGULECTOMY

The technique for this procedure is illustrated with the patient in the lateral position. It is assumed that this is a patient with bronchiectasis and that the lower lobe has already been removed.

Fig 8–1, A.—The first steps are dissection, ligation, and division of the lingular arteries, which arise either individually or, as shown, from a single trunk. The position of the lingular bronchus in relation to the artery is shown in the insert.

B.—The upper lobe is retracted posteriorly and the lingular veins, which enter the lowermost portion of the superior pulmonary vein, are ligated and divided. Only the lower portion of the hilum is dissected anteriorly and the pulmonary artery is not seen. Care must be taken to preserve the intersegmental vein, which drains into the anterior segmental vein. If there is doubt as to its position, it is advisable to defer ligation of the veins until after the bronchus is divided.

The lingular bronchus is most safely approached from below, following the inferior surface of the main basal bronchus upward until the lingular bronchus is encountered. It must be cleared sufficiently to allow room for the bronchial sutures and to differentiate the anterior segmental bronchus, which may also arise from the lower division of the upper lobe.

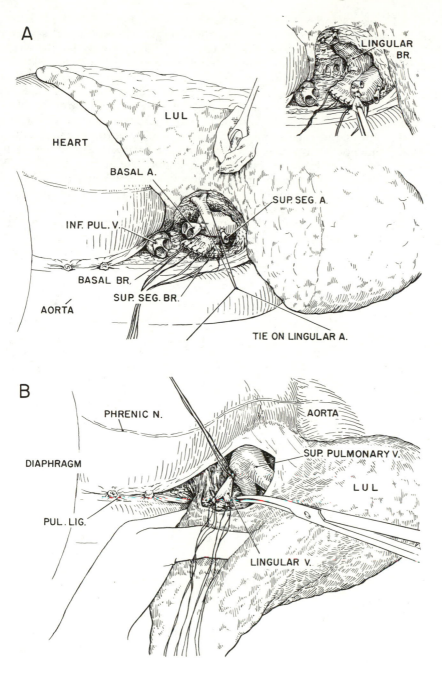

C.—Before clamping the lingular bronchus, the lung is deflated. After the clamps are applied, the lung is inflated, and the contrast between the airless segments and the expanded anterior segment is clearly seen. The dividing line between the segments is not always as clearly demarcated as shown here. Air frequently escapes from the anterior segment through the interalveolar pores into the lingula. Various methods of separating the intersegmental plane have been discussed. The illustration shows gentle squeezing of the parenchyma along the line of demarcation between the inflated and deflated segments and incision of the visceral pleura with a scalpel.

D.—An intersegmental vein on the inferior surface of the anterior segment is shown. A point not illustrated is that it is often necessary to divide one or more subpleural veins at the hilum to gain access to the intersegmental vein. A few air leaks may be seen on the remaining parenchymal surface of the anterior segment. The final steps are careful control of bleeding points and significant air leaks and covering the bronchial stumps with pleural flaps.

In some instances, particularly in patients with bronchiectasis, only the inferior lingular segment is diseased. It is a relatively simple matter to carry the hilar dissection a step farther and isolate and divide the inferior lingular artery, vein, and bronchus to remove only the diseased segment.

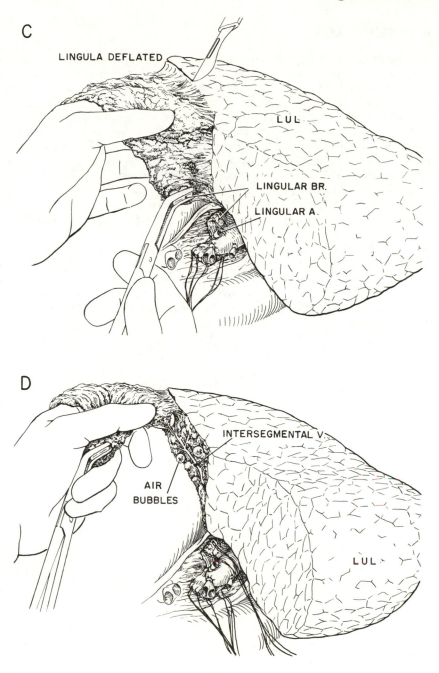

C

LINGULA DEFLATED

LUL

LINGULAR BR.

LINGULAR A.

D

INTERSEGMENTAL V.

AIR
BUBBLES

LUL

BASAL SEGMENTS, LEFT

Although the basal segments may be removed individually, the usual practice is to remove them as a group, because most, if not all, are usually involved. The pulmonary function which is conserved by individual removal does not warrant the greater difficulties in dissecting the more peripheral hilar structures and intersegmental planes. Removal of the left basal segments as a group is one of the most common segmental resections performed for bronchiectasis, because the superior segment is usually not involved. Segmental resection of the left basal group is illustrated, with the patient in the lateral position.

Fig 8–2, A.—The fissure is opened, and the interlobar portion of the pulmonary artery is exposed to the extent shown. In this instance the ligatures are placed on the basal segmental arteries because the main basal branch is very short. In this patient two separate arteries arise from the main trunk to supply the superior segment.

B.—The lung is permitted to fall forward, the pulmonary ligament is divided, and the posterior hilar pleura is incised to expose the inferior pulmonary vein. The basal segmental tributaries are ligated and divided, while branches from the superior segment are carefully preserved. Commonly, there are two main tributaries draining into the inferior pulmonary vein, one from the superior segment and one from the basal segments.

A

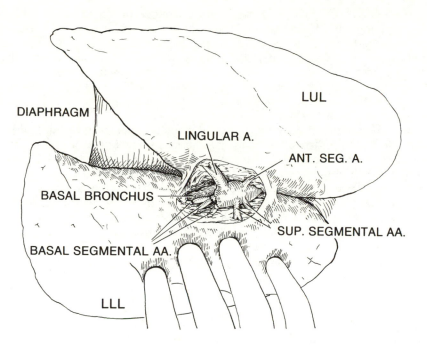

DIAPHRAGM

LUL

LINGULAR A.

ANT. SEG. A.

BASAL BRONCHUS

SUP. SEGMENTAL AA.

BASAL SEGMENTAL AA.

LLL

B

BASAL SEGMENTAL VV.

SUP. SEGMENTAL V.

LOWER LOBE BR.

PULMONARY LIG.

AORTA

INF. PULMONARY V.

C.—The main basal bronchus is most safely approached on its inferomedial surface, where it has been partially exposed during dissection of the arteries. It is freed sufficiently to allow clearance of the bronchial sutures below the superior bronchus, and it is clamped after the lung is deflated. Expansion of the lung then clearly demarcates the inferior surface of the superior segment. It is not customary to suture the bronchial stump until the segments have been removed. In this figure the stump is shown sutured, because the presence of the proximal bronchus clamp would obscure other anatomic features.

D.—Dissection of the intersegmental plane is begun at the hilum. With gentle traction on the distal bronchus clamp, the intersegmental veins are identified as the tissue at the line of demarcation between the inflated and deflated parenchyma is separated. Much of the dissection is done by gentle pushing with a gauze pledget. A second pledget is used to apply counteraction. The characteristic appearance of the intersegmental veins is illustrated. About two thirds of the separation of the inter-segmental plane has been completed in this view. Finally, bleeding points and significant air leaks are controlled, and the bronchial stumps are covered with pleural flaps.

C

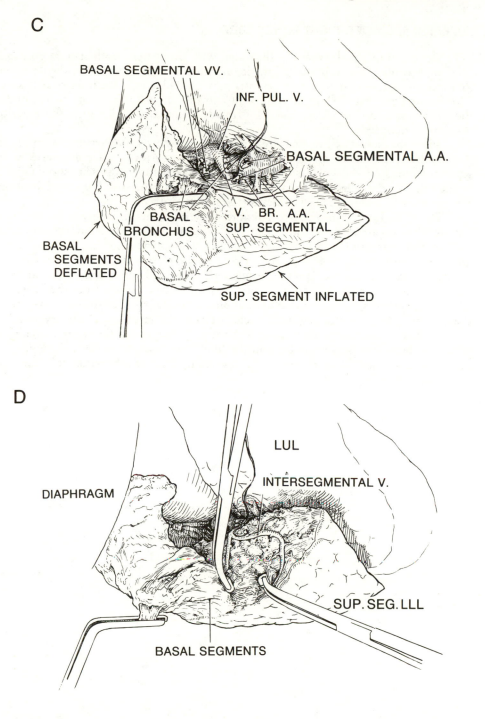

BASAL SEGMENTAL VV.

INF. PUL. V.

BASAL SEGMENTAL A.A.

BASAL
BRONCHUS

V. BR. A.A.
SUP. SEGMENTAL

BASAL
SEGMENTS
DEFLATED

SUP. SEGMENT INFLATED

D

LUL

INTERSEGMENTAL V.

DIAPHRAGM

SUP. SEG. LLL

BASAL SEGMENTS

SUPERIOR SEGMENT, RIGHT LOWER LOBE

Resection of this segment is illustrated with the patient in the lateral position. Not infrequently, the superior segment on either side is removed with the upper lobe because a lesion such as tuberculosis may extend across the interlobar fissure. The fissure between the superior segment and the upper lobe is not opened under these circumstances. In the instance illustrated, it is assumed that only the superior segment is diseased.

Fig 8–3, A.—The great fissure is opened, and the pulmonary artery supply to the superior segment is ligated and divided. Two superior segmental arteries with separate origins are shown. Also, two arteries with separate origins are shown going to the middle lobe. Ordinarily, only one artery goes to the superior segment of the lower lobe and only one artery goes to the middle lobe.

B.—The lung is allowed to fall anteriorly, and the inferior pulmonary vein and its branches are dissected sufficiently to determine which tributaries come from the superior segment. In this instance, there are two superior segmental veins. They are ligated and divided. The pulmonary ligament is not disturbed. The superior segmental bronchus is between the segmental arteries and veins, with little intervening tissue to obscure it. It is conveniently dissected and clamped from the posterior aspect. A bronchus clamp is about to be applied after deflation of the lung. As a rule, there is only one superior segmental vein entering the inferior pulmonary vein.

In this instance, it is assumed that the superior segment did not remain airless when the bronchus was occluded and the lung was reinflated. The intersegmental plane was not clearly demarcated, so the reverse method of differential inflation will be used.

A

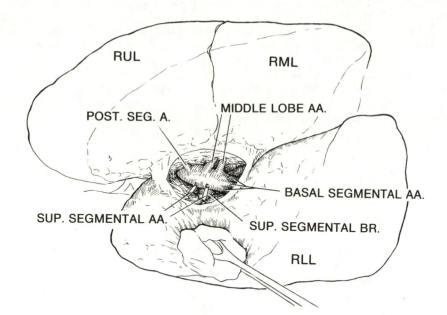

RUL

RML

POST. SEG. A.

MIDDLE LOBE AA.

BASAL SEGMENTAL AA.

SUP. SEGMENTAL AA.

SUP. SEGMENTAL BR.

RLL

B

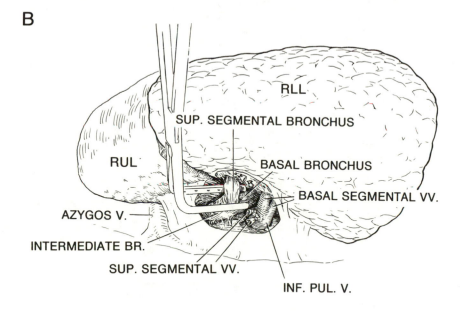

RLL

SUP. SEGMENTAL BRONCHUS

RUL

BASAL BRONCHUS

BASAL SEGMENTAL VV.

AZYGOS V.

INTERMEDIATE BR.

SUP. SEGMENTAL VV.

INF. PUL. V.

C.—The bronchus clamps are applied with the lung inflated. The bronchus is then divided and the lung is deflated. The superior segment remains expanded, and there is a clear-cut dividing line between it and the basal segments, which are collapsed. An intersegmental vein has been identified and is being followed into the intersegmental plane. The vein connecting this intersegmental vein with the superior segmental vein has been ligated and divided.

D.—Separation of the intersegmental plane is continued by the methods described. A subpleural vein at the periphery is about to be clamped. Branches on the superior surface of the intersegmental veins have been ligated and divided and removal of the superior segment is nearly completed.

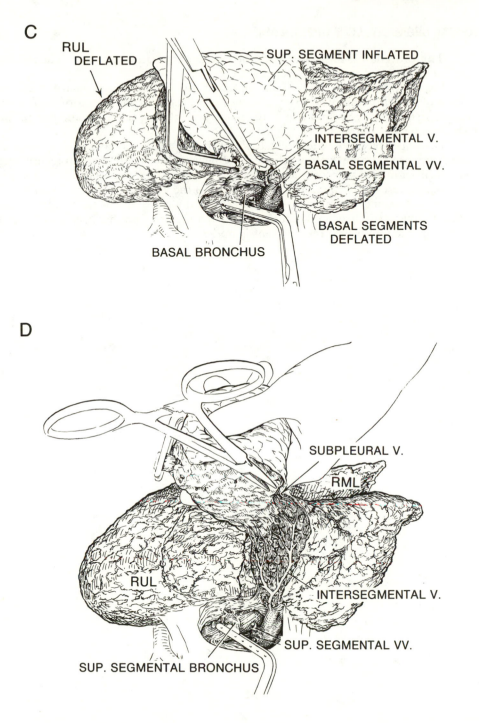

C

RUL
DEFLATED

SUP. SEGMENT INFLATED

INTERSEGMENTAL V.

BASAL SEGMENTAL VV.

BASAL SEGMENTS
DEFLATED

BASAL BRONCHUS

D

SUBPLEURAL V.

RML

INTERSEGMENTAL V.

RUL

SUP. SEGMENTAL VV.

SUP. SEGMENTAL BRONCHUS

APICAL SEGMENT, LEFT UPPER LOBE

This procedure is illustrated with the patient in the lateral position. The indication for resection is an apical tuberculoma.

Fig 8–4, A.—With the apex of the upper lobe retracted downward, the first branch of the left pulmonary artery is identified. The apical and posterior segmental arteries arise from a common trunk, the apical artery being the more anterior of the two. It is ligated and divided.

B.—The apical bronchus, which is a branch of the apical posterior division of the left upper lobe bronchus, is palpated just beneath the artery to aid in identifying the apical segmental vein on the anterosuperior surface of the hilum. The lung is retracted posteriorly for dissection and ligation of the vein. The posterior segmental vein lies just behind the apical segmental vein. If there is doubt as to the identity of the two, division of the vein is deferred until after the bronchus has been divided and the retrograde removal of the segment is under way.

A

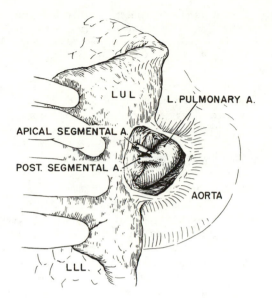

B

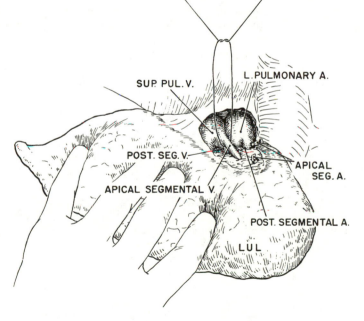

C.—The apex of the lung is again pulled downward, and the apical segmental bronchus is freed. The relation of this bronchus to both its segmental artery and vein and to the posterior segmental bronchus, which arises from the same bronchial trunk, is illustrated. A bronchus clamp is applied to the apical bronchus prior to division.

D.—The apical segment is excised in the usual way. The intersegmental veins in the planes between the apical segment and the anterior and posterior segments are carefully preserved. The bronchial stump has been sutured, and a pleural flap is advanced to cover the stump.

SEGMENTAL RESECTION: FINAL STEPS

After the specimen is removed, great care must be taken to control residual air leaks and bleeding points. The first step is to apply a sponge to the intersegmental surface for several minutes. This controls capillary bleeding. Larger bleeding points are clamped and ligated. Significant air leaks can usually be seen, and application of saline solution helps in determining their precise location. Babcock clamps are preferable to hemostats for controlling air leaks and bleeding points, because they can be applied effectively without penetrating the parenchyma and causing further damage.

If dissection in the intersegmental plane has been careful and accurate, air leaks are few and they seal over quickly. It must be emphasized, however, that small bronchi may be open if residual segments have been traumatized. Neglected bronchi of this caliber may not close for days or weeks, and empyema may result. Some surgeons have covered the remaining raw surface with pleural flaps or grafts, but this is not necessary and is probably not desirable because the covering tissue is almost certainly ischemic and may predispose to infection.

Adhesions between the parietal and visceral pleurae are freed so that the residual pulmonary tissue can expand uniformly to fill the chest. If adhesions remain within the fissure, however, they are not disturbed, because they tend to prevent rotation.

Finally, two tubes are always inserted into the pleural cavity at the close of a segmental resection. One is positioned at the apex, where it is anchored to the parietal pleura with a suture and is brought out through the anterior end of the incision. The other is led out through a separate stab wound in the seventh or eighth interspace, from the lower portion of the pleural cavity posteriorly. The tubes are then connected to a drainage system.

The incision is closed in the usual way. The lungs are expanded before closure is begun, and expansion is maintained so that the residual segments cannot rotate before negative intrapleural pressure is established.

C

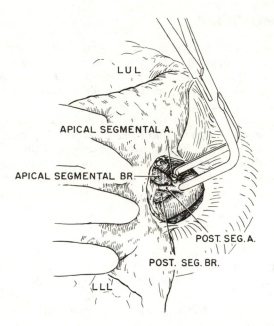

LUL

APICAL SEGMENTAL A.

APICAL SEGMENTAL BR.

POST. SEG. A.

POST. SEG. BR.

LLL

D

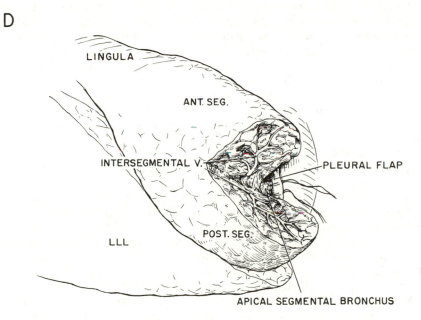

LINGULA

ANT. SEG.

INTERSEGMENTAL V.

PLEURAL FLAP

LLL

POST. SEG.

APICAL SEGMENTAL BRONCHUS

POSTOPERATIVE COMPLICATIONS

The principal complications of segmental resection are bronchopleural fistula and empyema. If the operative procedure is performed accurately and meticulously, the incidence of these complications is low. An incidence of approximately 25% has been reported in some series, however, and this should be regarded as evidence that, unless carefully performed, the operation is unduly risky.

Alveolopleura fistulas usually seal over within two to five days, but occasional small bronchopleural fistulas may remain open for weeks. A persistent leak should be treated with continuous suction for a reasonable length of time. Eventual thoracotomy, with suture of the fistula and decortication of the lung, may be necessary. Empyema usually responds to strong suction applied to a large catheter inserted into the cavity unless there is a persistent fistula, which may require suture and decortication.

WEDGE RESECTION

This was the procedure used routinely for resection of less than a lobe before the development of segmental resection. It is still the method of choice for certain small, well-circumscribed, benign tumors and for inflammatory lesions. The technique is not difficult. A wedge-shaped area of parenchyma, which includes the lesion, is resected without regard for the location of the intersegmental planes. Either the clamp–and–suture method, illustrated in Figure 8–5, or the open method may be used. Bleeding points and small bronchi are more accurately secured by the clamp–and–suture method, but considerable distortion of the remaining parenchyma may result if a large wedge is resected. In the open method, vessels and bronchi are clamped as they are divided, and the raw surface remains exposed. The relatively large bronchi, which may be divided when an intersegmental plane is not followed, must be either ligated or sutured to prevent a persistent air leak.

Wedge resection has been commonly employed in performing lingulectomy. Often, however, too much or too little tissue is resected, so segmental resection has become preferable. Wedge resection is frequently used for the removal of small, peripherally located lesions.

Fig 8–5, A.—Wedge resection of a hamartoma of the left upper lobe is illustrated. The patient is in the lateral position.

B.—Leaving a margin of normal tissue around the lesion, Kelly clamps are applied to outline the wedge for excision. It is then sharply excised, and a margin is left so that the remaining clamps do not slip.

C.—A 3–0 absorbable suture is used for double-layer closure. A basting stitch is placed behind the clamps before their removal.

D.—The crushed area is oversewn with a simple over-and-over suture. The pleural cavity is usually drained because of the possibility of an air leak.

The perfection of commercially available stapling instruments has made wedge resection a rapid and simple task. Several instruments can be used for the purpose, and an illustration showing the double application of a tool which staples both sides and divides in the center of the two staple lines is presented in chapter 5. The suture lines are generally hemostatic and air leaks are minimal, so that further suturing or reinforcement is not required. A thoracostomy tube is left in position until complete lung inflation has been documented and air leaks are no longer present.

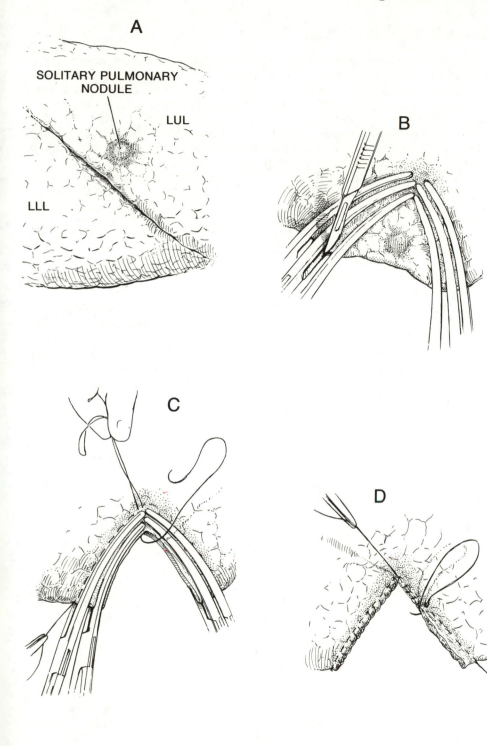

A

SOLITARY PULMONARY
NODULE

LUL

LLL

B

C

D

EXCISION OF BLEBS AND BULLAE

Spontaneous pneumothorax is frequently encountered and most often represents the spontaneous rupture of small blebs (almost always apically situated), which are congenital abnormalities. It is initially treated with tube thoracostomy and sometimes also with pleurodesis, using tetracycline or another agent injected into the tube. This problem tends to recur, however, and each time carries with it the risk of tension pneumothorax. Certainly, by the third occurrence, operative intervention should be offered to the patient. An attractive operation is the axillary thoracotomy, with oversewing or stapling of the apical blebs as illustrated.

Fig 8–6, A.—With the patient in the lateral position and the arm wrapped to the upper border of the anesthesia ether screen, a short (10-cm), oblique incision is made below the axillary hair line, between the palpable borders of the latissimus and pectoralis major. The fibers of the serratus are separated, and the chest is entered above the third or fourth rib. No attempt is made to dissect along the chest wall, and the intercostobrachiocutaneous nerve is therefore not endangered. The intercostal muscles can be divided above the rib for some distance in both anterior and posterior directions (beneath the pectoralis and serratus), so that a small self-retaining retractor can be inserted without breaking the ribs.

B.—With the use of the sponge sticks, lung clamps, and atraumatic forceps, the surfaces of all lobes are thoroughly inspected. One or several blebs are usually present at the apex of the upper lobe and are surrounded by thickened visceral pleura. This area is either oversewn or stapled off and excised, and pleurodesis is induced by the abrasion of both parietal and visceral pleural surfaces. Apical pleurectomy is also done through this small incision without difficulty. Closure of the wound is simple layered approximation of the serratus fibers, subcutaneous tissue, and skin. The chest tube placed before the operation is left in place until it can be removed safely.

If the pneumothorax is chronic or neglected, a fibrinous exudate will have formed over the visceral pleura, which will make reexpansion of the parenchyma difficult. The operation of choice in this circumstance is a standard thoracotomy, so that exposure is adequate to allow decortication. Two chest tubes should be used, as blood loss is invariably greater for this larger procedure.

An occasional patient will have giant lung cysts or localized gross emphysematous disease and can be helped with operation. These lesions, which reduce pulmonary function by their space-taking effect, are treated by either excising the lobe which they occupy or excising their walls. Excision of only the cyst itself may conserve a considerable amount of functioning lung tissue, which is a major consideration for patients who have impressive clinical obstructive lung disease. When this conservative option is exercised, all the bronchial openings into the cyst must be individually sutured. Portions of the cyst walls may be sutured over the exposed parenchyma.

A

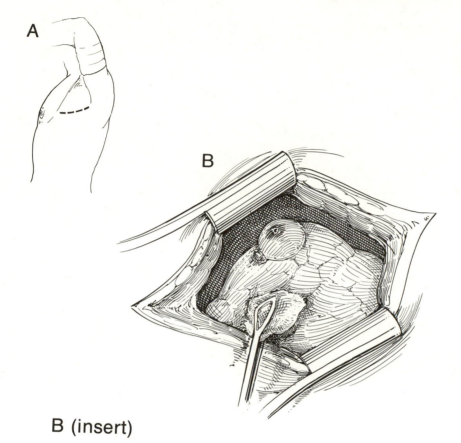

B

B (insert)

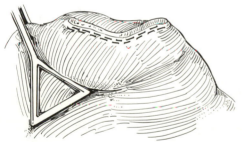

Beisel

CHAPTER 9

Superior Sulcus Tumors

THE SUPERIOR sulcus tumor is a particularly interesting form of lung cancer that has unique clinical signs and symptoms. This group of malignant tumors are primary lung malignancies that herald their presence by local effects, while pulmonary symptoms and complaints are notably absent. Its classic presentation is pain in the shoulder and along the vertebral border of the scapula. Complaints of ulnar nerve distribution arm pain and an ipsilateral Horner's syndrome (ptosis, dilated pupil, and hemianhydrosis of the face) are manifestations which are due to progressively higher invasion of the brachial plexus. Few other lesions are responsible for this group of symptoms.

Diagnosis is made by recognizing the combination of symptoms and findings on physical examination. The chest film may suggest only subtle thickening or roughening of the apical pleura; lordotic films may be required for clear demonstration. Erosion of the surface of the first or second ribs may be apparent on directed films. Computerized axial tomography is helpful in determining the true size and extent of the growth.

Any patient with an apical lung lesion and the classic symptoms described above is presumed to have this lesion. Bronchoscopy and sputum cytology are not usually helpful in diagnosis, but mediastinoscopy and scalene or supraclavicular node biopsy may be helpful in establishing the extent of the disease and determining its operability if either the chest film or physical examination shows gross abnormalities in these areas.

The tumor, which is most often slow growing, may be an epidermoid, large cell undifferentiated, or adenocarcinoma. The specific histology does not influence the therapeutic attack. Obtaining tissue for confirmation of diagnosis is not a simple task and at many institutions is considered unnecessary before the start of treatment. Needle biopsy with fluoroscopic control may be of help. When there is agreement on the diagnosis, the patient is given a short course of radiation therapy (3,000 rad over two weeks) to the apex of the lung. After an interval of three weeks, an extended resection involving the upper lobe, chest wall, and lower brachial plexus is performed.

Following combined therapy, the tumor can almost always be identified in the resected specimen. As in other lung tumors, the presence of involved lymph nodes has prognostic implications. In comparison to other primary lung cancers, however, survival of patients with superior sulcus tumors is much more prolonged. The palliation of pain is an important consideration in the selection of candidates for operation, since death does not come swiftly, and these individuals truly suffer intractable, excruciating pain.

The patient must accept a degree of postoperative neurologic deficit, for division of the first thoracic and eighth cervical nerve roots is often required. The loss of ulnar nerve function which ensues is usually readily accepted by the patient in exchange for control of the pain experienced before the operation. Sensory innervation to the inner aspect of the upper arm is also lost with the sacrifice of the intercostobrachiocutaneous nerve which emerges from the axillary aspect of the upper chest wall. The postoperative recovery from this operation is difficult because of discomfort, a component of paradox from loss of the upper chest wall, and the neurologic deficit.

RESECTION OF SUPERIOR SULCUS TUMOR

This operation is one of the most difficult and large-scale resections done in modern thoracic surgery. The following figures illustrate only the major steps of the procedure.

Fig 9–1, A.—With the patient in the lateral position, a generous posterolateral thoracotomy is made. The posterior extent of the incision is carried high and medial to the scapula, and the rhomboids are entirely divided, along with the lower portion of the trapezius (*insert*). The latissimus is sectioned and the serratus is detached from the upper rib insertions, allowing elevation of the scapula and axillary contents. The paravertebral muscles and fascia are sharply separated to expose the entire posteromedial extent of the upper ribs and transverse processes. The chest is entered in the fifth intercostal space for preliminary exploration and to determine whether resection should continue. Note is made of the extent of chest wall and vertebral involvement and hilar adenopathy. Extensive involvement of either the brachial plexus or vertebral bodies are contraindications to continued resection.

B.—En bloc resection is begun anteriorly by division of the first three ribs anterior to the tumor mass. The neurovascular bundles are ligated anterior to this point. This illustration shows how the structures at the apex of the chest are protected by passing the finger behind the anterior scalene muscle as it is divided. The same maneuver is used for section of the first rib anteriorly to protect the innominate vein and for division of the scalenus medius to protect the brachial plexus. After division of the costoclavicular ligament, the anterior portion of the first rib is pulled down, and the involved structures at the apex of the chest are seen from the posterior aspect.

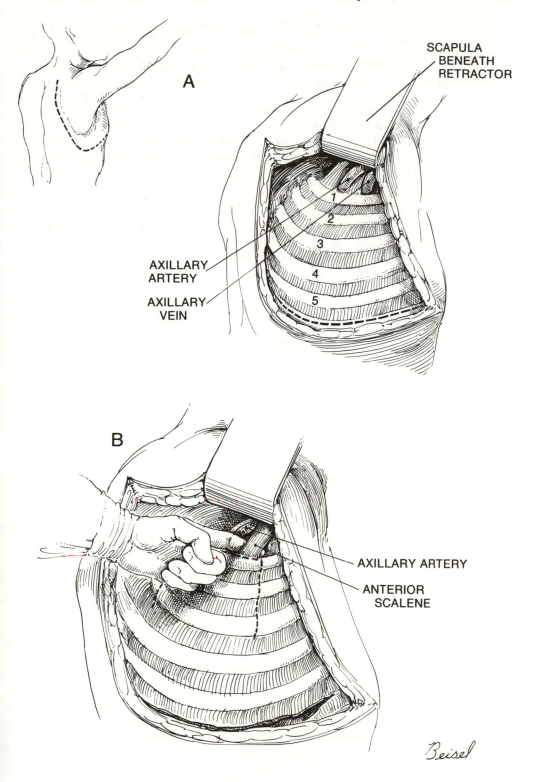

SCAPULA
BENEATH
RETRACTOR

A

1
2
3
4
5

AXILLARY
ARTERY

AXILLARY
VEIN

B

AXILLARY ARTERY

ANTERIOR
SCALENE

Beisel

C.—The subclavian artery within its sheath is identified laterally, and dissection is carried back toward the tumor. Involvement of the artery is a strong but relative contraindication to continued operation. The lower aspect of the brachial plexus is shown. Infiltration of the nerves is the reason for the symptomatic pain, and resection of the first thoracic nerve and, often, of the eighth cervical nerve is required. The tissues remaining above the mass are cleared from the posterior aspect. The inferior border of the tumor mass is defined from within the chest, and the lower limit of chest wall division is performed. The specimen is then tethered between the medial chest wall attachments and the hilum of the lung. The medial attachments are released by retracting the paraspinous muscles and ligaments and disarticulating the ribs from the upper transverse processes. Intercostal arteries are ligated, and intercostal nerves are divided. Transverse processes and segments of vertebral bodies that are involved can be removed with chisels.

D.—An upper lobectomy with mediastinal node dissection completes the en bloc resection. The subclavian artery and vein have been carefully preserved. The scapula and apical chest structures will drop down so that scapular motion is not restricted by the defect in the chest wall. Two chest tubes are placed, and anatomic closure of the divided muscles and soft tissues completes the procedure.

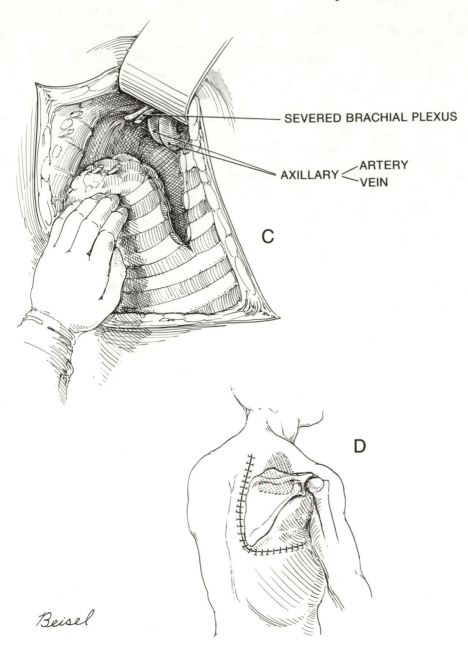

SEVERED BRACHIAL PLEXUS

AXILLARY — ARTERY
         — VEIN

C

D

Beisel

COMPLICATIONS

It is easy to appreciate that several significant problems can arise during this operation. Besides the predicted neurologic deficits and the risks inherent in upper lobe resection, there is the risk of injuring the major vessels at the apex of the chest. Protective maneuvers have been described with the illustrations, but if injury occurs, reconstruction of the artery with a prosthetic graft or of the vein with a patch is indicated.

Medial section of the intercostal nerves can encroach on the dural sleeve in which they exit the spinal cord, thereby causing leaks of cerebrospinal fluid. Suture ligature and muscle packing are used to control the leaks. Unipolar electrocautery should never be used near the spinal cord because of the risks of both electrical current and thermal injury.

CHAPTER 10

Surgical Treatment of Pulmonary Tuberculosis

THE TREATMENT of pulmonary tuberculosis is predominantly nonsurgical. Surgery is a supplementary rather than a competing form of therapy. Various antimicrobial agents are effective against tuberculosis and are now widely used, making ambulatory nonsurgical treatment of this once major health problem a reality.

In general, the surgical procedures used in the treatment of tuberculosis have been based on three principles: compression, drainage, and excision. Compression therapy essentially has been abandoned. Once very popular, temporary compression by induced pneumothorax, phrenic nerve paralysis, or pneumoperitoneum is no longer employed. Thoracoplasty was used to collapse permanently an involved lung, but currently its indications are infrequent. Likewise, drainage alone (intracavitary suction, cavernostomy) is seldom used except in poor-risk patients with bilateral disease. Pulmonary resection is now the most common surgical procedure for tuberculosis, yet the indications for this form of treatment continue to diminish as time passes.

Operation is now undertaken in two groups of patients. The first group consists of patients who are found to have abnormal chest films and who undergo operation for diagnosis when this disease is either not suspected or not demonstrated before operation. This group of patients will probably increase as tuberculosis becomes less commonly suspected by newer generations of physicians. The second group is made up of individuals with advanced stages of pulmonary tuberculosis which has been refractory to drug treatment. In underdeveloped countries, it is unfortunate that the size of this group of patients remains impressive.

SELECTION OF PATIENTS

General Condition

The age of the patient is not in itself a contraindication to any form of mechanical therapy, except that deforming procedures, such as thoracoplasty, are undesirable in growing children. Tuberculous infection and coexisting diseases may have caused an overall deterioration in the clinical condition of the patient and thus increase the risk of major operation.

173

Nutrition and Immune Competence

Any patient selected for operative intervention should evidence an ability to resist dissemination of the tuberculous infection. There should be no demonstrable tuberculous lesions elsewhere in the body. Recent spread of tuberculosis or exacerbation of the pulmonary lesion is an indication for vigorous antibiotic treatment before operation. Skin tests to evaluate anergy and laboratory determinations of reduction in absolute lymphocyte count, albumin, and transferrin confirm the clinical impression of inadequate nutritional status. In such cases, supplemental alimentation before operation can result in fewer postoperative complications.

Size and Location of the Lesion

The destruction of a large portion of the pulmonary parenchyma is a strong indication for pulmonary resection. Large cavities are not as reliably controlled by compression procedures as small ones are. Antimicrobial therapy dictated by appropriate culture and sensitivity tests should be given in all cases before operation, and an apparently extensive exudative lesion may clear considerably with only a small residual focus remaining. Thoracoplasty is not appropriate treatment for lesions in the lower lobes or apical or paravertebral areas because they cannot be effectively compressed. When a lesion is restricted to a single bronchopulmonary segment, segmental resection may be a suitable method of treatment.

Endobronchial Disease

Tuberculous bronchitis is present in a significant percentage of patients with parenchymal disease. Bronchial lesions may cause obstruction with secondary bronchiectasis, mixed infection, and atelectasis. If there is a check-valve mechanism, a tension cavity may develop. Careful bronchoscopic evaluation of the endobronchial disease is essential to planning therapy. Compression procedures are usually contraindicated in the presence of obstructive bronchitis.

TUBERCULOSIS: PULMONARY RESECTION

In recent years, administration of the antimicrobial agents has made it possible to control the disease in a great many instances, and the surgical procedure is designed to remove the ravages of the previously active disease. At present, therefore, pulmonary resection is considered to be the standard form of surgical therapy, but even this has decreased greatly in the recent past.

Extent of Resection

The scope of operation required for control of disease can be determined preoperatively on the basis of the chest film. In general, the tendency is to conserve as much lung as possible when the disease is well controlled with drug therapy. The size of the lesion and whether it is an inflammatory mass, abscess, or cavity will dictate whether segmentectomy, lobectomy, or pneumonectomy is the best resection. In the presence of a drug-resistant organism, it may be wise to avoid segmental resections.

General Operative Considerations

The technique of resection requires no special elaboration beyond previous descriptions. Hilar dissection may be more difficult than usual because of matting of tuberculous nodes in the primary, secondary, or tertiary hilum. The peripheral part of the dissection is often the most difficult, but it is greatly simplified by dissecting extrapleurally wherever there are dense adhesions. This maneuver is also helpful in avoiding contamination of the pleural cavity.

THORACOPLASTY

Thoracoplasty is an operation in which collapse of the lung is produced by removing the supporting framework; i.e., removing the ribs from the chest wall. An effective collapse of the diseased area cannot be produced without partial collapse of undiseased areas; however, the removal of ribs causes paradoxical motion, and the classic procedure is done in stages to minimize this effect.

Indications

In the past, some type of thoracoplasty was almost always done following a lobectomy or pneumonectomy for tuberculosis. The purpose was to minimize over-distention of the remaining pulmonary parenchyma and thereby provide a less favorable environment for the growth of the tubercle bacillus. An additional advantage was that dead space was more rapidly obliterated, thus decreasing the risk of bronchopleural fistula and tuberculous empyema. Currently, the necessity for thoracoplasty is dubious, and it is not performed unless more than a single lobe has been resected for tuberculosis. The issue of either concomitant or delayed thoracoplasty has been discussed in chapter 6.

Thoracoplasty is sometimes indicated in the surgical treatment of postoperative complications, such as empyema and bronchopleural fistula following a previous resection. Air leaks following resections for tuberculosis seem to be more difficult to control than those which occur following operations for other indications. Thoracoplasty will eliminate a persistent air space which is chronically infected. As a primary operation, thoracoplasy is reserved for patients in whom resection seems too hazardous because of their poor condition or in whom the disease remains uncontrolled by drug therapy. When the organisms are resistant to all drugs, the incidence of complications following resection is sufficiently high to justify the use of thoracoplasty as the primary procedure. Again, with the current medical armamentarium, this situation is rare.

Contraindications

A great deal has been learned about lesions in which there is a high incidence of thoracoplasty failure. Among these are tension cavities, giant cavities extensively destroyed areas of parenchyma, and lesions associated with various types of tracheo-bronchial disease.

General Operative Considerations

The number of ribs resected depends on the location and size of the cavity. As a general rule, at least two ribs are resected below the lowermost border of the cavity. Often, three or four ribs must be resected below the cavity to ensure complete collapse. Most lesions which are suitable for thoracoplasty require a six- or seven-rib resection. Resection of five ribs will sometimes suffice for small lesions at the apex.

The ribs are resected subperiosteally so that regeneration can occur in the collapsed position. This prevents prolonged paradoxical motion and a tendency toward reexpansion. Except for the head of the first rib, the entire first three ribs and their costal cartilages are resected. The costal cartilages and progressively longer anterior segments of the ribs are left intact below that level because of the normal downward slope of the ribs. This gradual tapering of the level of resection anteriorly decreases paradoxical motion and reduces the extent of collapse of healthy lung tissue. Preservation of the anterior rib segments on the left side of the chest also preserves protection for the heart.

Posteriorly, the paravertebral groove is eradicated as completely as possible by disarticulation of the ribs and resection of the transverse processes. The latter maneuver undoubtedly increases the tendency toward scoliosis, but it must be accepted in the interest of obtaining a more complete collapse. The first transverse process and the head of the first rib are usually not removed because they are above the apex of the lung and there is risk of injury to the stellate ganglion during their removal.

Types of Thoracoplasty

Many techniques of performing thoracoplasty have been described. Most of them are minor modifications which influence their overall effectiveness only slightly. Only the well standardized techniques will be given on the following pages. No other methods are required for the routine treatment of tuberculous lesions. The modified types of thoracoplasty which are performed concomitantly with or following pulmonary resection have been described previously.

POSTEROLATERAL THORACOPLASTY

First Stage

This is the conventional thoracoplasty which has been used for many years. It is assumed in this discussion that a seven–rib resection is required. The procedure is performed in three stages. General anesthesia is preferable, but either spinal anesthesia or a combination of local and regional anesthesia may be used.

Fig 10–1, A.—With the patient in the lateral position, an incision, made midway between the spinous processes and the scapula, is curved around the tip of the scapula. The portions of the trapezius, rhomboid, and latissimus dorsi muscles which lie beneath the skin incision are divided.

A scapula retractor is inserted, and the rib cage is widely exposed. The attachments of the scalene muscles are divided to provide free access to the first and second ribs. Posteriorly, the paraspinal muscle group is mobilized and retracted to expose the head and neck of the ribs and the transverse processes. The third and second ribs are resected before the first rib so that the chest wall falls inward, providing better exposure of the extreme apex. Periosteal elevators are used to resect the ribs subperiosteally. Every effort is made to keep the internal periosteum intact and to avoid opening the parietal pleura.

Two steps require special comment: resection of the first rib and disarticulation of the other ribs.

B.—The flat surfaces of the first rib are nearly at a right angle to the spine, and the lower border is the portion closest to the surgeon. The usual maneuvers with periosteal elevators are dangerous because an accidental slip might cause serious injury to either the subclavian vessels or the brachial plexus. The attachments to the outer border are cut with scissors, as illustrated, and the inferior surface is freed by careful dissection. A portion of the inner border, posteriorly, is freed so that a finger may be interposed to protect the neurovascular structures during the remainder of the dissection.

C.—The first rib is divided with first rib shears.

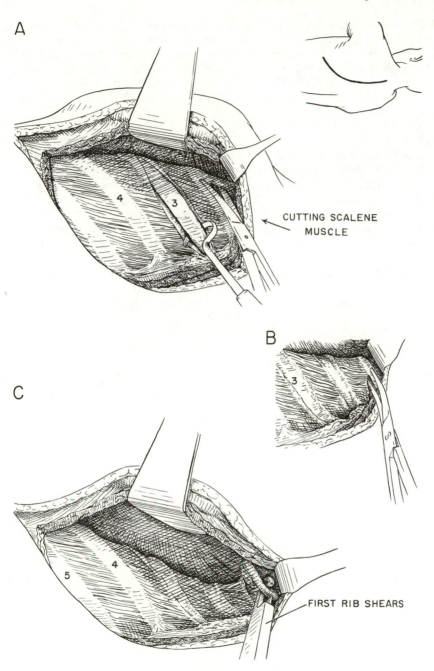

A

CUTTING SCALENE
MUSCLE

B

C

FIRST RIB SHEARS

D.—In disarticulating a rib, the internal periosteum is readily stripped down to the head with the fingers. Superior and inferior attachments are cleared away with a periosteal elevator. The articulation between the transverse process and the tubercle of the rib is opened with a heavy scalpel, and the neck of the rib is pried away from the transverse process with a periosteal elevator. The neck of the rib is grasped with a bone-holding forceps and rotated, first in one direction and then the other, to rupture the remaining ligamentous attachments. The head of the rib with its articular surface is then pulled away from the spine. The head of the first rib is usually not disarticulated because it lies above the dome of the pleura and the stellate ganglion can be injured during its removal.

E.—Resection of a transverse process is accomplished by clearing away the ligamentous attachments with a periosteal elevator and then cutting across the base of the process with a large rongeur. The first transverse process is not removed.

F.—These skeletal diagrams show the extent of resection at the first stage. All of the first and second ribs (except the head of the first rib) and their costal cartilages, the posterior half of the third rib, and the second and third transverse processes are resected.

After the resection is completed, the chest wall is closed in layers in the usual way.

D

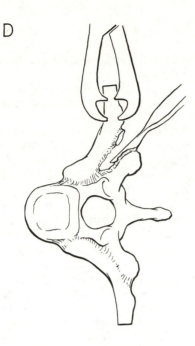

E

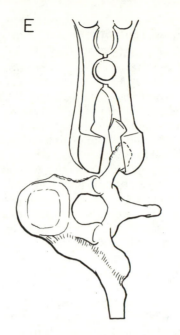

F

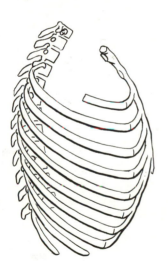
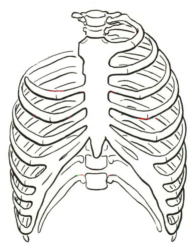

Second and Third Stages

In performing the second stage, 10 to 14 days later, the cutaneous scar is excised and the muscle layers are opened as in the first stage.

Fig 10–2, A.—The skeletal diagrams show the additional resection performed at the second stage. The anterior half of the third rib and its costal cartilage are removed, and the fourth rib is resected almost to the costal cartilage and the fifth rib to slightly beyond the anterior axillary line. The fourth and fifth transverse processes are resected. The wound is closed in layers in the usual way.

B.—The seven-rib thoracoplasty is completed at the third stage. It is not necessary to reopen the entire wound. Excision of the lower half of the cutaneous scar with separation of the previously divided muscles at that level usually provides adequate exposure. It may be necessary to extend the lower end of the incision anteriorly and to divide the rest of the latissimus dorsi muscle. Relatively short segments of the sixth and seventh ribs and the sixth and seventh transverse processes are resected. The chest wall is closed in layers in the usual way.

It is usually advisable to perform a partial scapulectomy with five- and six-rib thoracoplasties. If this is not done, the tip of the scapula can either "ride" in and out over the top of the highest intact rib, causing pain, or be held outward by the intact ribs, limiting the effectiveness of the collapse. The technique of partial scapulectomy is not difficult. All muscular attachments are freed from the lower portion of the scapula. This must be done almost entirely by sharp dissection. The scapula is then transected with rib shears.

A

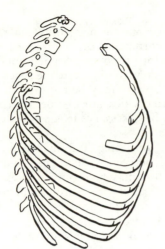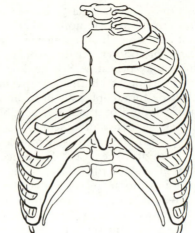

B

SCHEDE THORACOPLASTY

This type of thoracoplasty is used to close chronic empyema cavities, both tuberculous and nontuberculous, when decortication or extrapleural pneumonectomy is not advisable. If an empyema develops following a pneumonectomy and, for one reason or another, the thoracoplasty done to obliterate the space is delayed, a chronic space may persist. A Schede thoracoplasty may be required to correct it. If all efforts are made to eliminate empyema cavities during the acute or subacute stages, a Schede thoracoplasty will seldom be necessary. It is a bloody, mutilating operation and should be avoided if possible.

In the classic Schede thoracoplasty, as illustrated, the thickened rigid parietal pleura along with the intercostal muscles, nerves, vessels, ribs, and periosteum overlying the cavity, is excised. The procedure may be modified to excise only the rigid parietal pleura and ribs, allowing the remaining structures to fall in and obliterate the space if a thoracoplasty has not been done previously.

Fig 10–3, A and B.—An eight-rib thoracoplasty, done previously, did not eliminate the empyema cavity because the parietal pleura was too thick to allow total collapse. The persistent sinus is excised, and a midaxillary line incision is carried down to the regenerated ribs.

C.—The regenerated ribs, along with the rigid parietal pleura, intercostal muscles, nerves and vessels, are excised to unroof the empyema cavity completely (leaving no overhanging edges). The intercostal vessels are best controlled with suture ligatures.

D.—Gauze packing may be inserted for a few days, and then the chest wall flaps of skin, subcutaneous tissue, and muscle are allowed to fall in to adhere to either the mediastinum or visceral pleura. Complete healing may require several weeks or months.

A

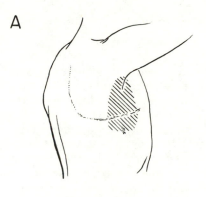

B

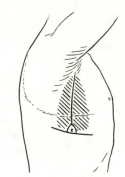

C

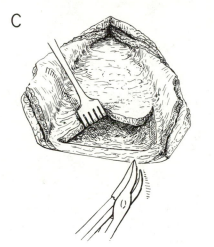
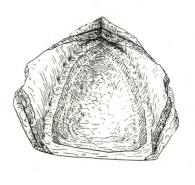

D

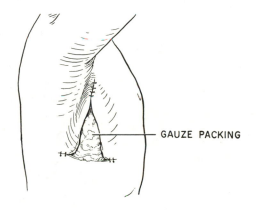

GAUZE PACKING

COMPLICATIONS OF THORACOPLASTY

Paradoxical Motion

The ill effects of paradoxical motion have been previously discussed, and it has been mentioned that only a limited number of ribs are resected at each stage so that the paradoxically moving area will not be large. Suitable adhesive strapping is helpful to partially immobilize the decostalized area. In particular, the support is needed anteriorly, because the scapula and large back muscles provide relative immobility posteriorly. Large gauze pads are placed beneath the clavicle and in the axilla and are held firmly in place with 2-in. adhesive strips. The adhesive strapping is extended well over the back and shoulders, so that tension on the skin will be widely distributed. Paradoxical motion can be almost eliminated if the strapping is applied tightly enough. Blistering of the skin is a definite limiting factor.

Scoliosis

Curvature of the spine, with the convexity toward the side of operation, invariably follows thoracoplasty. The degree of scoliosis can be limited by proper positioning postoperatively. The patient lies on the operated side with a pillow under the upper portion of the chest for eight to ten hours daily. A head pillow is omitted so that upper thoracic and lower cervical portions of the spine curve toward the side of operation. In addition, the patient is instructed to attempt to assume the same position frequently when sitting up. These measures are continued for about three months.

Frozen Shoulder

If exercising the shoulder is begun within three to four days after each stage of the thoracoplasty and approximately 75% of normal motion is attained before the performance of the next stage, full motion is usually achieved within a few weeks after the final stage. The patient must be made to realize that the result is dependent on his own efforts.

CHAPTER **11**

Tracheobronchial Resections

TRACHEAL RESECTION AND RECONSTRUCTION

SEVERAL uncommon conditions require resection of major parts of either the trachea or the main bronchi. In light of unsatisfactory tracheal prostheses and substitutes, tracheal resection with primary end-to-end reconstruction has emerged as an acceptable method of dealing with tracheal strictures, selected tumors, and trauma. The most frequent indication for tracheal surgery is a complication of endotracheal intubation that has resulted in stenosis or malacia.

Tracheal resections are not often easy operations. Resection for stenosis at the site of a previous tracheostomy is actually a reoperation, and the major vessels of the neck and the recurrent nerves can be damaged. In centers where these operations are done with relative frequency, there is a generous supply of patients who have been referred after the initial operation failed. Excellent results, however, are reported by those with a specific interest and expertise in this problem.

Preoperative Considerations

Patients with an inflammatory component to a critically obstructing lesion may have improvement by preoperative steroid treatment. Antibiotic therapy is started before operation and continued for 48 hours afterward. The trachea is approached through the neck for high lesions and through the right side of the chest for lesions closer to the carina; both incisions may be necessary for adequate control of the airway during operation. Few operative procedures require such close cooperation between the surgeon and anesthesiologist, and the surgeon must have available a supply of sterile endotracheal tubes, tracheostomy tubes, and ventilator extension tubing to maintain ventilation. High-frequency jet ventilation is not usually necessary during the operation. For patients with critical tracheal narrowing, however, heliox (helium and oxygen mixture) allows easier breathing and superior ventilation because the helium is less viscous than nitrogen.

General Operative Considerations

Successful tracheal surgery depends on an accurate assessment of the lesion by bronchoscopy and biopsy. Tomograms of the trachea help to determine the extent of the lesion when there is major airway obstruction and a bronchoscope cannot be passed through the narrowed area. Establishing the upper margin of resection may require that a bronchoscope be used with a needle passed through the anterior trachea as a marker to ensure that the trachea is not resected at too high a level.

A wide, transverse collar incision, as used for thyroidectomy, enables adequate access to the upper trachea for resection of postintubation stenosis. The lower trachea and carina can be safely approached only through the right side of the chest; a fourth interspace thoracotomy provides excellent exposure. To avoid thoracotomy, some surgeons have advocated splitting the upper sternum to provide access to the upper mediastinal trachea. However, mobilization of the trachea must be wide enough to permit resection of the diseased area, but not so extensive as to place the blood supply in jeopardy. The blood supply of the trachea is, for the most part, laterally oriented, and the lateral "wings" are best left intact until after the trachea is divided.

Several maneuvers may be used to gain length of trachea and thus decrease tension on the anastomosis. Table 11–1 lists the lengths of trachea which can be resected and the various maneuvers required to obtain the additional length. Animal studies have shown that the trachea will heal satisfactorily if the tension on the ends

TABLE 11–1.—GAINING TRACHEAL LENGTH

TRACHEAL LENGTH	MANEUVER
Operations in the neck	
3 cm	No special dissection
4.5 cm	Cervical flexion with chin fixation
6.5 cm	Flexion plus hyoid release
Operations in the chest	
3 cm	Dividing inferior pulmonary ligament and mobilizing the right hilum
4 cm	Above, plus intrapericardial release of the right pulmonary artery and veins
6.5 cm	All the above, plus division and reimplantation of the left main-stem bronchus into the (right) bronchus intermedius

of the trachea to be approximated is less than 1,000 grams. Division of the anular ligaments between the tracheal rings is of limited use, because further dissection will compromise the supply of blood.

Tracheal suture technique is identical to bronchial suture technique; 3–0 or 4–0 synthetic absorbable suture material is used in simple, interrupted fashion. Permanent suture material has been associated with the formation of granulations within the trachea after otherwise successful surgery. Multiple sutures are placed in simple fashion around the cartilaginous rings, with the knots outside the lumen. Some surgeons advocate keeping the sutures in the submucosal plane rather than taking full-thickness bites. The sutures are first placed and then tied after the neck is flexed to allow approximation of the ends of the trachea under little or no tension. Enough sutures should be used to make a leak-proof anastomosis, but an excessive number can compromise blood supply.

Postoperative Care

Postoperative tracheostomy should be avoided because of associated contamination and the risk of further late complications caused by the tube. Prolonged endotracheal intubation is not desirable because positive-pressure ventilation stresses the anastomosis, can spread infection, and can cause subcutaneous emphysema when the cuff of the tube is located above the anastomosis. Following a cervical resection, flexion of the neck is maintained for seven days, effected by a sturdy suture affixing the chin to the sternum on completion of the operation.

TRACHEAL RESECTION: CERVICAL APPROACH

The illustrated operation is performed for critical airway stenosis following tracheostomy. Preoperative studies showed an involved length of 3.5 cm, with the stenosis at the level of the tracheostomy (rather than the cuff).

Fig 11–1, A.—A collar incision is made to include the stoma of the previous tracheostomy. Dissection is carried through the platysma, and if retraction requires much further dissection, the strap muscles are divided. The surgeon quite purposefully keeps the dissection on the wall of the trachea in order to protect the recurrent laryngeal nerves, which are not dissected out.

B.—In the case of benign disease, the surgeon incises the lesion and resects up and down to normal tissue. When this is not possible, the trachea is divided below the lesion, and a tube is inserted quickly into the distal trachea and attached to sterile ventilator tubing. The lesion is then carefully evaluated and resected with an appropriate upper margin. Tracheal tissue which has either excessive scar tissue or malacia should be removed to prevent recurrence.

The margins of resection may be submitted for frozen section examination when the indication for operation is tumor.

C.—Simple sutures are placed so that when they are tied, the knots will be outside the tracheal lumen. The suture ends are tagged with hemostats and kept in sequential order.

D.—With the patient's neck flexed, the sutures are tied down securely, under little tension. If an auxiliary tube was used, it is removed just before the final few sutures are tied; the patient receives no ventilation during these few seconds. Leaks are evaluated by flooding the operative field with saline solution. The wound is closed in layers, avoiding tracheostomy if at all possible.

Complications

Dehiscence of the anastomosis is rare when there is only moderate tension on the ends of the tracheal segments. The most frequent difficulty is restenosis. Again, the use of appropriate resection of all the diseased trachea and techniques for decreasing tension minimize the likelihood of this complication. Meticulous suture technique and testing of the completed suture line ensure that there is no leak. Adequate postoperative drainage, with passive drains for neck procedures and chest tubes for transthoracic operations, prevents minor leaks from developing into major problems.

Vocal cord paralysis is an infrequent problem, even though the recurrent nerves are not routinely identified. Keeping the dissection close to the trachea minimizes the risk of damage to these nerves and to the major neck vessels.

Chronic granulations with irritation and intermittent bleeding often occurs following the use of permanent suture material for airway anastomoses. Complete endoscopic removal of these foreign bodies is difficult for the surgeon and unpleasant for the patient. Synthetic absorbable suture made of polyglycolate or polydioxanone is strong and is not associated with granulation formation.

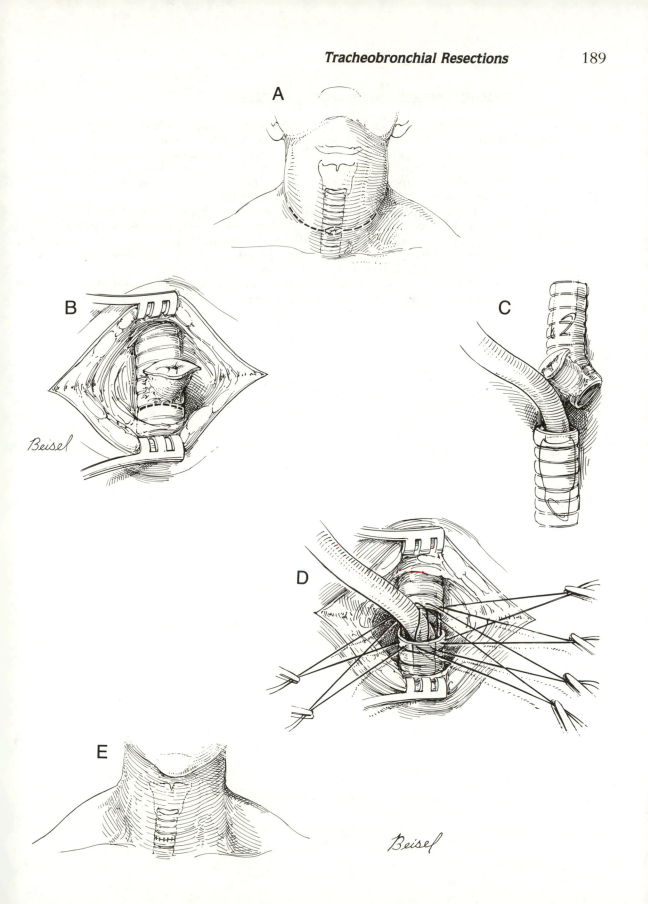

TRACHEAL RESECTION: LARYNGEAL RELEASE

The larynx is suspended from the hyoid bone, and an additional length of 2 cm can be gained by dividing the attachments of the larynx to the hyoid bone at a level either above or below the hyoid. The figures show release of the larynx through a small, separate superior neck incision, but mobilization of a large subplatysmal flap can allow access from the primary incision. This operation results in few postoperative difficulties with either swallowing or speech.

Fig 11–2, A.—The suprahyoid release of the larynx is accomplished by exposure of the hyoid bone and division of the muscle attachments on the superior surface. The lateral extent of this division is the tendinous sling of the digastric muscle. Mylohyoid, geniohyoid, and genioglossus fibers are sectioned, and the body of the hyoid is transected at either end.

B.—The central portion of the hyoid and the entire larynx and upper trachea then drop to allow further inferior mobilization of the upper tracheal segment.

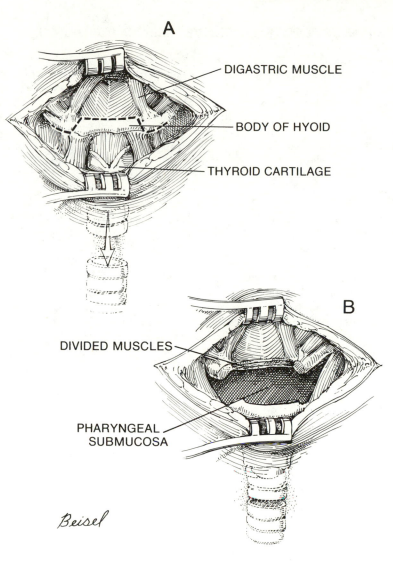

A

DIGASTRIC MUSCLE

BODY OF HYOID

THYROID CARTILAGE

B

DIVIDED MUSCLES

PHARYNGEAL
SUBMUCOSA

Beisel

BRONCHOPLASTIC RESECTIONS: "SLEEVE" RIGHT UPPER LOBECTOMY

A variety of resections that save parenchyma, collectively called "bronchoplastic" procedures, require section and reanastomosis of either the primary or the secondary bronchi. The suture technique has been presented, and operative concerns regarding ventilation are similar to those for tracheal resections. Indications for these operations include benign intrabronchial tumors, trauma, and some malignancies. Carinal reconstruction is an extension of both tracheal and bronchoplastic procedures.

In this example, the right upper lobe and adjacent right main-stem and intermediate bronchial segments are removed. The indication for removal is a bronchial carcinoid of the right upper lobe bronchus which protrudes into the right main-stem bronchus.

Fig 11–3, A.—The atelectatic right upper lobe is shown following dissection and division of the arteries and veins. The lobe is rotated forward, and the bronchus is cleared posteriorly from the carina superiorly to beyond the superior segment bronchus below. The inferior pulmonary ligament is released to allow superior mobilization of the hilar structures.

B.—The specimen has been removed, and simple interrupted 4–0 absorbable sutures are placed so that the knots will be outside the lumen. During this phase of the operation, the double-lumen tube ventilates only the left lung.

The sutures are tied, and the repair is tested by reinflation of the right lung at 30–40 cm H_2O pressure with the anastomosis under water. The anastomosis is wrapped with a viable pleural or intercostal flap before closure of the chest.

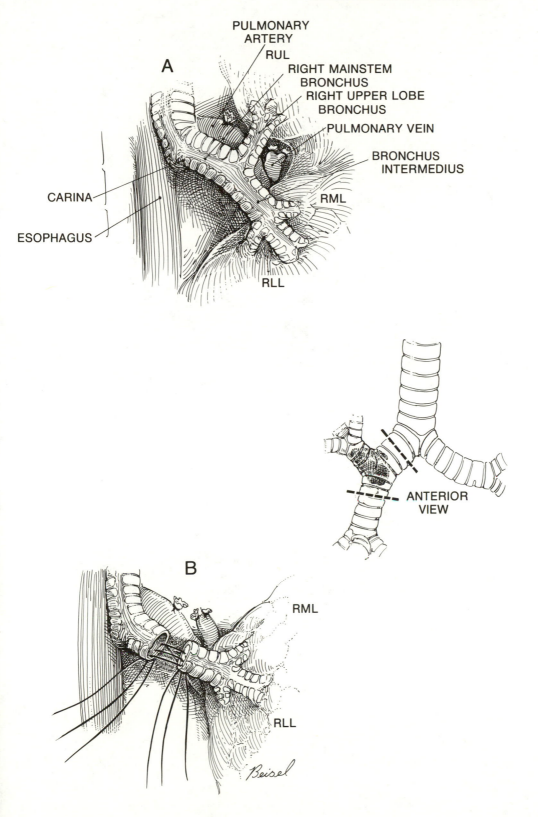

CHAPTER 12

Surgery of the Esophagus

ESOPHAGEAL ATRESIA AND TRACHEOESOPHAGEAL FISTULA

ESOPHAGEAL atresia, which is usually accompanied by tracheoesophageal fistula, is encountered in approximately one of every 5,000 live births. Most of the malformations are incompatible with life and must be recognized and corrected in the neonatal period if the infant is to survive.

Fig 12–1.—The five recognized types of malformations are shown with their frequency and the letter classification which was developed by Gross.

Diagnosis

Most of the patients have respiratory symptoms such as cough and pneumonia. The nurses' notes usually describe excessive drooling of saliva and vomiting. If not diagnosed early, severe pneumonia with respiratory failure may develop.

An air esophagogram, enhanced by placing a feeding tube into the stomach and having it curl within the proximal pouch of the esophagus, is the easiest way to make the diagnosis. In general, radiopaque media should not be used. It is especially important to avoid using hypertonic water-soluble contrast media, since, if aspirated, they are poorly tolerated by the epithelium of the bronchial tree. The presence of air in the gastrointestinal (GI) tract documents the presence of a fistula.

Preoperative Preparation

In most cases, an emergency gastrostomy should be performed under local anesthesia prior to the thoracotomy so that aspiration of gastric acid and enzymes through the fistula will not occur. This allows the infant's pulmonary status to improve until an appropriate time for thoracotomy. We have waited for as long as 13 days before performing primary esophagoesophagostomy. During this time, the proximal pouch should be aspirated with a nasoesophageal tube, and the child should be maintained in a head-up position. Parenteral nutrition is not required during the staging process.

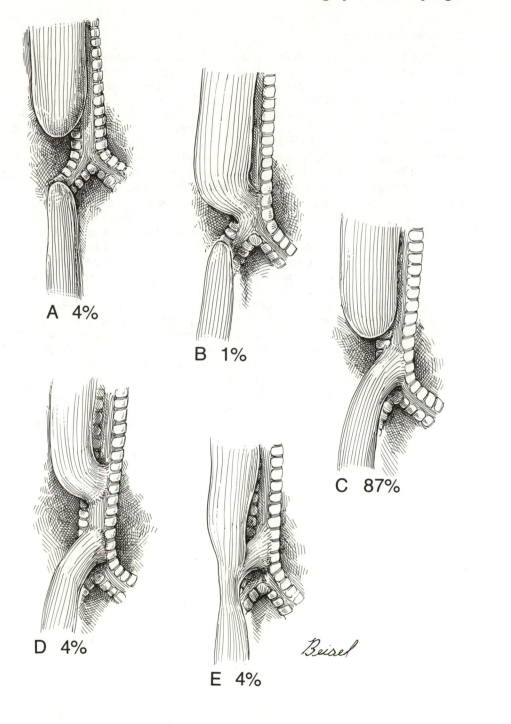

A 4%

B 1%

C 87%

D 4%

E 4%

Beisel

Operative Treatment

Fig 12–2, A.—The infant is placed in the left decubitus position (right side up), and a fourth–interspace lateral thoracotomy is performed. If the infant has been stable prior to operation, an extrapleural dissection is preferred to minimize the risk of empyema. The transpleural approach is more direct but leads to adhesions.

B.—The azygos vein is identified, ligated, and divided. At the carina, nearly always medial to the azygos vein, the fistula is identified and divided. This should be done without the use of clamps so that the distal esophagus is not damaged. The anesthesiologist should be warned that the fistula is going to be opened and that there will be a resultant air leak. Traction sutures are placed on the distal segment, and the fistula is closed with interrupted sutures of nonabsorbable material. Care is taken not to narrow the trachea. The operation may be terminated at this point if the infant's condition is unstable, in which case the distal segment is oversewn, and a traction suture is placed to maintain its position as far superior as possible.

C, D.—The esophagoesophagostomy may be performed in a number of different ways. It is of primary importance to reduce tension on the anastomosis so that neither stenosis nor a leak occurs. The anesthesiologist places downward pressure on the nasoesophageal tube, making identification of the proximal pouch easy. It is elevated from the surrounding tissues, and a no. 4F Fogarty embolectomy catheter is placed through a pursestring suture and into the pouch. When the balloon is inflated, one has a nice traction device for further mobilization of the esophagus. Since the blood supply to the proximal pouch is based on the inferior thyroid artery, this portion of the esophagus may be mobilized up to the thoracic inlet. Care must be taken to avoid creating an inadvertent tracheotomy, which may lead to significant narrowing of the trachea when such a defect is closed. It is better to narrow the esophagus.

If adequate length cannot be obtained, an esophagomyotomy may be performed as shown in Figures 12–2, C and D. The longitudinal and circular muscle fibers are divided down to the submucosa, which carries the blood supply to the distal esophagus.

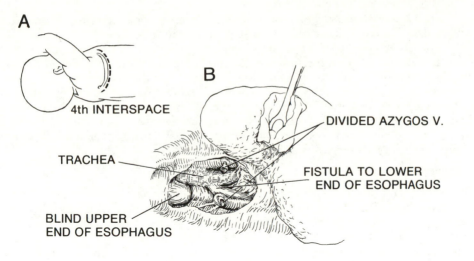

A

4th INTERSPACE

B

DIVIDED AZYGOS V.

TRACHEA

FISTULA TO LOWER
END OF ESOPHAGUS

BLIND UPPER
END OF ESOPHAGUS

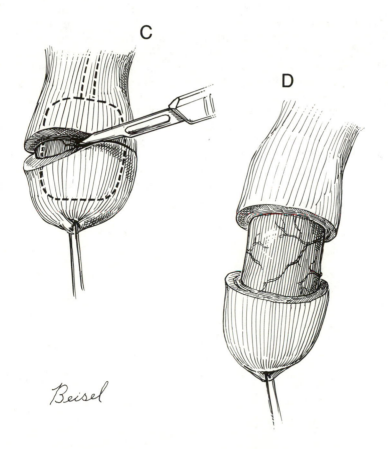

C

D

Beisel

Fig 12–3.—Some surgeons prefer a single-layer esophagoesophagostomy, believing that this reduces the risk of subsequent stricture.

Fig 12–4.—We prefer the "telescoping anastomosis" which was devised by Cameron Haight. In this anastomosis, the mucosa and submucosa of the proximal pouch are sutured to all layers of the distal segment, and then the muscularis, which was previously elevated away from the submucosa, is brought down over the first suture line to protect it. We prefer the newer absorbable suture materials such as Vicryl and Dexon, believing that the stricture rate is lower. A small chest tube is sutured to the chest wall near the anastomosis to facilitate drainage if a leak should occur. The thoracotomy is closed in the usual manner.

Postoperative Care

At the end of the procedure, the anesthesiologist accurately measures the distances to the carina and to the anastomosis by the insertion of nasotracheal and nasoesophageal tubes. Nurses are instructed not to suction beyond these lengths. In the postoperative phase, the infant is nursed in the head-up position, and the proximal esophagus is continuously aspirated with a sump tube. Seven days postoperatively, a barium swallow is obtained before any feedings are begun. If there is no leak, oral feedings may be started immediately. In the event of a leak, parenteral nutrition is continued, and a barium study, performed one week later, will usually show that the leak has closed. If there is no leak, the chest tube may be removed.

Three weeks following operation, a dilating string is placed through the anastomosis in the following manner: a no. 5 F feeding tube is passed through the nose and into the stomach. Under fluoroscopic control, the tip of the catheter is grasped through the gastrostomy and brought through the gastrostomy site. A no. 2 nonabsorbable ligature is then attached to the feeding tube and brought out through the nose. The two ends are tied together, making a continuous ligature. The dilating string may be taped to the infant's back and also to the upper lip to avoid damage to the lateral nasal ala. At six weeks following surgery, the esophagus is calibrated and then dilated periodically in the office with Tucker dilators attached to the string. When the esophagus accommodates a 30–36 F dilator without restricturing, the dilating string may be removed and the gastrostomy closed, after which the child may be treated as a normal infant. No special diet is necessary.

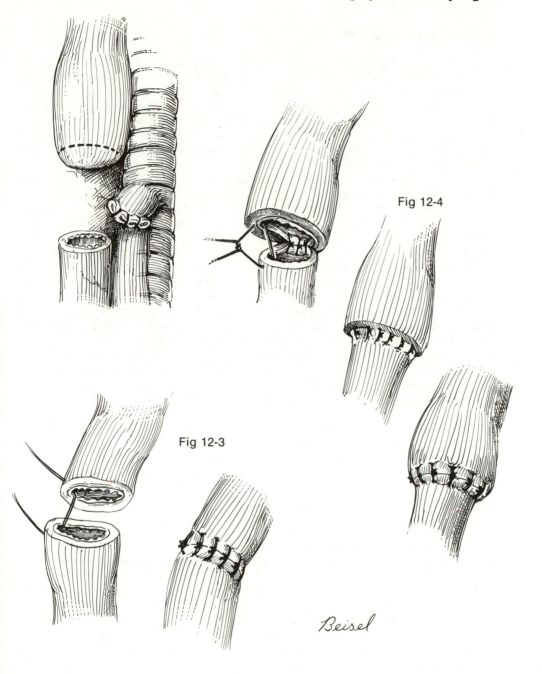

Fig 12-4

Fig 12-3

Beisel

SPECIAL CONSIDERATIONS

In the type A anomaly (proximal pouch–distal pouch) the distance between the two pouches is usually greater than three vertebral bodies, which is the generally accepted maximum separation for primary anastomosis. It has been shown that the length of the proximal pouch may be extended by regular bougienage, during which time the infant may be fed by gastrostomy. However, the infant must be maintained in the hospital to provide good pharyngeal toilet. A primary esophagoesophagostomy, which is certainly a better choice than esophageal replacement with some other intestinal organ, may then be anticipated.

Occasionally, in spite of all attempts at primary repair, approximation of the two ends of the esophagus is not possible. The surgeon is left with two possibilities: (1) The two ends of the esophagus (the fistula has been divided) may be approximated as closely as possible and, after one week, bougienage reinstituted. The additional length that is obtained allows primary esophagoesophagostomy at a second thoracotomy. (2) The other option is to bring out a cervical esophagostomy, close the distal end, and allow the child to grow and gain weight while being fed entirely via gastrostomy. Our preference is to bring out the "spit fistula" between the heads of the sternocleidomastoid. In this position, a stoma bag is placed on the infant's neck to aid in the handling of secretions. It is of particular psychological importance that the infant be fed by mouth during this phase, even though all of the food passes through the spit fistula and into the stoma bag.

At approximately 12 months of age, the infant may be returned to the operating room for an esophagoplasty. The selection of jejunum, right colon, left colon, or the greater curvature of the stomach for esophageal replacement, will depend on the surgeon's assessment of the infant's anatomy at the time of operation.

Associated anomalies are common with tracheoesophageal fistula. The most significant ones are associated cardiac anomalies, such as atrial and ventricular septal defects, patent ductus arteriosus, and tetralogy of Fallot. Imperforate anus and vertebral anomalies may also be seen and should be documented during the patient's initial hospitalization.

ACQUIRED ESOPHAGEAL DISEASE

Esophageal surgery offers some of the most formidable operative challenges for the thoracic surgeon. This 8-in. organ is one of the least accessible in the body, and its anatomic peculiarities and continuous alimentary function demand superb operative planning and technique if excellent results are to be achieved. It is intimately related to many other vital intrathoracic organs, including the trachea, the recurrent laryngeal nerves, the thoracic duct, the aorta and its great branches, and the pulmonary hila. Grave complications can follow operation, and all available efforts must be put forth to ensure an optimal outcome the first time.

Surgery of the adult esophagus is directed at correcting a number of acquired disorders of widely differing pathologies. The number of operations which can be offered, however, is limited, consisting of plastic procedures such as myotomy as well as resection and reconstructive operations.

Preoperative Considerations

Transthoracic esophageal operations are almost invariably major in their scope, and thus the patient should be well prepared before surgery. In addition to the routine preoperative considerations for other organ systems, it will be remembered that mechanical embarrassment to both heart and lung function will likely occur during surgical manipulation.

Many patients, particularly those with cancer, will have evidence of malnutrition and anergy. Preoperative preparation with total parenteral nutrition for 10–14 days has found favor with some surgeons. Postoperative complications, particularly infection, may be reduced in patients who convert anergy status, but the influence on survival is unsettled. Protocols in which preoperative radiation therapy has been used have failed to demonstrate any favorable impact on resectability, operative mortality, or long-term survival. The role of preoperative chemotherapy alone or in combination with radiation therapy is currently being defined.

Indications for Resection

The most frequent indication for esophageal resection is cancer. Carcinoma of the esophagus itself is nearly always squamous, but either stomach adenocarcinoma around the esophagogastric junction or laryngeal cancer will require that at least a portion of the length of esophagus be resected. Benign stricture secondary to caustic ingestion or reflux is much less commonly an indication for removal of all or part of this organ. Resection of the esophagus is not done for variceal disease. Benign esophageal tumors, such as leiomyoma, can often be locally enucleated so that resection is not required.

General Operative Considerations

With regard to reconstructive operations of the esophagus, two factors are of particular importance. First, sufficient tissue must be mobilized to allow the reconstruction to lie without tension. Excessive stretch can cause early anastomotic breakdown and leakage. Less tension can embarrass the blood supply to the anastomosis and lead to stricture. Complicating this concept, however, is the consideration that the esophagus, particularly over its lower extent, has a segmental blood supply. Excessive mobilization can lead to an inadequate blood supply at its transected margin. The second consideration is that of technical skill in performing the anastomosis itself. Precise approximation of tissues, with enough sutures to prevent leaks but not so many as to cut off blood supply, is required. A variety of stapling instruments is currently available, capable of creating superb end-to-end anastomoses. The use of these devices is recommended.

During the operation, it is often helpful to have some sort of tube or bougie within the esophagus to aid in its identification and dissection from surrounding structures. It is customary to pass a Penrose rubber drain around the esophagus at the point of initial mobilization. Traction on this can aid in safely freeing the remainder of the required length.

Postoperative Care

Following major reconstructive operations of the esophagus, most surgeons follow a postoperative protocol designed to provide the best chance of healing and to maximize the patient's safety. Following esophagogastrectomy, for example, it is customary to maintain the patient with IV alimentation during the first seven to ten days after surgery. The nasogastric and chest tubes are left in place during this interval, and prophylactic broad-spectrum antibiotic therapy is continued. The tubes are removed only after a barium swallow examination has demonstrated patency and an absence of leaks. The patient is then allowed to advance his diet as tolerated.

PHARYNGOESOPHAGEAL (ZENKER'S) DIVERTICULUM: MYOTOMY

The pharyngoesophageal diverticulum represents an acquired aneurysmal dilatation of the posterior lower pharyngeal wall secondary to dysfunction of the upper esophageal sphincter and obstructive spasm of the cricopharyngeus muscle. Symptoms are primarily those of dysphagia, and regurgitation and its complication are often responsible for the condition of the sickest patients. Respiratory complications such as pneumonia and lung abscess can be grave in these patients, particularly when the swallowing difficulties have led to malnutrition. Diagnosis is best made by barium swallow before instrumentation.

When a diverticulum is small and broad based, surgical correction can be successfully accomplished by release of the tight transverse cricopharyngeus fibers.

Fig 12–5, A.—The incision is made parallel to the anterior border of the sternocleidomastoid muscle, is carried down through the plastysma and lateral to the thyroid and strap muscles. The carotid sheath is retracted laterally. One or two traction sutures in the lobe of the thyroid will allow elevation and rotation of these anterolateral structures, providing better exposure of the posterior pharyngoesophageal junction. The area of the tracheoesophageal groove is not dissected.

B.—The operation consists of division of the spastic fibers of the cricopharyngeus muscle below the diverticulum. These fibers are elevated with an angled clamp and cut. Care is taken to avoid perforation of the mucosa as this incision is carried down the esophagus 3 cm.

C.—Relief of the obstruction is ensured when the mucosa of the upper esophagus is seen to protrude into this area.

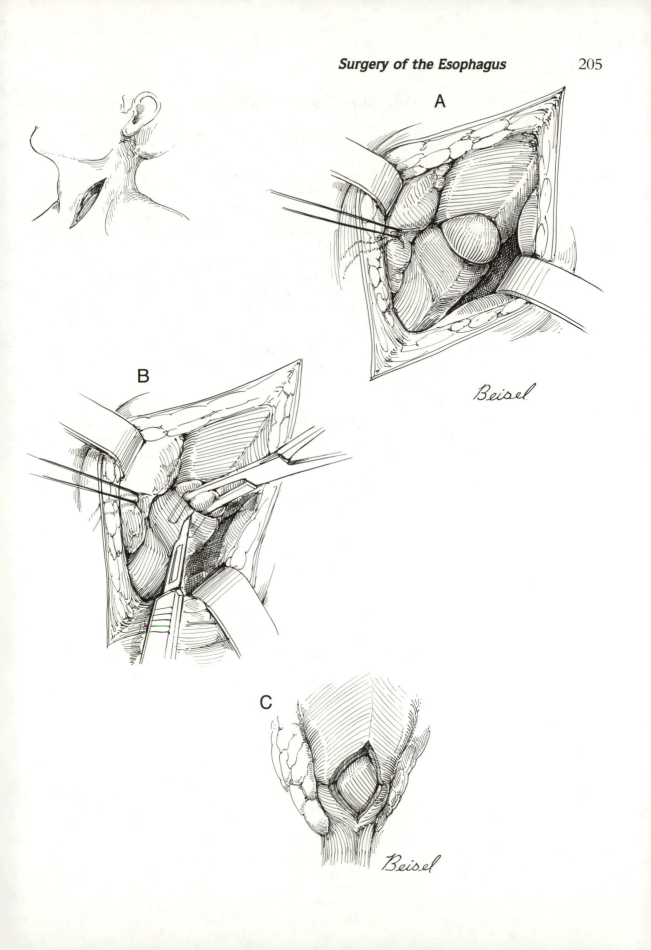

A

Beisel

B

C

Beisel

PHARYNGOESOPHAGEAL (ZENKER'S) DIVERTICULUM: DIVERTICULECTOMY

When a diverticulum is large, excision and repair is an acceptable method of treatment. Myotomy is performed along with the removal of the diverticulum to ensure that the problem does not recur.

Fig 12–6, A.—A long-standing diverticulum can be quite adherent to the posterior wall of the esophagus below the mouth of the diverticulum, but the sac can be delineated with careful sharp and blunt dissection. It is shown here with the transverse fibers of the cricopharyngeus muscle below the origin of the sac. The offending muscle fibers are elevated above the submucosal layer with a right-angle clamp and divided.

B.—The sac is divided at its mouth after application of an angled clamp. Special care is taken to avoid constriction of the esophagus. The use of an intralumenal bougie ensures a lumen of adequate size. Division is by cutting and suturing in several steps so as to minimize contamination. A transverse repair offers the greatest protection against stricture. With generous exposure, the surgical stapler can be used as well. A 30-mm instrument with 3.5-mm staples is ideal.

C.—A few interrupted sutures are used to approximate muscle fibers over the closure. A soft suction drain or simple Penrose drain is left in place at this level and closure is the same as for myotomy alone.

Postoperative Care

A nasogastric tube is not used, and a contrast study is done the day following surgery. If satisfactory, an oral diet is begun immediately and advanced. Drains are removed over the first three postoperative days. Complications are infrequent. Injury to the thoracic duct is recognized at operation and treated with ligation. Evidence of leak or excess drainage is treated conservatively, avoiding oral intake and utilizing parenteral alimentation if the fistula does not close promptly.

A

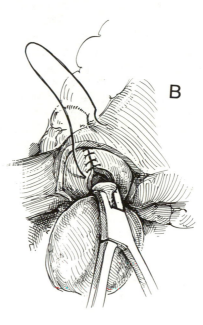

B

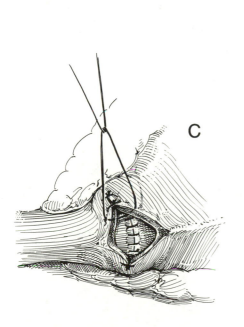

C

Beisel

ESOPHAGEAL MYOTOMY

Longitudinal incision of the muscular layers of the esophagus has become an accepted method of treatment for a variety of disorders of the esophagus. In the treatment of achalasia, the operation is often done from an abdominal approach, but when a longer myotomy is required, as for diffuse spasm, entry through the left chest is necessary. The most critical point in the operation is determining where the incision should end distally. Severe reflux may follow complete destruction of the lower esophageal sphincter, which can result from too long an extension onto the stomach.

Fig 12–7, A.—An extended myotomy for diffuse esophageal spasm is shown through a left sixth interspace thoracotomy. With the inferior pulmonary ligament sectioned, the esophagus is mobilized by sharp and blunt dissection. Ties or surgical clips are used on the short esophageal vessels. The vagus nerve fibers and the thoracic duct are preserved.

B.—With the esophagus grasped with the hand and the index finger behind the organ, an anterior myotomy is made. The posterior finger aids in putting the muscle fibers on tension, allowing them to be split down to the submucosal layer. This maneuver also controls bleeding during this part of the operation.

C.—The myotomy has been carried up the esophagus to the level of the inferior pulmonary veins. The inferior extent is onto the stomach a distance of less than 1 cm.

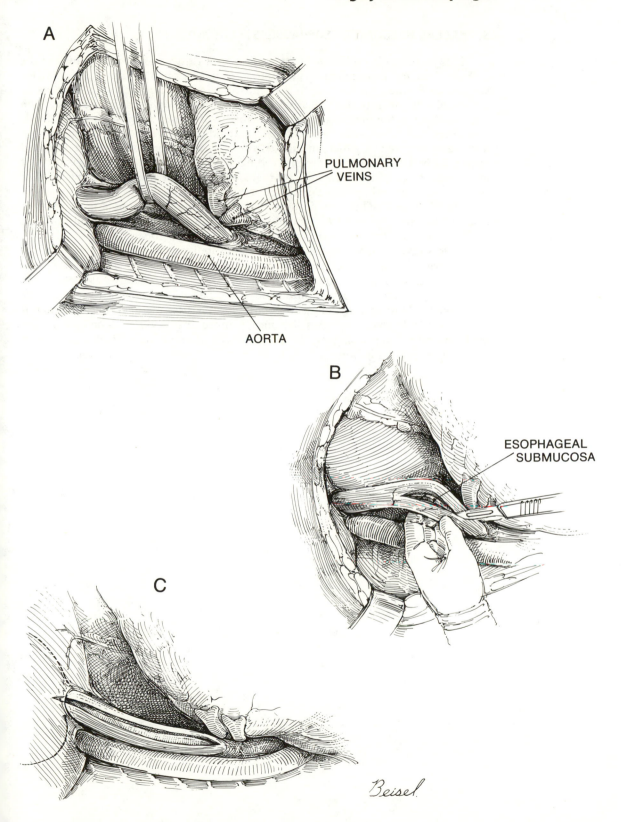

A

PULMONARY
VEINS

AORTA

B

ESOPHAGEAL
SUBMUCOSA

C

Beisel.

ESOPHAGEAL RESECTION: ESOPHAGOGASTRECTOMY

This resection is applicable in the treatment of tumors of the lower third of the esophagus and gastroesophageal junction. Consideration of reflux control is not generally warranted in the case of cancer, for it most often becomes obvious at surgery that the operation is palliative. The procedure, however, should include en bloc dissection of the mediastinal and para-aortic soft tissue and lymph nodes down to the celiac axis when there appears to be limited disease. When there is doubt about the stage of disease in a patient at high risk, it may be prudent to perform a limited upper midline laparotomy before proceeding with the major resection. Fixation of the stomach to the aorta may indicate that palliative intubation is a better form of treatment, as survival in such cases is quite limited.

Fig 12–8, A.—This tumor, above the esophagogastric junction, is approached through a left sixth interspace thoracotomy. A thoracoabdominal incision provides somewhat wider exposure at the expense of increased postoperative pain. The diaphragm is shown opened radially, allowing mobilization of the upper stomach. Short gastric vessels are clamped and ligated along the greater curvature, and the branches of the left gastric artery on the lesser curvature are cleared as well.

B.—The esophagus is mobilized above and below the level of the mass. Since this tumor tends to spread along submucosal lymphatics, the operative specimen is transected at rather wide margins (>5 cm). A more or less vigorous en bloc dissection is indicated, depending on whether the operation offers a chance of cure or simply represents palliation.

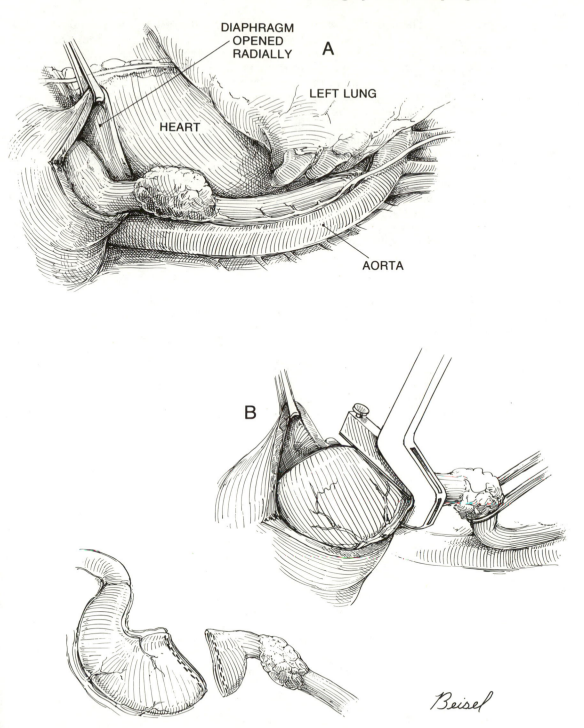

DIAPHRAGM
OPENED
RADIALLY

A

LEFT LUNG

HEART

AORTA

B

Beisel

C.—Through a short anterior gastrotomy, the end-to-end stapling device is introduced and its shaft brought out the posterior wall of the stomach. A full-thickness pursestring suture of strong monofilament polypropylene is placed and tied down securely around the instrument. The proximal (esophageal) pursestring suture is then placed, using the specimen to apply traction. Because the esophagus tends to retract superiorly, the specimen is not excised until the pursestring and a few traction sutures around the proximal line of division are placed.

D.—The anvil of the stapling instrument is then secured to the exposed shaft and inserted into the lumen of the esophagus. After the pursestring suture is tied securely, the device is tightened, opposing the staple cartridge and anvil. The area is inspected once again before the instrument is fired. After firing, it is then removed and disassembled to ensure that a complete ring of tissue was excised from each end. If the surgeon elects, either formal pyloroplasty or pyloromyotomy is performed next. Despite the vagotomy which occurs in this resection, the necessity of pyloroplasty is unclear.

E.—The gastrotomy is closed, the diaphragm is repaired with nonabsorbable suture, and chest tubes are placed before thoracotomy closure.

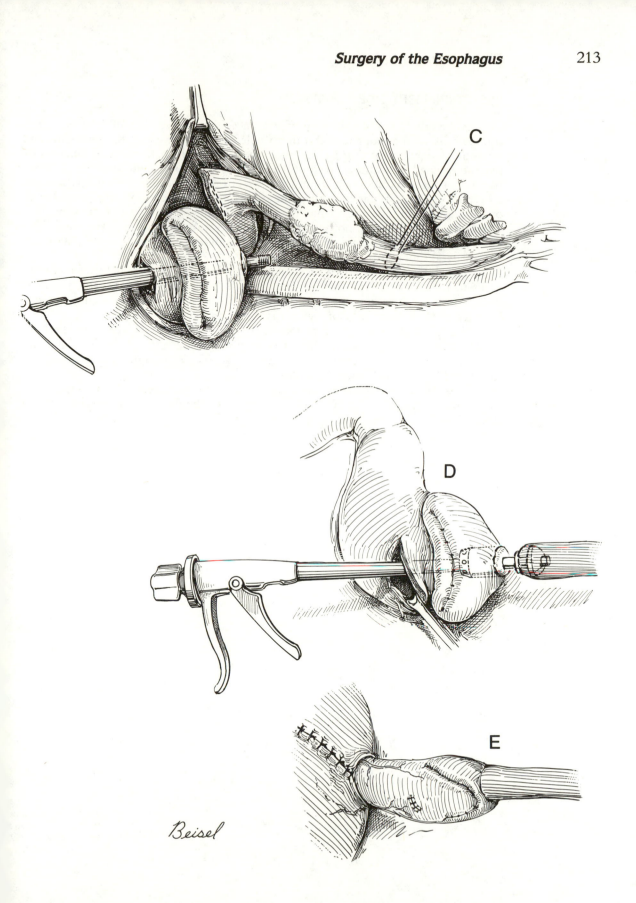

Beisel

RESECTION: RIGHT-SIDED APPROACH

Although it is possible to perform an adequate resection of lesions of the middle third of the esophagus through the left side of the chest, the problems and potential dangers of having to deal with the aortic arch make the combination of laparotomy and right thoracotomy ("Ivor Lewis resection") quite attractive. Obese patients or those with lesions around the level of the aortic arch are safely managed by repositioning and redraping the patient for formal thoracotomy after completion of the stomach mobilization from within the abdomen. If the patient is slim, it is often possible to perform both phases of this operation without repositioning. The buttocks are kept supine, while the chest and shoulders are rotated up 45°, allowing anterolateral thoracotomy.

The abdomen is explored for evidence of widespread disease before a commitment to major resection is made. The stomach is then freed, with blood supply preserved from the right gastric and right gastroepiploic vessels. Vascular arcades are preserved. Pyloroplasty or pyloromyotomy may be performed.

Fig 12–9, A.—A right fifth interspace thoracotomy is shown with the lung retracted forward. The azygos vein has been suture ligated and divided, and the esophageal lesion evaluated as to its resectability. The esophagus is mobilized and the stomach passed through the hiatus.

B.—An end-to-end anastomosis has been performed between the upper portion of the body of the stomach and the esophagus. The right side of the chest is then drained with two tubes, and both incisions are closed.

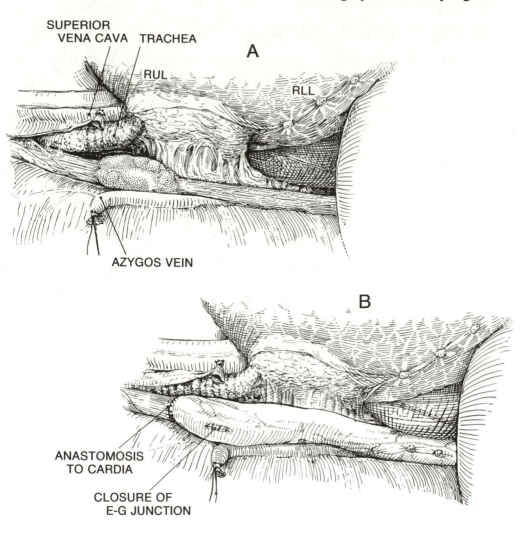

SUPERIOR
VENA CAVA   TRACHEA

A

RUL

RLL

AZYGOS VEIN

B

ANASTOMOSIS
TO CARDIA

CLOSURE OF
E-G JUNCTION

RESECTION: SUBSTERNAL COLON INTERPOSITION

Reconstruction of the esophagus is most commonly performed with the stomach, but colon can be used when this is not acceptable. All manner of variations—isoperistaltic, antiperistaltic, right colon, left colon, orthotopic, substernal—have been used with success. This operation, however, is tedious, and it requires three anastomoses as well as a thorough bowel preparation before surgery. Some surgeons recommend the reconstruction as an initial step followed by esophagectomy after an interval. One method of performing the entire operation follows.

Fig 12–10, A.—The minimal incisions required to perform the operation are demonstrated. Although the esophagus can be removed without thoracotomy, in the classic resection the patient is first placed on the left side, and the right chest is opened through the fifth interspace. The tumor and esophagus are freed as for the Ivor Lewis resection just described. The esophagus is divided just above the diaphragm and the lower end inverted. The upper esophagus is divided near the level of the thoracic inlet. The thoracotomy is then closed, and the patient positioned as shown. One problem with resecting the esophagus as an initial step is that the surgeon is then committed to reconstruction. Removal of the esophagus can be performed just as well as the final step in this procedure, after the surgeon is satisfied with the colon pedicle.

B.—A generous midline laparotomy is made and the colon examined. Following division of the gastrocolic, lienocolic, and lateral descending colon attachments, transillumination will help to define the vascular anatomy, and the colon pedicle then prepared.

C.—The transverse colon is divided just to the right of the middle colic vessels, upon which the colon pedicle will be based. The colon is then reconstructed with repair of the mesenteric defect, and the colon gently wrapped in a moistened towel and protected from further manipulation.

Some surgeons clamp the vessels along the intended lines of resection early in the procedure in order to assess the adequacy of both arterial supply and venous drainage. If the colon segment becomes dusky over the observed period, it should not be used. Stomach substitution then becomes the operative strategy.

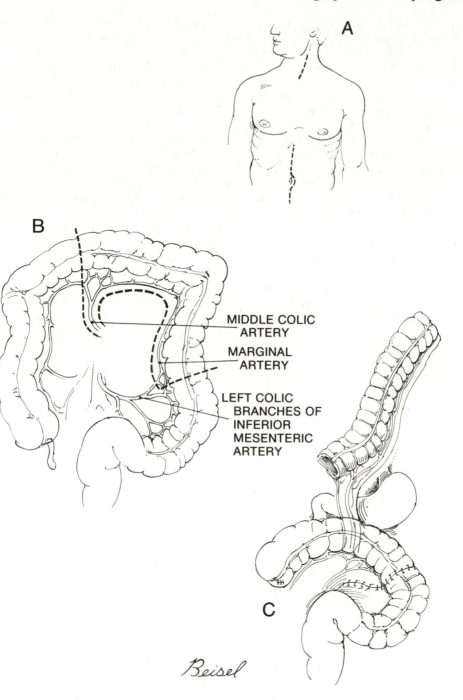

A

B

MIDDLE COLIC
ARTERY

MARGINAL
ARTERY

LEFT COLIC
BRANCHES OF
INFERIOR
MESENTERIC
ARTERY

C

Beisel

D.—The esophagus is then freed in the neck and controlled with a Penrose drain. If the esophagus was resected first, the proximal esophageal segment is simply delivered through the cervical wound.

E.—The diaphragm is detached from the abdominal end of the sternum, staying close to the bone in order to avoid entry into the pericardium. With one hand in the cervical incision and one working in the mediastinum through the abdominal incision, a tunnel can easily be established behind the sternum for passage of the colon.

F.—The colon pedicle is passed behind the stomach so that obstruction of the stomach or compromise of the vascular pedicle by a distended stomach cannot occur. The colon must be treated very gently, for its blood supply is precarious. The distal anastomosis of transverse colon to stomach is then made.

G.—The colon pedicle is then very gently passed up through the substernal tunnel without stretch, kink, or twist. Some surgeons advocate resection of the medial clavicle and adjacent sternum to open up the thoracic inlet and aid in decreasing problems with edema and venous engorgement, both of which may jeopardize the upper anastomosis. The proximal anastomosis is then created, sewing the sigmoid colon to the proximal esophageal stump. These two structures are usually well matched in size. The neck incision is then closed with passive drainage of the area of anastomosis. The laparotomy is also closed, after performing either a tube or catheter jejunostomy for enteral alimentation.

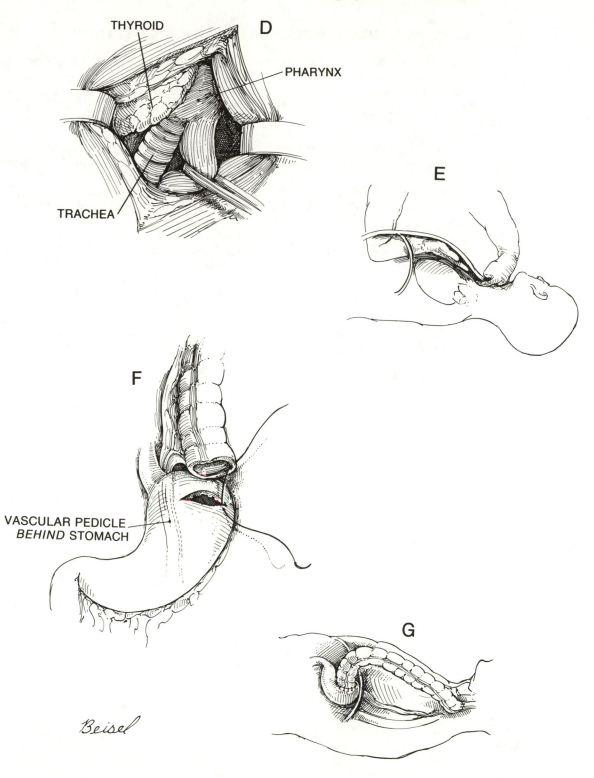

THYROID

D

PHARYNX

TRACHEA

E

F

VASCULAR PEDICLE
BEHIND STOMACH

Beisel

G

RESECTION: SEGMENTAL REPLACEMENT (WATERSTON OPERATION)

Corrosive or severe peptic strictures of the esophagus can often be successfully managed by repeated dilatation. Intractable areas of narrowing, however, can be successfully managed by resection and interposition of a segment of transverse colon. This operation is also applicable in cases of long-segment esophageal atresia.

Fig 12–11, A.—A sixth or seventh interspace posterolateral thoracotomy is made.

B.—An anterior circumferential incision in the diaphragm allows the transverse colon to be delivered into the chest after dividing attachments to the stomach and spleen.

C.—A segment of colon has been isolated and resected distal to the middle colic vessels, basing the vascular supply on the ascending branches of the left colic artery.

D.—The pedicle has been passed behind the stomach through a small posterior incision in the diaphragm. The colon is then anastomosed after resection of the diseased esophageal segment, providing an orthotopic reconstruction.

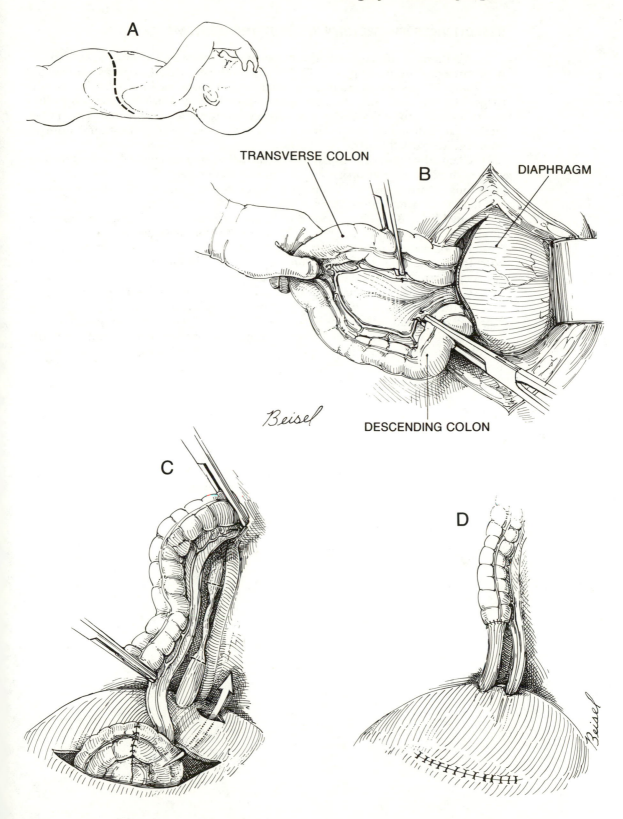

A

TRANSVERSE COLON

DIAPHRAGM

B

Beisel

DESCENDING COLON

C

D

Beisel

RESECTION: ESOPHAGECTOMY WITHOUT THORACOTOMY

All thoracic surgeons recognize the dismal prognosis of unselected patients with carcinoma of the esophagus. This fact, combined with the operative mortality attending the rather substantial reconstructive operations just covered, has led some surgeons to conclude that the best operation is the one which has a low operative mortality and morbidity and yet results in comfortable swallowing. This rather fatalistic attitude has led to the development of the trans-hiatal ("non-thoracotomy") esophagectomy with gastric substitution.

Claimed advantages of this operation over those previously described include similar survival, shorter operation, less postoperative pain, fewer respiratory complications, shorter hospitalization, and better control of the area of anastomosis should a postoperative leak occur.

Fig 12–12, A.—The patient is positioned supine, with the head angled to the right. The surgical preparation includes all of the abdomen, chest, and neck.

B.—Generous upper midline laparotomy allows access to the stomach, and both the greater and lesser curvatures are mobilized. The right gastric and right gastroepiploic arteries provide a reliably adequate blood supply.

C.—The use of a sturdy, overhanging mechanical retractor optimizes exposure of the esophageal hiatus as the gastroesophageal junction and progressively more of the intrathoracic esophagus are freed from the surrounding soft tissue. Surgical clips are applied to the vessels encountered, but hemostasis is not ordinarily a problem in this operation. It is possible to free the esophagus, with visualization, almost to the level of the carina.

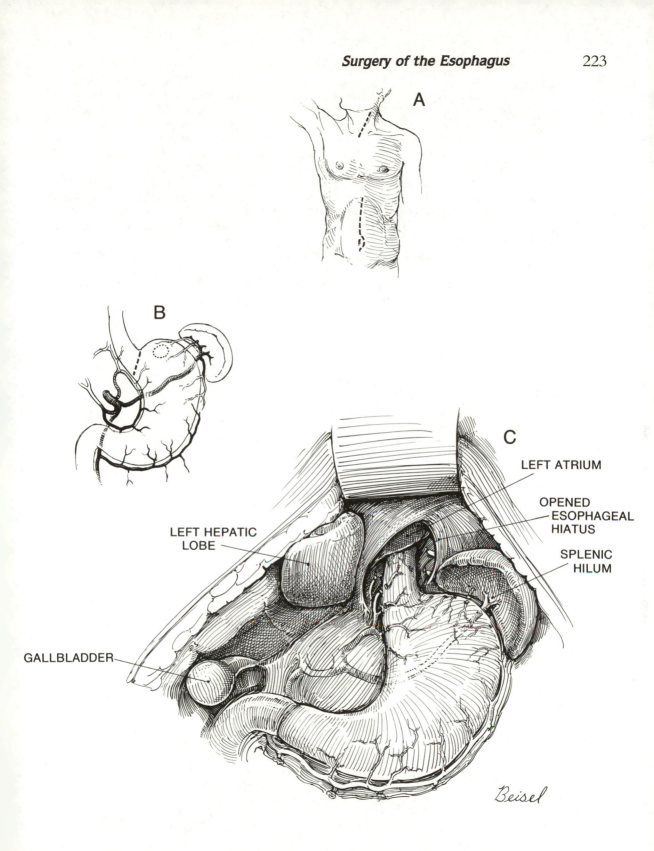

A

B

C

LEFT ATRIUM

OPENED
ESOPHAGEAL
HIATUS

SPLENIC
HILUM

LEFT HEPATIC
LOBE

GALLBLADDER

Beisel

D.—A second incision is made along the anterior border of the sternocleido-mastoid muscle, and the upper esophagus is encircled. Working from both top and bottom, it is possible to complete mobilization of the esophagus.

E.—The stomach is divided at a conservative level after the esophagus is delivered from the cervical incision. The uppermost part of the fundus is passed up through the chest in the esophageal bed, ensuring that no torsion occurs.

F.—It is frequently possible to use the end–to–end stapling instrument for the cervical anastomosis when there is enough redundant stomach delivered in the neck. At the completion of the cervical anastomosis, the fundus of the stomach above this level is anchored to the prevertebral fascia, ensuring that there is no tension on the anastomosis.

The stomach can also be brought up through a nonanatomic route, either through the chest or a substernal tunnel. Because of the bulk of the tissues, resection of the medial clavicle and sternum is advised when a cervical anastomosis is performed in a heterotopic fashion.

D

E

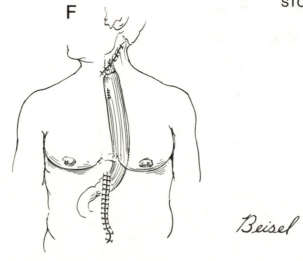

PULLED UP
STOMACH FUNDUS

F

Beisel

ESOPHAGEAL PERFORATION

Esophageal perforation is now more frequently iatrogenic. With remarkable regularity, the most common site of perforation is just above the gastroesophageal junction on the left side. The patient frequently complains of pain early after the event. Fever, neck swelling, crepitus, and increasing shortness of breath from increasing left pleural fluid and sepsis develop within a few hours. This subject is included at this point because the surgical considerations for treating esophageal perforation and anastomotic leaks which occur within the thorax are similar. As has been mentioned, leaks which occur in the cervical area are easy to deal with because drainage alone is generally adequate intervention.

The single most important factor in determining the success of primary closure of a perforation is the time interval between the perforation and operation. When surgery is delayed beyond six to eight hours, the failure rate of simple repair increases dramatically. Other, much less desirable alternatives, such as exclusion and drainage of the perforation, cervical esophagostomy, and gastrostomy must sometimes be used to achieve survival. Secondary reconstruction is undertaken much later, when the condition of the patient permits. The operative principles of immediate primary repair include wide mediastinal drainage, accurate visualization of the perforation, and closure in a single layer. An intense inflammatory reaction occurs with surprising speed, spreading throughout the mediastinum. The pleura overlying the mediastinum, therefore, is widely opened to effect drainage. Vigorous debridement is usually ill-advised, for there is no excess tissue. Still, the necrotic tissue around the perforation should be removed and the margins identified. Satisfactory closure is achieved by full-thickness, single-layer closure of the edges of the defect, using synthetic absorbable suture. It is not usually possible to do a satisfactory double-layer repair. Since the mediastinum has been widely opened into the pleural cavity, chest drainage with two tubes is appropriate.

The patient is fed nothing by mouth until a contrast study has proved the adequacy of repair at seven to ten days after operation. The chest tubes are left in place until after the patient begins to eat, and antibiotics are continued during this interval. Parenteral nutrition is reasonable for some patients, determined by their preoperative status and the findings at surgery. A small leak on the barium swallow examination can be treated by continued IV caloric support alone, if the fistula seems controlled and chest drainage is adequate.

THE SURGERY OF REFLUX

The several operations which are currently performed for gastroesophageal reflux and its complications are not included in this book. The majority of these procedures are done through abdominal incisions. Although a transthoracic approach is often required for reoperation or particularly complex primary repairs, such operations demand extraordinary judgment and deserve discussion which cannot be made available here.

CHAPTER 13

Surgery of the Diaphragm, Mediastinum, and Chest Wall

CONGENITAL DIAPHRAGMATIC HERNIA

CONGENITAL diaphragmatic hernia occurs about once in every 6,500 live births. The infant has a scaphoid abdomen, a barrel-shaped chest, and respiratory insufficiency, all of which may be noted in the delivery room.

Fig 13–1, A.—The most common congenital diaphragmatic hernia is a defect in the foramen of Bochdalek. Ninety percent of these defects occur on the left side, while 5% are bilateral and 5% occur on the right side. Incomplete development of the diaphragm may or may not be associated with incomplete development of the pleuroperitoneal membrane. If the pleuroperitoneal membrane is intact, there is a better chance of survival.

Preoperative Care

Surgical repair is a dire emergency, and transportation to a fully-equipped neonatal nursery should be arranged at once. The insertion of an endotracheal tube for ventilation and good pulmonary toilet is essential. A nasogastric tube to remove air and secretions from the GI tract should be placed as soon as the diagnosis is established. Physician-attended transport is mandatory. During the transport, the major risk is a contralateral pneumothorax. The attending physician must not hesitate to insert a chest tube in the unaffected chest if the infant's condition deteriorates. Resuscitation and stabilization are usually accomplished in the operating room. If possible, preductal and postductal PaO_2 monitoring should be undertaken. Transcutaneous oxygen monitoring is adequate for this, although an umbilical artery catheter also provides physiologic monitoring.

Operative Care

After all monitoring has been established and the patient is relatively stable, the operation may be undertaken. The most important steps are to reduce the intestines out of the chest and to effect closure of the defect. This is best performed through the transabdominal route.

Fig 13–1, B.—We use a paramedian incision for this operation.

C.—Because of the negative intrathoracic pressure, it is often helpful to introduce a small red rubber catheter through the defect to allow air to replace the mass of intestines which will be removed. If a pleuroperitoneal membrane is found, it should be excised.

D.—The anterior and posterior rims of the hernia are then approximated with nonabsorbable mattress sutures and reinforced with a running suture of similar material. Often, there will be immediate improvement in the patient's condition. A chest tube is placed but it is not connected to suction—only to underwater seal drainage. In the least favorable form, there is diaphragmatic atresia and there may be no tissue available for repair. In this instance, polypropylene mesh is sutured circumferentially to the margin of the defect.

In these infants the intra-abdominal volume is reduced, and the intestines have lost their "right of domain." Thus, replacement of the viscera may lead to significant upward compression on the repaired diaphragm and may make closure of the abdominal wall difficult. In most cases, this is circumvented by developing skin flaps medially and laterally and intentionally creating a ventral hernia. The fascia may be closed at a subsequent operation when the infant is approximately 6 months of age. In rare instances, the creation of an abdominal prosthesis, utilizing silicone rubber sheeting, may be indicated if it is impossible to raise adequate skin flaps.

Postoperative Care

The infant should be nursed with the affected side dependent, since the ipsilateral lung is usually hypoplastic and relatively nonfunctional. All efforts must be directed toward improving oxygenation through the contralateral lung and reversing the persistent fetal circulation (elevated pulmonary blood pressure) usually seen with congenital diaphragmatic hernia. Pharmacological manipulations and ventilatory assistance are often required. If the infant survives for four to five days, the outcome is usually favorable, and there are no long-term sequelae.

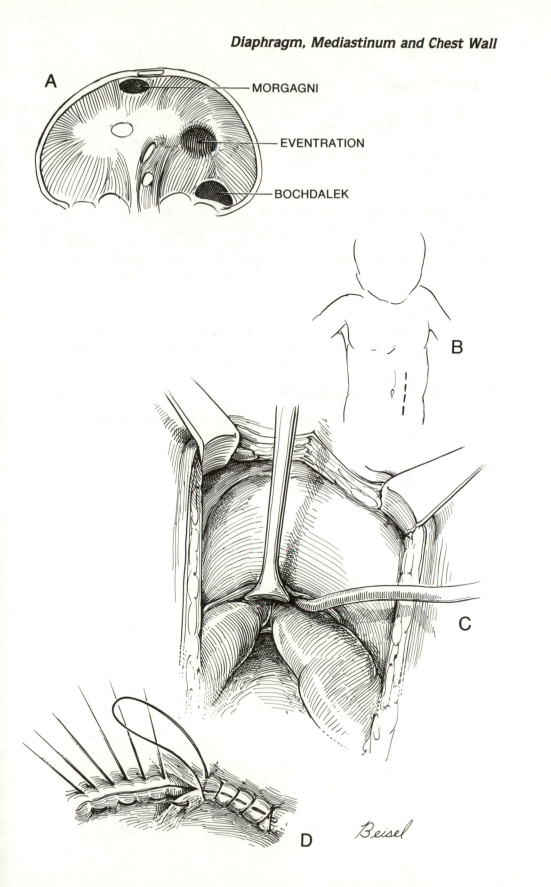

A — MORGAGNI — EVENTRATION — BOCHDALEK

B

C

D

Beisel

EVENTRATION OF THE DIAPHRAGM

Eventration (Fig 13–1, A) is usually congenital and may be related to a phrenic neuropraxia. In the infant with increasing CO_2 retention and respiratory effort, the diagnosis is best established by fluoroscopy. Endotracheal intubation for stabilization is often required prior to surgery. The improvement in the infant's condition after artificial ventilation is usually quite striking.

Operation

Fig 13–2.—The condition as seen in a right-sided anteroposterior roentgenogram of the chest and demonstrates the eventration of the dome of the diaphragm. A low, lateral thoracotomy is performed. Plication of the dome with nonabsorbable sutures to transform the diaphragm from a baggy, passive membrane into a rigid structure is usually a sufficient operation. Excision of the eventrated diaphragm is to be avoided. Nonabsorbable sutures should be used.

Postoperative Care

A chest tube is placed at the time of surgery and may be removed shortly thereafter. These infants usually may be advanced rapidly to formula and may be discharged within a few days of surgery.

HERNIAS OF THE FORAMEN OF MORGAGNI

Figure 13–1, A, shows the anterior, parasternal foramen of Morgagni. This defect is rare and is seldom life-threatening, although occasionally bowel may become trapped within the hernia sac. Sometimes the defect is so large that the liver herniates into the anterior part of the chest and causes respiratory embarrassment. Surgical repair is facilitated by a subcostal abdominal incision, which readily allows reduction of the viscera and primary closure of the fascia surrounding the hernia defect. Prosthetic material may be required.

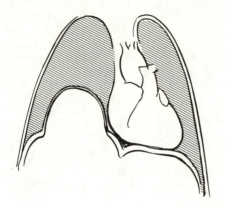

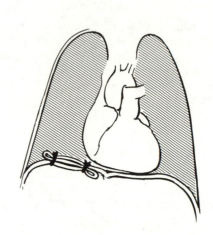

MEDIASTINAL TUMORS

Fig 13–3.—The mediastinum can be divided into superior, anterior, middle, and posterior compartments. Tumors can originate from structures present in any of these areas, and the likelihood of their being either malignant or benign is usually a function of the patient's age and of the location of the tumor.

Superior Mediastinal Masses

These are usually a type of hemolymphangioma and are often called cystic hygromas. The cystic hygroma may have the predominant amount of mass above the clavicles and cause a significant deformity of the neck. Careful exploration for an intrathoracic element is imperative, however, because these tumors may have a hemangiomatous component. There may be significant intrathoracic hemorrhage if the tumor is inadvertently torn at operation. In addition, compression of the airway at the thoracic inlet may occur with any of these lesions. Teratoma, rhabdomyosarcoma, and neuroblastoma may occur in this location as well.

Anterior Mediastinal Masses

Thymomas, thyroid tumors and dermoids (teratomas) may occur in this location. A lateral thoracotomy or median sternotomy can be used with almost equal exposure for complete excision of these tumors.

Middle Mediastinal Tumors

Lymphoma predominates in this location, although foregut anomalies, benign cysts, and congenital lesions of the tracheobronchial tree may be seen as well. Careful evaluation for metastatic lesions may obviate a thoracotomy in some cases. A lateral thoracotomy gives adequate exposure for diagnosis and also for excision of localized lesions. In rapidly enlarging mediastinal tumors that are associated with respiratory distress, an emergency thoracotomy with biopsy and emergency radiation therapy in combination with appropriate chemotherapy may be required. In such cases, endotracheal intubation and mechanical ventilation prior to operation should not be delayed.

Posterior Mediastinal Tumors

Neurogenic tumors are most common in this area. Neuroblastoma and its more benign variants (ganglioneuroblastoma and ganglioneuroma) are the most typical. A thoracotomy and excision of the tumor for staging purposes is indicated in most cases. Because of the frequency of "dumbbell" tumors, in which the lesion extends into the spinal canal through the foramen, a careful neurologic examination is a prerequisite to thoracotomy. If there is any neurologic deficit, either a formal myelogram or a metrizamide computerized tomographic scan of the spinal column should be undertaken prior to thoracotomy. Occasionally, a decompressive laminectomy should either precede or be performed at the same time as the thoracotomy. Most of these lesions may be approached through a lateral thoracotomy and excised. Care must be taken to mark the foramen from which the tumor arises and to be sure that adequate hemostasis is obtained in this area. Hemorrhage into the spinal canal can be as devastating as the growth of the tumor itself.

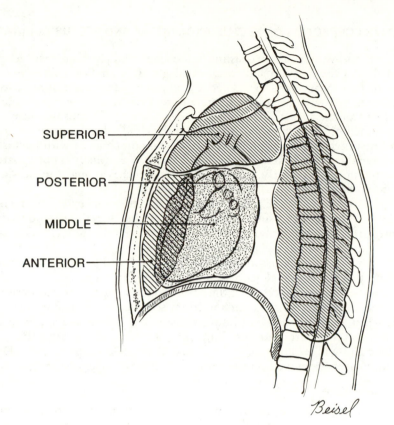

SUPERIOR

POSTERIOR

MIDDLE

ANTERIOR

Beisel

OPERATIVE CORRECTION OF PECTUS EXCAVATUM AND PECTUS CARINATUM

Pectus excavatum and carinatum (funnel chest and pigeon breast) are congenital anomalies of the sternum and costal cartilages. It is rarely possible to document any specific pulmonary or cardiac defect by pulmonary function testing. Most of the abnormalities that have been demonstrated are a result of the defect which causes displacement of the mediastinal content. Nonetheless, the conspicuousness of the defect and the impact of the abnormalities on the child's development are indication enough for surgery. It is our preference to operate on children with pectus excavatum between the ages of 2 and 6 years. Pectus carinatum usually is not apparent until the growth spurt of the early teens. When the defect is thought to be significant, repair should be performed as soon as possible.

Figs 13–4, A–C.—The usual appearance and the usual extent of the defect are demonstrated. A transverse submammary incision that does not extend to the nipple line is preferred. The pectoral muscles are elevated from the thoracic wall, and every effort is made to keep the operative field dry.

D.—In turn, the perichondrium of each deformed cartilage is elevated. We have found that the Welch elevator works well for this purpose. The cartilages are removed usually in two pieces from the costochondral junction to the sternum. Care must be taken to preserve the perichondrium so that the ribs may reform.

E.—Just below the angle of Louis, the sternum is fractured and bent upward. Overcorrection is important at this point, since the pectoral muscles will be closed in the midline and will lead to appropriate convexity as healing progresses. Drains are placed and may be removed on the third or fourth postoperative day.

Postoperative Care

Limited supervised activity is permitted during the postoperative course of these children. Although they will not suffer difficulty with normal activity, significant damage to the repaired chest wall may occur as a result of a fall or a blow to the chest. We prescribe limited activity for six weeks and then gradually allow an increase as circumstances warrant. Approximately 10% of these repairs have some degree of recurrence. However, reoperation should be approached with some caution because the scar tissue makes a satisfactory result extremely difficult. In reoperative cases, the use of a supporting substernal bar is often indicated.

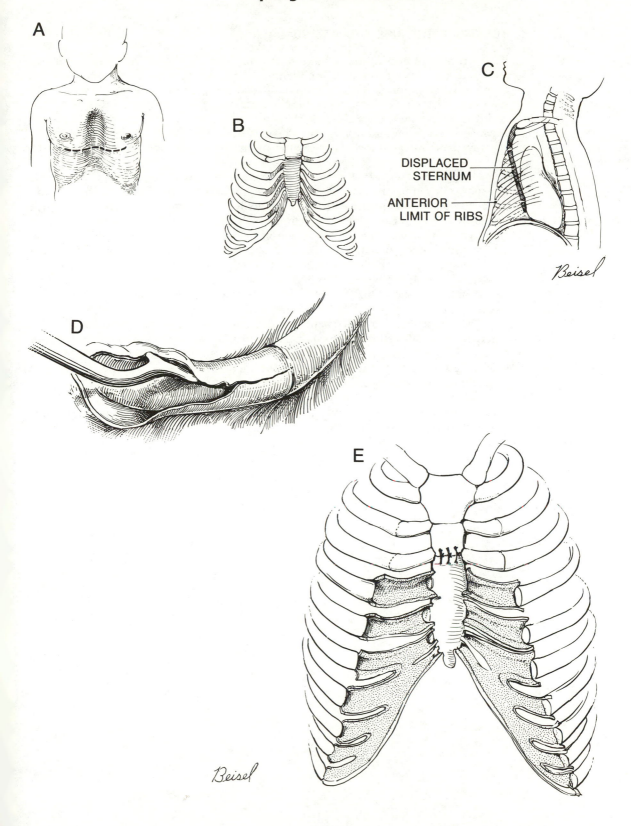

TUMORS OF THE RIBS AND STERNUM

Primary tumors of the ribs and of the sternum may be either benign or malignant and some have a characteristic roentgenographic appearance. Chondrosarcoma is the most common malignant tumor. Chondromas of the anterior chest wall are seen in young adults. Sometimes there is confusion concerning the exact cell type, and it is usually best to treat either one with wide excision. Fibrous dysplasia is the most common benign tumor but may be locally invasive. If the rib lesion is not part of a systemic disease, such as myeloma or metastatic disease, resection is appropriate.

Fig 13–5, A.—Whether or not a significant area of skin must be excised depends on its apparent involvement. Resection of involved ribs with adjacent and attached muscles and pleura en bloc is best achieved by entering an interspace above or below the area of involvement. This affords the benefit of palpation and inspection to determine the extent of the resection to be done. The line of resection should, where practicable, include a normal rib above and below the lesion and several centimeters, posteriorly and anteriorly, of grossly normal tissue. This usually leaves a wide defect subject to paradoxical motion when covered only with skin and subcutaneous tissue. This is especially true anteriorly, where the overlying soft tissue is thin.

B.—A prosthetic replacement provides some immediate stability and provides a matrix into which fibroblasts can grow to form a fairly rigid wall to substantially protect the underlying viscera. Knitted polypropylene mesh (Marlex) has been very useful. It should be sutured firmly to the pleural surface of the chest wall with polyethylene or polypropylene sutures passed full-thickness through the chest wall.

C.—If the overlying skin is inadequate for coverage, a plastic closure, using skin shifted from an area overlying normal tissue may be used, which in turn may be covered by using a skin graft.

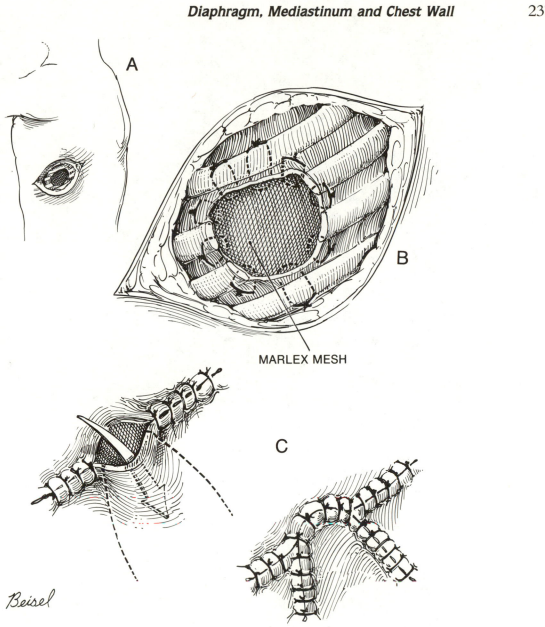

MARLEX MESH

Beisel

CHAPTER 14

Thoracic Outlet Syndrome

THE EXACT role of operative intervention in the management of the thoracic outlet syndrome is not firmly established. Indications for operation include subjective and objective evidence of the disorder. Opinions differ widely regarding the selection of candidates for operation. Some experienced physicians believe that physiotherapy will suffice in most instances.

This notwithstanding, operation is frequently employed, and the transaxillary approach has been widely accepted. Anterior and posterior approaches have been employed, but their complexity has caused them to be used infrequently. Because of this, we limit our description to the transaxillary approach.

TRANSAXILLARY APPROACH

Fig 14–1, A.—The patient is placed in the lateral thoracotomy position, and the table is tilted backward about 30°–40°. The entire arm is prepared and included in the operating field. The assistant plays a vital role in providing exposure by applying perpendicular traction on the arm.

A transverse incision is made at the lower border of the axillary hairline, and dissection between the latissimus dorsi and pectoralis major is deepened to the rib cage. Dissection is then extended upward to the level of the axillary vessels where they course over the first rib. The intercostohumeral nerve crosses the operative field and may be sacrificed; doing so may avoid neuritic pain, which is usually more bothersome than the resultant numbness along the medial aspect of the arm.

B.—Because of the limited exposure, palpation affords a most reliable guide to safe conduct of the procedure. The first rib is dissected extraperiosteally and, using an Overholt elevator (or similar one), great care is taken to avoid injury to the vessels and plexus. The anterior scalene muscle is divided at its attachment to the superior border of the first rib.

C.—It is important to remove as much of the first rib as possible, being careful to include its posterior aspect where the major nerve compression takes place.

D.—The result is a widened portal through which vessels and nerves may exit without compression. The skin and subcutaneous tissues are closed without drains.

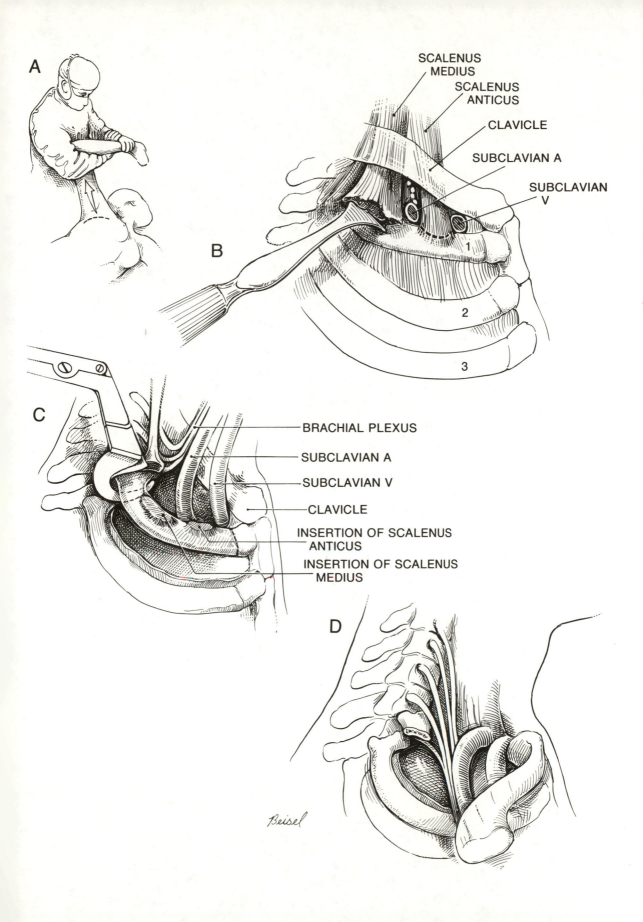

A

B

SCALENUS
MEDIUS

SCALENUS
ANTICUS

CLAVICLE

SUBCLAVIAN A

SUBCLAVIAN
V

1

2

3

C

BRACHIAL PLEXUS

SUBCLAVIAN A

SUBCLAVIAN V

CLAVICLE

INSERTION OF SCALENUS
ANTICUS

INSERTION OF SCALENUS
MEDIUS

D

Beisel

Part II

Cardiac Support Techniques

CHAPTER 15

Pump Oxygenators, Techniques of Cardiopulmonary Bypass

THE PUMP OXYGENATOR

With the use of the pump oxygenator, blood is removed from the venous system, oxygenated, and pumped into the arterial system. While the bypass apparatus has myriad components and tubing, it is readily understood when it is studied as a series of functional units.

Fig 15–1.—Venous blood is drained by gravity from the right atrium or venae cavae into an oxygenator of either the bubble or microporous membrane type. Most modern oxygenators have a reservoir and heat exchanger as an integral component. Thus, as blood leaves the oxygenator unit, the temperature is adjusted as required by the surgeon. The blood is pumped from the reservoir into the arterial system by the use of a roller pump whose speed directly controls the flow rate. We use a 40-μ filter in the arterial line to remove particulate matter such as fibrin strands.

Two additional roller pumps are used to remove shed blood from the pericardial sac and from within the cardiac chambers (cardiotomy suckers). This blood is returned to a separate reservoir (cardiotomy reservoir) and then the oxygenator unit. A remaining pump is used with an intracardiac vent. Blood from the vent is returned to the cardiotomy reservoir.

Special attention must be directed to maintain the integrity of the venous syphon that drains blood from the patient into the oxygenator. If the venous drainage line is allowed to fill with air, blood can no longer drain from the patient. When this happens, the cardiotomy suckers may be used to draw blood from the atrium and the venous drainage line must be clamped, disconnected, reprimed with blood or saline solution, and reconnected. Standard cardiopulmonary bypass then can be resumed.

The perfusionist must constantly observe the level of blood in the oxygenator reservoir. If the level falls, the surgeon is notified, and the arterial pump rate is slowed as required. If the reservoir is allowed to empty, as during kinking of the venous return line, air can be drawn into the line and pumped into the arterial system, with disastrous results. A variety of safety systems have been used over the years, but a simple ball-in-cage mechanism,* positioned in the arterial line just under the oxygenator, fulfills all of the requirements. During bypass, the ball floats in the cage and allows drainage of the reservoir. If the reservoir is emptied, the ball seats and occludes the drainage port, preventing air from entering the arterial tubing. When the venous reservoir again contains blood, the ball must be loosened by briefly reversing the arterial pump and then resuming normal bypass. The surgeon and perfusionist should ensure that the oxygenator reservoir is never allowed to empty.

---

* Automatic Shut-off Valve: Delta Medical Industries.

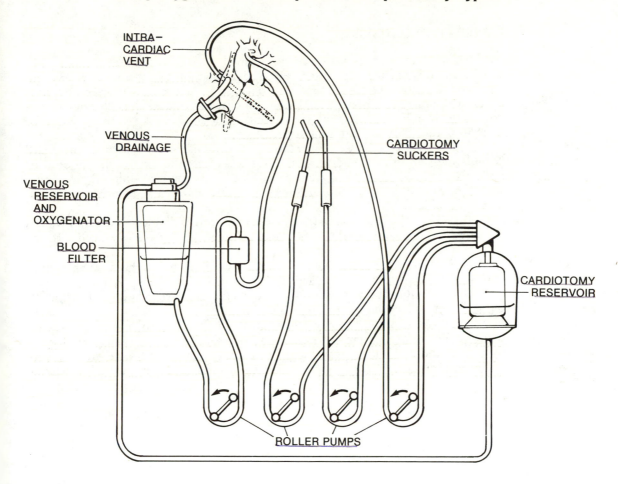

CANNULATION TECHNIQUES

Most open heart operations are performed through a midline approach. The venous blood is drained from either the cavae or the right atrium and, after oxygenation and filtration, is returned to the arterial system. Generally, the arterial cannula is inserted prior to venous cannulation, so that any blood shed during venous cannulation can be reinfused into the patient. Heparin (3 mg/kg) must be administered intravascularly prior to cannula insertion.

Fig 15–2, A.—Aortic cannulation is accomplished by inserting an angled cannula high into the ascending aorta, which is cleared to expose the innominate vein. Two pursestring sutures are inserted just below the vein, thus allowing adequate space on the aorta for the cardioplegia cannula and, when required, the attachment of grafts.

B.—The adventitia within the pursestring suture is divided, and a stab wound is made. A saline solution-filled, bevel-tipped aortic cannula is advanced into the aorta.

C.—The aortic cannula is then secured by tightening the pursestring sutures with rubber keepers, which are held to the cannula with a heavy ligature.

Venous cannulation is accomplished through pursestring sutures placed in the right atrium. When the right atrium is to be opened, as for the repair of an atrial septal defect or tricuspid valve replacement, it is helpful not to "cross" the venous cannulae. For most coronary artery operations, a single two-stage cannula,★ having right atrial and inferior vena caval drainage ports, provides both excellent exposure and venous drainage, even when the ventricles are tipped out of the pericardial sac.

★ Two-Stage Venous Return Catheter: Sarns, Inc.

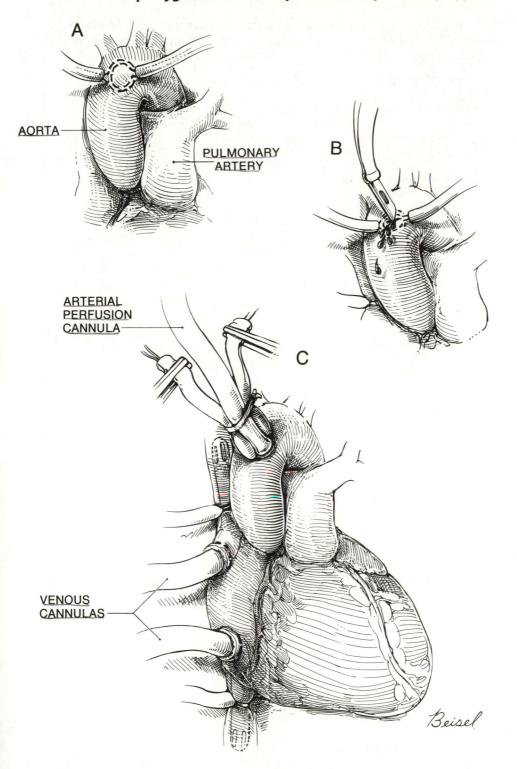

A

AORTA

PULMONARY
ARTERY

B

ARTERIAL
PERFUSION
CANNULA

C

VENOUS
CANNULAS

Beisel

In patients having an inadequate length of ascending aorta and in reoperative patients, when there is a risk of bleeding during opening of the sternal incision, the arterial cannula can be inserted into either the common femoral or the external iliac artery.

Fig 15–3, A.—The common femoral artery is exposed using a self-retaining retractor.

B.—The cannula is inserted and secured with cotton tape.

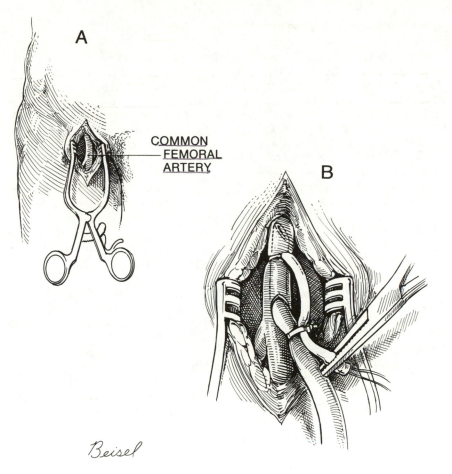

A

COMMON
FEMORAL
ARTERY

B

Beisel

VENTING OF THE LEFT VENTRICLE

An elevated left heart pressure in the nonbeating heart may result in lung damage and injurious left ventricle distention. Regurgitation of blood across the aortic valve as well as Thebesian and bronchial venous drainage contribute to an elevated left heart pressure. Cross-clamping the ascending aorta markedly reduces but does not eliminate the tendency for blood to accumulate in the left heart. Left ventricular venting prevents the elevation of left heart pressure, aids in de-airing the heart, and generally increases the safety of cardiac operations.

Fig 15–4.—Several types of venting procedures that are commonly employed in open heart operations are shown.

A vent can be inserted through the left atrium directly into the left ventricle. This is best accomplished by placing a 3–0 pursestring suture in the anterior surface of the right superior pulmonary vein. The perfusionist temporarily restricts venous drainage and thereby elevates the left atrial pressure. A stab wound is made in the pulmonary vein. The slit is dilated and a no. 20 F curved vent* is inserted. It is easily guided into the left ventricle by a hand positioned behind the heart. The vent is attached to a suction line of the pump oxygenator. Excessive negative pressure in the vent line is avoided by introducing an 18-gauge needle into the side of the vent tubing.

The optimal visualization needed for coronary artery operations requires left ventricular venting. This is most readily accomplished by a small cannula positioned in the ascending aorta and attached to a needle-vented suction line. The use of a branched cannula† as shown allows the cardioplegia solution to be administered through the same aortic puncture site. The vent tube is clamped while the cardioplegia solution is being administered. This type of vent is helpful also in de-airing the heart after repairing a ventricular septal defect or replacing an aortic valve.

---

* Curved Left Heart Vent Catheter: Sarns, Inc.
† Aortic Root Cannula with Attached Vent Line: DLP Inc.

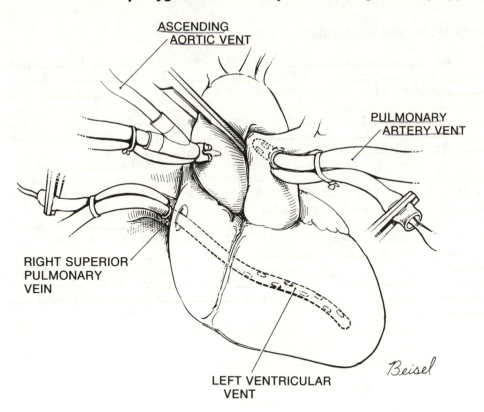

ASCENDING
AORTIC VENT

PULMONARY
ARTERY VENT

RIGHT SUPERIOR
PULMONARY
VEIN

Beisel

LEFT VENTRICULAR
VENT

MYOCARDIAL PRESERVATION

Safe myocardial preservation is achieved by the use of systemic hypothermia, topical myocardial cooling, and cold potassium cardioplegia solution. Topical myocardial cooling is achieved and maintained by the use of a myocardial cooling pad, intermittent bathing of the heart with 4°C saline solution, and by ensuring that the cardioplegia solution is cold (4°C). The cardioplegia solution consists of a balanced electrolyte solution (Plasmalyte 148* [1,000 ml]), potassium bicarbonate (20 mg), heparin (2,500 units), and calcium chloride (100 mg).

Fig 15–5.—The cardioplegia delivery system consists of a reservoir having an integral cooling coil, a roller pump, and appropriate valved tubing to permit recirculation and delivery. The solution is cooled to 4°C and is delivered to the proximal aortic root after aortic cross-clamping. In patients with aortic regurgitation, it is introduced directly into the coronary ostia. The initial cardioplegia dose is usually 10 ml/kg, and subsequent doses are given every 15–25 minutes in an amount of 3–4 ml/kg. The rate of infusion is governed by either the aortic root or coronary artery pressure, as measured from the delivery cannula; the mean infusion pressure should not exceed 90 mm Hg. The goals of cardioplegia infusion are to maintain zero electrical activity of the ventricles and maintain a myocardial septal temperature below 12°C.

---

* Baxter-Travenol Laboratories.

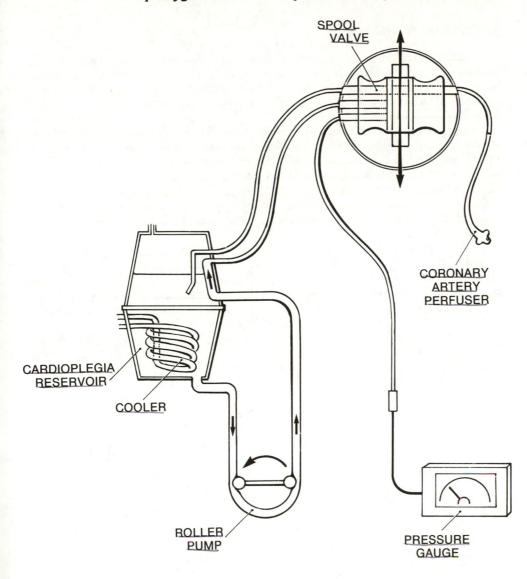

SPOOL
VALVE

CORONARY
ARTERY
PERFUSER

CARDIOPLEGIA
RESERVOIR

COOLER

ROLLER
PUMP

PRESSURE
GAUGE

MONITORING TECHNIQUES

Safe cardiac surgery is dependent on the use of modern monitoring of cardio-vascular parameters. Those parameters monitored include ECG, direct intra-arterial blood pressure, pulmonary arterial capillary wedge pressure, pulmonary artery pressure, central venous or right atrial pressure, and cardiac output and urine output.

Intra-arterial pressure is most often monitored through a no. 18 plastic catheter inserted percutaneously into one radial artery, although the brachial artery in the antecubital fossa can be employed. When upper extremity sites are not available, or when use of the intra-aortic balloon is contemplated, we insert a plastic catheter percutaneously into the common femoral artery. This site provides both an accurate measurement of pressure not subject to stenosis by spasm, as is the radial artery, and vascular access for subsequent percutaneous intra-aortic balloon insertion should this be required.

We have found the Swan–Ganz flow-directed pulmonary artery catheter to be most helpful in adults undergoing open heart operations. This catheter is inserted percutaneously through the right internal jugular vein and "floated" into the distal pulmonary artery. Use of this catheter provides continuous accurate monitoring of the pulmonary artery systolic and diastolic pressures and central venous pressure. Intermittent balloon inflation with a properly positioned Swan–Ganz catheter provides an accurate measurement of the pulmonary capillary wedge pressure, generally a good indication of the left atrial pressure. Furthermore, the Swan–Ganz thermodilution catheter allows intermittent, reasonably accurate determination of cardiac output and cardiac output index prior to initiation of cardiopulmonary bypass and as required following bypass.

In critically ill patients and in infants and children, a catheter is inserted directly into the left atrium to ensure the availability of continuous, accurate left atrial pressure measurements during separation of the patient from cardiopulmonary bypass and throughout the postoperative period. The small-diameter vinyl catheter is inserted in much the same way that a vent is inserted into the left atrium (and then ventricle) through the right superior pulmonary vein. Indeed, in operations where such a vent is employed, the monitoring catheter can be inserted through the same pursestring suture.

Fig 15–6, A.—The right atrium is retracted to the left side by an assistant, putting the right pulmonary vein on "stretch."

B.—A pursestring suture of 4–0 Prolene is placed at the junction of the vein and the left atrium. The 17-gauge epidural needle with a long vinyl catheter contained within it is inserted through the pursestring and into the left atrium. The catheter is advanced approximately 5 cm into the left atrium; the needle is carefully withdrawn, leaving the catheter in place. The pursestring suture is tied.

C.—A separate but longer needle is then passed from the skin into the pericardial space. The free end of the vinyl catheter is passed through this needle onto the skin.

D.—The proper catheter length is ascertained, and the catheter is cut and attached to a stopcock. Blood is aspirated to ascertain proper placement of the catheter. The stopcock is sutured to the skin. An additional suture used to secure the catheter to the pericardium is helpful in preventing inadvertent removal during pacing wire and chest tube insertion.

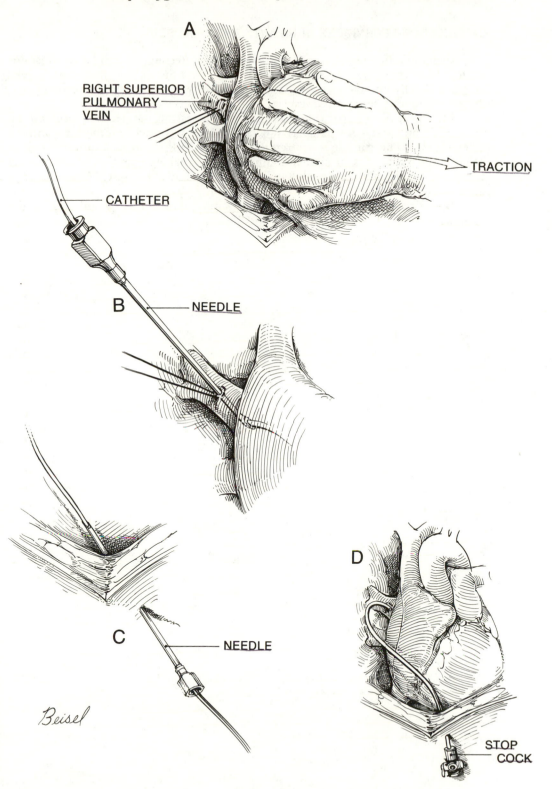

A

RIGHT SUPERIOR PULMONARY VEIN

TRACTION

CATHETER

B

NEEDLE

C

NEEDLE

D

STOP COCK

Beisel

CANNULATION TECHNIQUES IN INFANTS AND CHILDREN

Older children are managed with cannulation techniques similar to those for adults, using two caval cannulas introduced through the right atrium. The arterial inflow is usually into the ascending aorta. However, in smaller children and infants, these techniques require modification.

Fig 15–7, A.—Aortic cannulation. Two pursestring sutures are placed on the distal ascending aorta. A small partial occlusion clamp is placed on the aorta and the latter incised. The cut edges are retracted with 5–0 Prolene stay sutures. This is helpful, since the aorta in infants is quite pliable, making insertion of the arterial cannula more difficult than in adults. The arterial cannula* is inserted as the clamp is removed.

B.—The keepers on the pursestring sutures are tightened and tied to the cannula.

---

* High Flow Aortic Arch Cannula: Sarns, Inc.

A

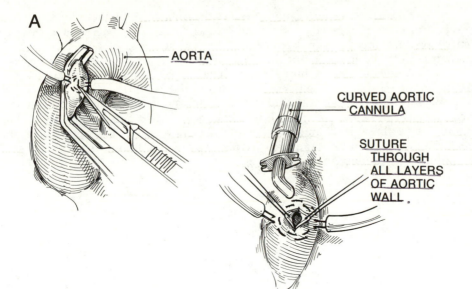

AORTA

CURVED AORTIC CANNULA

SUTURE THROUGH ALL LAYERS OF AORTIC WALL .

B

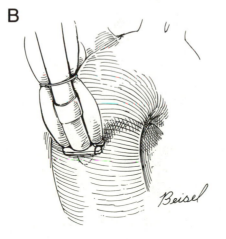

Beisel

C.—To keep the venous cannulas out of the right atrium (especially important in repair of cases of transposition of the great arteries), the superior and inferior venae cavae are directly cannulated. A 4–0 Prolene suture is placed as a "square" pursestring into the adventitia of the vena cava.

D.—A stab wound is made and a metal-tipped cannula* is inserted. The keeper on the pursestring is tightened and tied to the cannula.

E.—The left ventricle is vented with a cannula† placed into the left atrium near the right superior pulmonary vein. It is held in place with a pursestring suture. The cannula passes through the mitral valve into the left ventricle. Postoperatively, the left atrial pressure can be monitored by placing pressure tubing through the stab wound used for venting the left ventricle.

---

* Pacifico Caval Cannula: DLP Inc.
† Left Ventricular Vent Cannula: DLP Inc.

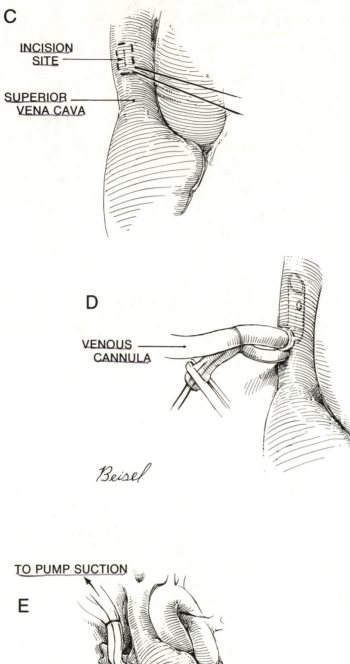

C

INCISION
SITE

SUPERIOR
VENA CAVA

D

VENOUS
CANNULA

Beisel

TO PUMP SUCTION

E

LEFT
VENTRICULAR
VENT

Beisel

CHAPTER **16**

Pacemakers

C ARDIAC pacing is a dependable mode of therapy for a variety of cardiac rhythm disturbances, and the transvenous route of electrode placement is favored by most physicians. The reliability of transvenous leads is established, and remarkable advances in the capabilities of pulse generators continue to add to the therapeutic applications. Sophisticated systems that have pacing and sensing capacities in both the atrium and ventricle require the placement of two leads and are being used with increasing frequency. Multiprogrammability is the standard, even for single-lead pacing systems. Discussion of the different types and features of pulse generators and the indications for pacing are beyond the scope of this chapter.

In the typical adult patient, permanent transvenous pacing is instituted with the aid of local anesthesia and fluoroscopy. In the past the cephalic vein in the deltopectoral groove was chosen as the point of entry, but the subclavian vein is used now and has several advantages.

The placement of epicardial electrodes, usually during cardiac operations, in patients at risk of developing a high-grade heart block is required less frequently. When required, special atrial hook and ventricular screw electrodes are placed easily. Elective epicardial lead placement is rarely necessary. An abbreviated left anterior thoracotomy provides optimal access to the ventricle if it is needed. In most such cases, two leads are placed so that a second major operation can be avoided if problems develop with the primary lead.

In patients without an existing pulse generator, it is entirely safe to use electrocautery during the operation until the time the generator is brought onto the field and connected. Then, or if the patient has an existing pacemaker, the use of electrocautery in the vicinity of the unit is dangerous. Under certain circumstances, excessive currents, which can be picked up by the generator, have been transmitted down the electrode. Arrhythmias and actual myocardial burns have resulted.

Fig 16–1, A.—After infiltrating the skin with 1% lidocaine, a transverse incision is made where the pocket is to be developed. This should be in an area that is comfortable for the patient, taking care that the position chosen is neither too lateral nor too high. A unit placed too close to the axilla is painful; it interferes with arm motion and may lead to skin breakdown and infection. Movement near a generator placed too close to the clavicle results in pain, particularly when the arm is elevated or when the patient is supine. These problems are more frequent in obese persons, and preoperative marking ensures optimal placement. A pocket, slightly larger than the pulse generator, is developed just above the level of the pectoralis fascia, and meticulous hemostasis is achieved. The pocket is loosely packed with a gauze sponge soaked in antibiotic solution.

B.—With the patient in the Trendelenburg position and the head turned to the opposite side, the subclavian vein is punctured through the upper margin of the wound and a J-tipped guidewire is introduced.

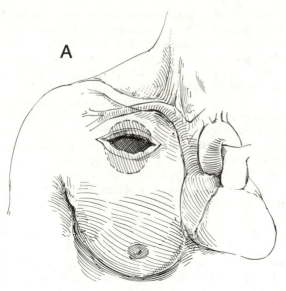

A

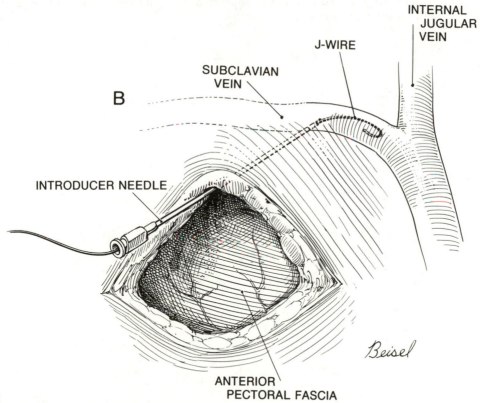

B

INTERNAL
JUGULAR
VEIN

J-WIRE

SUBCLAVIAN
VEIN

INTRODUCER NEEDLE

Beisel

ANTERIOR
PECTORAL FASCIA

C.—A dilator-sheath assembly has been advanced over the guide wire. The illustration shows the introduction of one transvenous lead through the sheath after removal of the wire and dilator. The sheath can then be withdrawn and discarded as pressure is briefly applied around the cannulation site. Stylets are then used to manipulate the tips of the pacing leads. Initially, it is advisable to advance the ventricular lead across the tricuspid and pulmonary valves to avoid placement in the coronary sinus. If a curved stylet is used for this preliminary maneuver, it is exchanged for a straight stylet as the tip of the electrode is withdrawn into the body of the right ventricle and then advanced to a suitable apical position as determined by electrical threshold testing. In dual-chamber applications, the atrial lead can be introduced either through the same introducer (if large enough) or through a second small introducer. A permanently formed J-shaped electrode is positioned with the aid of a straight internal stylet, which is withdrawn to permit engagement within the trabeculae of the right atrial appendage. Atrial threshold and retrograde conduction determinations are then made.

D.—In the finished implantation the ventricular lead is in a good apical position, and the atrial lead is placed solidly in the appendage. The redundant portion of the lead has been withdrawn and the permanent leads firmly anchored to the pectoralis fascia at their point of entry. After checking the pulse generator, the excess length of electrode is coiled behind the implanted unit, and the incision is closed in layers with absorbable suture.

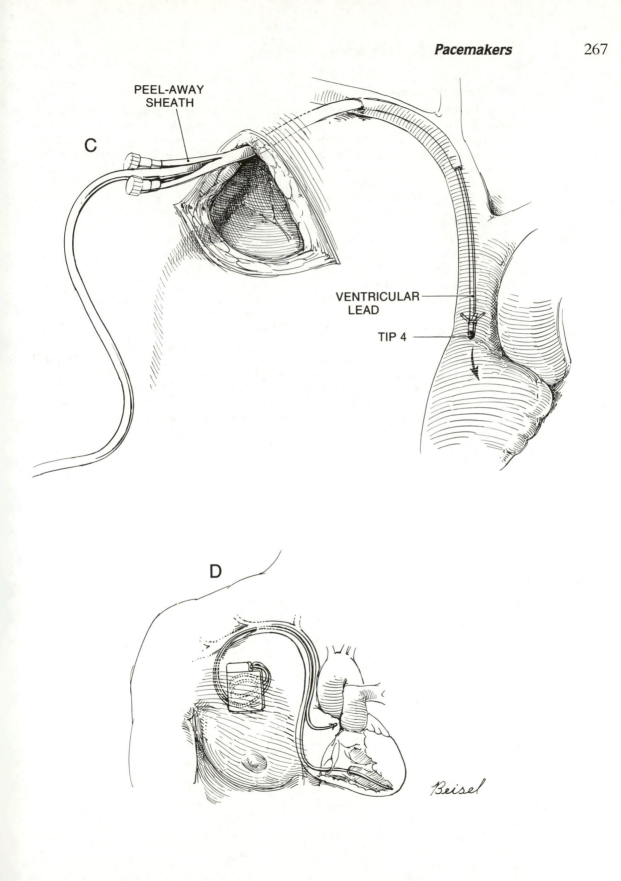

C

PEEL-AWAY
SHEATH

VENTRICULAR
LEAD

TIP 4

D

Beisel

Postoperative Care

In either the intensive care or ambulatory ward setting, continuous ECG monitoring is used to evaluate the function of the new implants during the first few postoperative days. Antibiotic therapy, started before operation, is continued for five days. Those patients with dual-chamber generators are best evaluated by 24-hour ECG monitoring in the perioperative period and at intervals after operation. The function of most ventricular pacemakers can be followed with periodic rhythm strips obtained in the clinic or with transtelephonic monitors.

Complications

The two major complications of this method of inserting a transvenous pacemaker are pneumothorax and ventricular perforation. Malpositioned or unstable leads can be avoided by attention to the details of insertion and placement. An occasional patient will have ventricular irritability and require treatment of arrhythmias. With familiarity, the technique of subclavian vein catheterization carries an extremely low incidence of pneumothorax. Perforation of the right ventricle is best avoided by gentle lead manipulation and the use of the most flexible stylets available. As the lead is positioned at the apex of the ventricle, continuous fluoroscopic monitoring allows the operator to assess the amount of stress on the lead. Modern tined and active fixation leads require less "wedging" than the older (and stiffer) ball or cylindrical tipped leads. Tactile feedback cues, fluoroscopic appearance, characteristic threshold values, and, occasionally, diaphragmatic pacing can be diagnostic of perforation, in which case the lead should be withdrawn and repositioned. Careful observation is all that is required in most instances, but clinical or roentgenographic signs of tamponade will require urgent operative drainage.

CHAPTER 17

Mechanical Circulatory Assistance

INSERTION OF THE INTRA-AORTIC BALLOON

A SMALL but definite percentage of patients cannot be weaned from cardiopulmonary bypass after an open heart operation, even with the use of inotropic and vasodilator drugs. Introduction of the intra-aortic balloon provides a safe technique to increase the cardiac output index by as much as $0.5 \ L/min/m^2$ and may permit separation of the patient from cardiopulmonary bypass.

Fig 17–1, A.—Insertion of a plastic catheter into one femoral artery prior to initiation of cardiopulmonary bypass provides an arterial pressure monitoring site as well as ready access to the femoral artery in case an intra-aortic balloon is required at the completion of the cardiac operation.

B.—For balloon insertion, a flexible guide wire is passed into the artery through the catheter; the plastic catheter is then removed. The overlying tissue and anterior artery wall entrance site are dilated to a no. 12 F diameter using graduated dilators. The balloon sheath fits snugly over the larger dilator. After the balloon sheath has been inserted, the dilator is removed.

C.—The carefully furled balloon is inserted through the sheath and is advanced gradually. Excessive resistance to advancement generally indicates atherosclerosive arterial occlusive disease and is a contraindication to balloon advancement. If this occurs, the balloon must be withdrawn. Depending on the location of the blockage, a passage may be attempted through the opposite groin or, if infeasible, the balloon may be inserted directly into the transverse aortic arch and positioned appropriately.

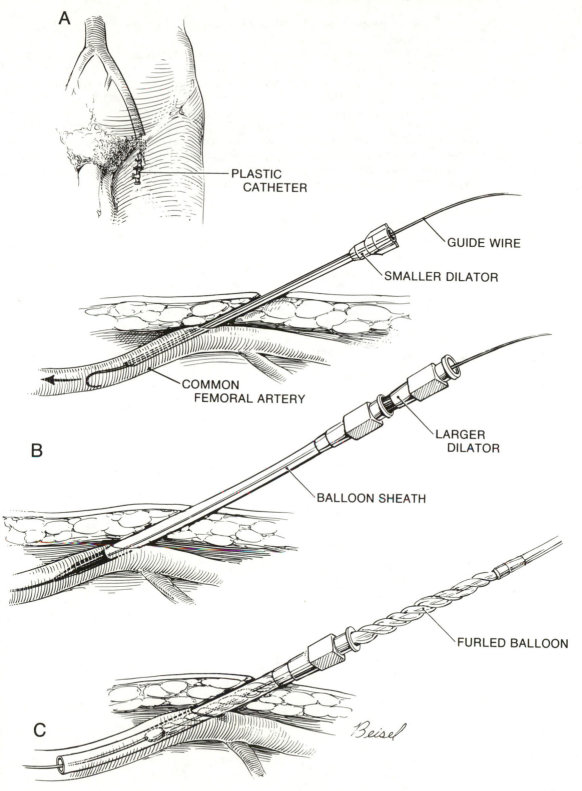

A

PLASTIC CATHETER

GUIDE WIRE

SMALLER DILATOR

COMMON FEMORAL ARTERY

LARGER DILATOR

B

BALLOON SHEATH

FURLED BALLOON

Beisel

C

D.—When properly positioned, the balloon tip rests just below the left subclavian artery orifice.

Following percutaneous balloon insertion and activation, the surgeon must assess the arterial circulation to the lower extremity. Any evidence of insufficient arterial circulation (cyanosis, pain) must be considered a risk to the viability of the limb and should be treated by balloon removal, by removal with reinsertion at another site, or by the appropriate arterial reconstructive operation.

E.—For optimal effectiveness, the balloon must be deflated during cardiac systole and inflated during diastole. This sequence lowers the left ventricular systolic pressure (unloading the left ventricle) while increasing the diastolic pressure (increasing coronary blood flow). The proper timing sequence can be based on either the R wave of the ECG or the leading edge of the patient's arterial pressure pulse contour.

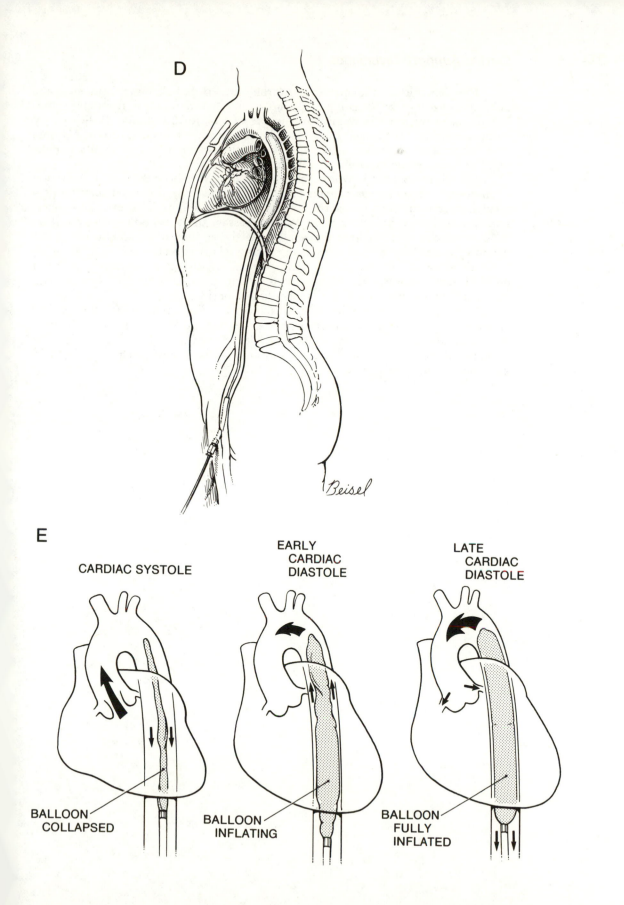

D

E

CARDIAC SYSTOLE

EARLY
CARDIAC
DIASTOLE

LATE
CARDIAC
DIASTOLE

BALLOON
COLLAPSED

BALLOON
INFLATING

BALLOON
FULLY
INFLATED

F.—When it is no longer required, the intra–aortic balloon is removed in the intensive care unit by deflating the balloon and withdrawing it from the groin. Manual pressure must be applied to the site of exit for 20 minutes, followed by sandbag pressure for the next six hours. The patient must remain in bed for 24 hours after removal of the balloon. Periodic observation of the lower extremity is indicated to detect evidence of inadequate arterial circulation.

G.—In the patient in whom the femoral artery has been exposed at operation or in whom percutaneous balloon passage is not feasible, insertion may be performed directly through an arteriotomy in the common femoral artery. This is best accomplished in the operating room. Prior to passage of the balloon, an 8-cm section of 10-mm woven Dacron graft is carefully passed over the balloon and the stem. The balloon plus the length of stem needed to permit its insertion to the level of the angle of Louis is marked on the balloon stem. Again, significant resistance encountered during passage indicates that atherosclerotic vascular disease is present. Removal and reinsertion at an alternative location should be considered.

When circulatory stability has been achieved, balloon removal is accomplished in the operating room. At that time, the groin wound is opened, the balloon is removed, and the artery is repaired. Complete removal of the prosthetic graft is desirable. If the femoral artery is small, a saphenous vein onlay patch may be helpful in reconstructing the artery.

F

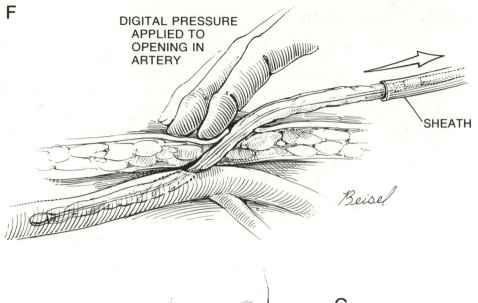

DIGITAL PRESSURE
APPLIED TO
OPENING IN
ARTERY

SHEATH

Beisel

G

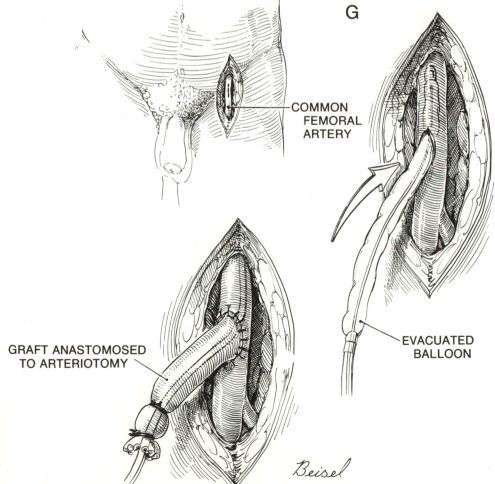

COMMON
FEMORAL
ARTERY

GRAFT ANASTOMOSED
TO ARTERIOTOMY

EVACUATED
BALLOON

Beisel

VENTRICULAR ASSIST PUMP

Patients who cannot be separated from cardiopulmonary bypass either with inotropic and vasodilator drug therapy or with use of the intra-aortic balloon can be helped with a left atrial-to-aortic assist system. In our experience, about 50% of the patients who require such a device will have enough return of cardiac function after four to eight days of ventricular bypass for the assist pump to be removed.

Prior to use of the ventricular assist device, the surgeon must ascertain that all mechanical problems have been satisfactorily repaired and that major coronary artery stenoses have been bypassed. Cardiopulmonary bypass is required for the safe insertion of the left ventricular assist pump.

Fig 17–2, A.—Before inserting the left ventricular assist device, the surgeon must palpate the atrial septum to ensure that the foramen ovale is closed. A patent foramen ovale will permit right-to-left atrial shunting and significant arterial blood desaturation. Closure requires superior and inferior vena caval cannulation, placement of superior and inferior vena caval "tapes," and a right atriotomy. In preparation for placement of the arterial and atrial cannulas, tunnels are developed from the pericardial space to the skin, just below the left costal margin.

A

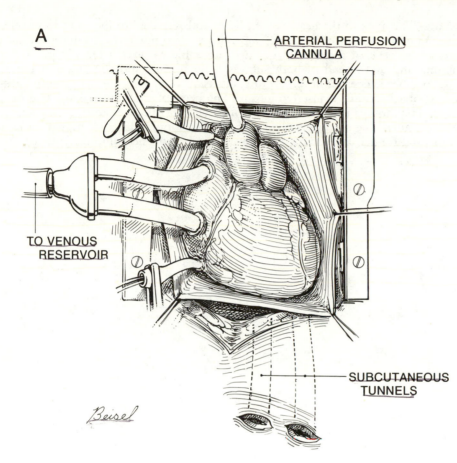

ARTERIAL PERFUSION
CANNULA

TO VENOUS
RESERVOIR

SUBCUTANEOUS
TUNNELS

Beisel

B.—The apex of the heart is then lifted and retracted to the right to provide maximum exposure of the left atrial appendage. Two pursestring sutures are then placed at the neck of the appendage. It is advisable to place a felt pledget at the beginning and at the end of both sutures. The sutures are left long and passed through rubber keepers. The left atrium is incised, and an appropriate-length lighthouse tip atrial cannula is inserted into it. The keepers are tightened and tied over buttons. The cannula is further secured with a tape ligature tied around each keeper and the cannula. The cannula is filled with saline solution, clamped, passed through the subcostal tunnel, and attached to the suction line of the pump oxygenator.

B

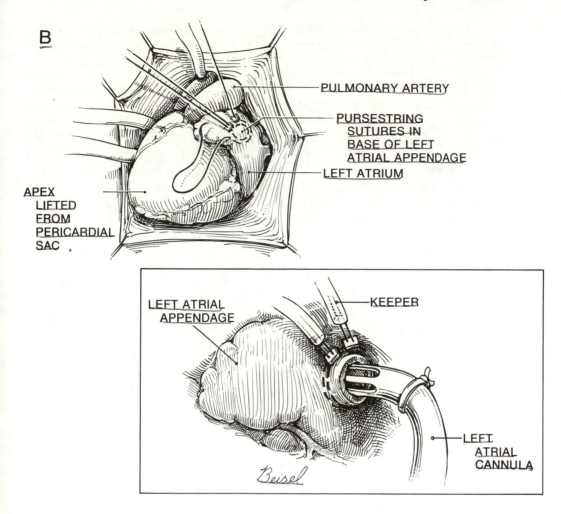

PULMONARY ARTERY

PURSESTRING SUTURES IN BASE OF LEFT ATRIAL APPENDAGE

LEFT ATRIUM

APEX LIFTED FROM PERICARDIAL SAC.

LEFT ATRIAL APPENDAGE

KEEPER

LEFT ATRIAL CANNULA

Beisel

C.—The Dacron graft portion of the composite arterial cannula is then anastomosed to the side of the ascending aorta. The cannula is filled with saline solution, clamped, and passed through the medial subcostal tunnel.

D.—The pump is attached and carefully de-aired. Pumping is initiated and cardiopulmonary bypass is discontinued slowly. After hemostasis is achieved, the chest is closed in a routine fashion.

When the assist pump support is no longer required, the patient is returned to the operating room and the sternotomy is reopened. Pumping is discontinued and the cannulas are clamped. The atrial cannula is withdrawn from the left atrium, and the previously placed pursestring sutures are tied. The arterial cannula graft is clamped near the aortic anastomosis. The graft is divided and the stump is oversewn. The pump and attached cannulas are then removed from the operative field. The pericardial end of the cannula tunnel sites are oversewn, chest tubes are inserted, and the chest is closed in the standard fashion.

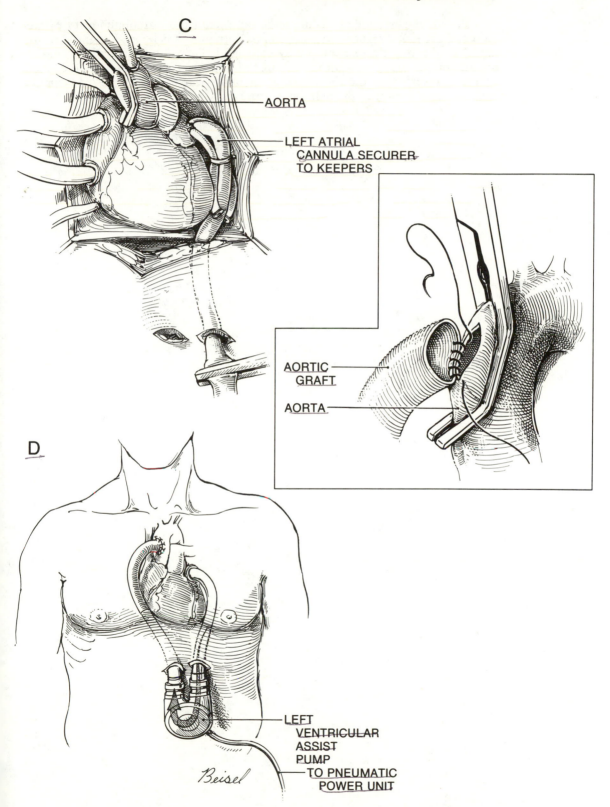

C

AORTA

LEFT ATRIAL
CANNULA SECURER
TO KEEPERS

AORTIC
GRAFT

AORTA

D

Beisel

LEFT
VENTRICULAR
ASSIST
PUMP
TO PNEUMATIC
POWER UNIT

222222222222222

E.—In certain patients, failure to be separated from cardiopulmonary bypass is a manifestation of right ventricular failure. Intra-aortic balloon assistance may be helpful in improving cardiac output by reducing left atrial pressure and thus reducing pulmonary artery pressure and by augmenting coronary artery flow. If balloon support is insufficient, the ventricular assist pump can also be employed to pump from the right atrium to the pulmonary artery.

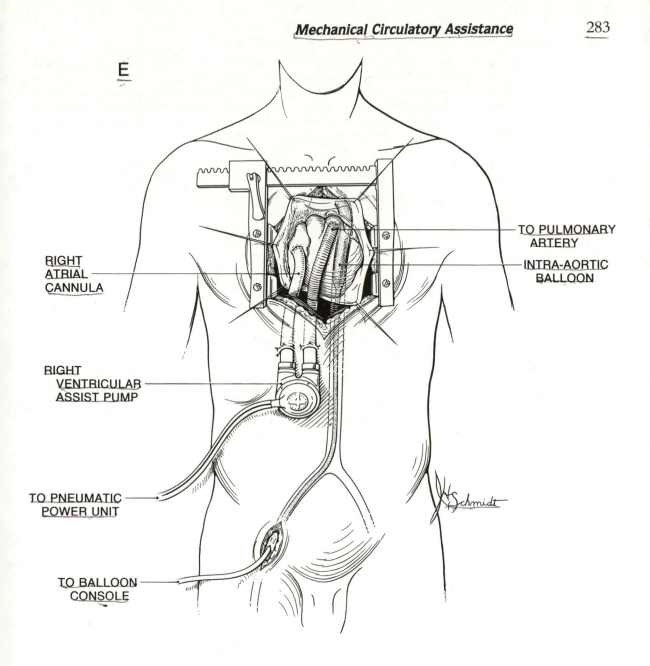

E

TO PULMONARY
ARTERY

INTRA-AORTIC
BALLOON

RIGHT
ATRIAL
CANNULA

RIGHT
VENTRICULAR
ASSIST PUMP

TO PNEUMATIC
POWER UNIT

TO BALLOON
CONSOLE

Part III

Congenital Heart Disease

CHAPTER **18**

Congenital Heart Disease

PATENT DUCTUS ARTERIOSUS

A PATENT ductus discovered after the newborn period should be closed, with few exceptions, as soon as practicable after the diagnosis is made. In infants we usually wait until they are 1 year old, except when there is congestive heart failure, in which case ductal ligation is carried out promptly.

Division of a Patent Ductus Arteriosus

Fig 18–1, A.—The patient is placed in the right lateral decubitus position, and the chest is opened through the fourth intercostal space. The apex of the lung is retracted downward and forward. The mediastinal pleura is opened over the aortic isthmus, and the incision is continued up along the left subclavian artery. The highest intercostal vein must be divided.

B.—Dissection is then carried out over the anterior surface of the aorta to the patent ductus, then across the ductus toward the pulmonary artery. In this fashion, the patent ductus will be exposed without injury to the recurrent laryngeal nerve. As the pulmonary artery adjacent to the ductus is approached, the vagus nerve comes into view. Not infrequently, this nerve can be seen clearly through the pleura. The recurrent laryngeal nerve leaves the vagus nerve just below the ductus and curves posteriorly around the ductus and aorta.

The pericardial sac usually extends over the anterior surface of the patent ductus. This pericardial extension should be mobilized and reflected medially.

C.—Dissection of the posterior wall of the ductus is the most critical part of the operation and should be attempted only after preparation has been made to occlude the aorta in the event of hemorrhage. Tapes are placed around the aorta, both above and below the ductus arteriosus, and around the left subclavian artery. Exposure of the posterior wall of the ductus may be obtained by retracting the aorta upward and anteriorly and dissecting out the isthmus as well as the posterior wall. Tissue behind the ductus may be relatively dense. The recurrent laryngeal nerve is not apt to be injured if it is adequately visualized and maintained on the pulmonary artery side.

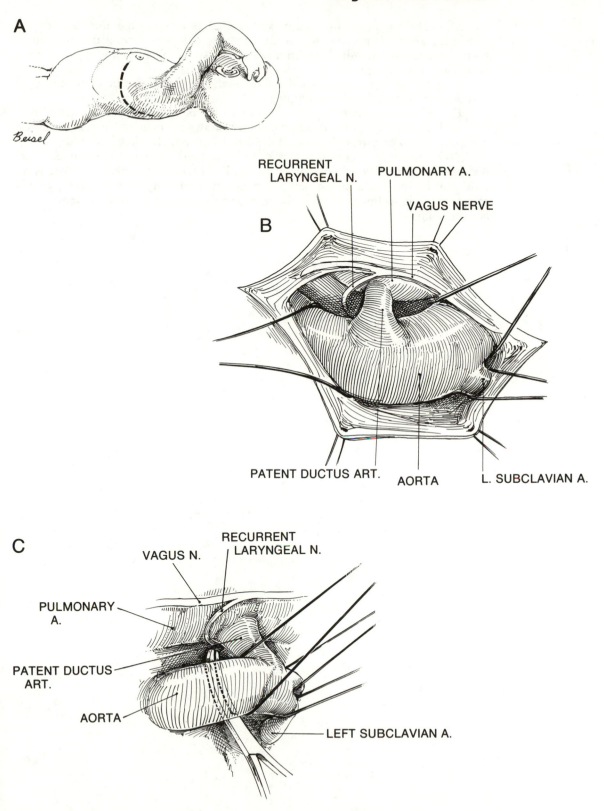

A

Beisel

B

RECURRENT
LARYNGEAL N. PULMONARY A.

VAGUS NERVE

PATENT DUCTUS ART. AORTA L. SUBCLAVIAN A.

C

VAGUS N. RECURRENT
LARYNGEAL N.

PULMONARY
A.

PATENT DUCTUS
ART.

AORTA

LEFT SUBCLAVIAN A.

D.—The patent ductus clamps are applied as close to the aorta and to the pulmonary artery as possible so that an adequate cuff will be available for suture when the ductus is divided. Additional length can be obtained by applying four clamps and removing the middle two.

E.—The ductus is divided halfway through and partially sutured, as shown, as a precaution against the clamp slipping.

F.—A running mattress suture, followed by an over-and-over suture of 6–0 Prolene, is used to close each end of the ductus. Stay sutures at each end of the aortic suture line allow easy reapplication of the arterial clamp, should hemorrhage occur.

When suturing is completed, the pulmonary artery clamp is removed first, since this is a generally low-pressure area and hemorrhage is unlikely. If there is no significant bleeding, the aortic clamp is then removed. Any oozing is readily controlled by placing a finger between the aorta and the pulmonary artery to tamponade the suture line.

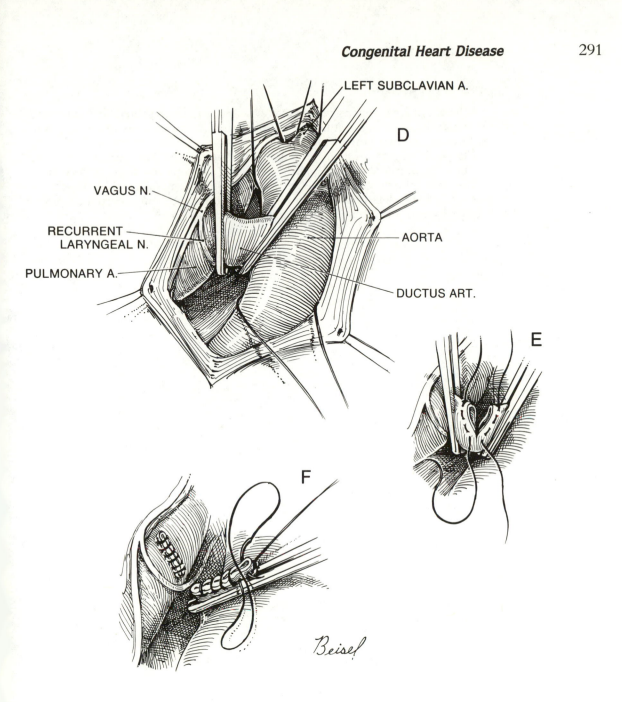

LEFT SUBCLAVIAN A.

D

VAGUS N.

RECURRENT
LARYNGEAL N.

AORTA

PULMONARY A.

DUCTUS ART.

E

F

Beisel

Ligation in the Newborn

Whereas many surgeons believe that every patent ductus should be divided and the ends sutured, we think that ligation alone is satisfactory in newborns as well as in infants during the first year of life.

Fig 18–2, A.—In the neonate, the ductus is often quite large and appears to be in continuity with the descending aorta, while the isthmus and arch are smaller.

B.—After the ductus is adequately exposed, a no. 1 nonabsorbable ligature is placed around the ductus and tied carefully. The ligature must be pulled down tightly enough to make certain that the lumen is occluded.

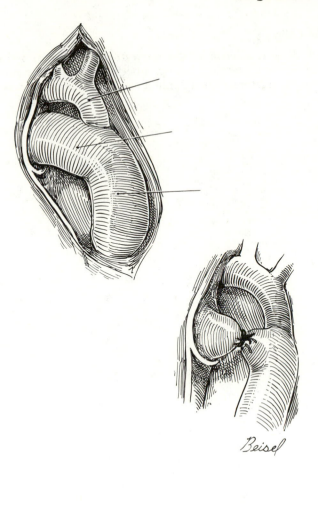

Beisel

Ligation in the Child

Fig 18–3, A.—In older infants, a pursestring ligature of 3–0 nonabsorbable suture is placed on the aortic side, taking superficial bites in the aortic wall.

B.—A second ligature is then applied to the pulmonary artery.

A

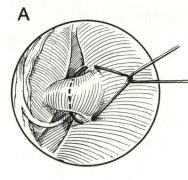

B

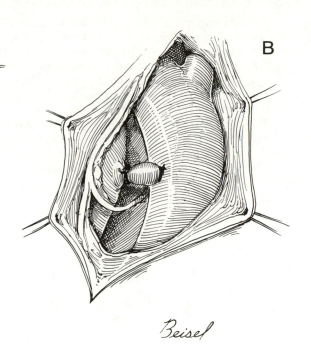

Beisel

Closure of Calcified Patent Ductus Arteriosus with a Gott Shunt

In older patients with a patent ductus arteriosus, there may be calcification of both the ductus and the aorta at the orifice of the ductus. This makes the usual operation more precarious. A Gott shunt is placed between the ascending aorta and either the descending aorta or the femoral artery.

Fig 18–4, A.—This is done by placing two pursestring sutures in the ascending aorta and inserting the shunt proximally. Distally, the shunt is inserted in a similar manner after all air from the shunt has been removed.

B.—The aorta is now clamped above and below the patent ductus arteriosus. A clamp is placed on the pulmonary artery side of the ductus, and the ductus is incised. The pulmonary artery side is oversewn as is the aortic side. The clamps are removed, and if there is no bleeding, the Gott shunt is removed and the pursestring sutures are tied.

A

B

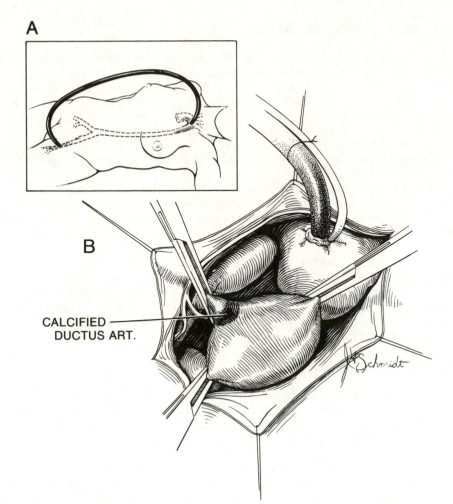

CALCIFIED
DUCTUS ART.

AORTOPULMONARY SEPTAL DEFECT

These uncommon defects may be clinically confused with a large patent ductus arteriosus because of the continuous murmur. Angiography of the aortic root is essential for the diagnosis. Type I defects are the most common and are characterized by a communication between the ascending aorta and the main pulmonary artery just distal to their valves. In type II defects, the communication is at the junction of the right and the main pulmonary arteries, where they are crossed by the ascending aorta. In type III defects, the right pulmonary artery arises from the ascending aorta and requires reanastomosis to the main pulmonary artery. Type I and type II defects are repaired through the aorta.

Fig 18–5, A.—Through a median sternotomy the heart is exposed. Cardiopulmonary bypass is instituted, with transatrial vena caval cannulation and return to the ascending aorta, as far distally as possible. The left ventricle is vented with a catheter placed through the right superior pulmonary vein. The aorta is cross-clamped.

B.—The aortic root is incised. The heart is stopped by injection of cold cardioplegia solution into the coronary arteries. The defect is exposed.

C.—An appropriate-sized Dacron patch is sutured into the defect, using continuous 4–0 Prolene sutures. The aorta is closed with 4–0 or 5–0 Prolene sutures. After proper de-airing of the aortic root and heart, the aortic clamp is removed and cardiopulmonary bypass discontinued.

COARCTATION OF THE AORTA

The correction of coarctation of the aorta is usually an elective procedure and can be carried out at almost any age. However, operation performed at an early age is far more likely to prevent long-term hypertension than when operation is carried out later. We usually wait until a child is 3 years old, when maximum growth of the aorta has taken place. Furthermore, at this age, the vessels are still pliable, and neither sclerotic changes nor sequelae to arterial hypertension have yet occurred. Every possible maneuver should be used to obtain a satisfactory anastomosis without a graft, especially in childhood. A graft is frequently required in adults, whose vessels have lost much of their elasticity.

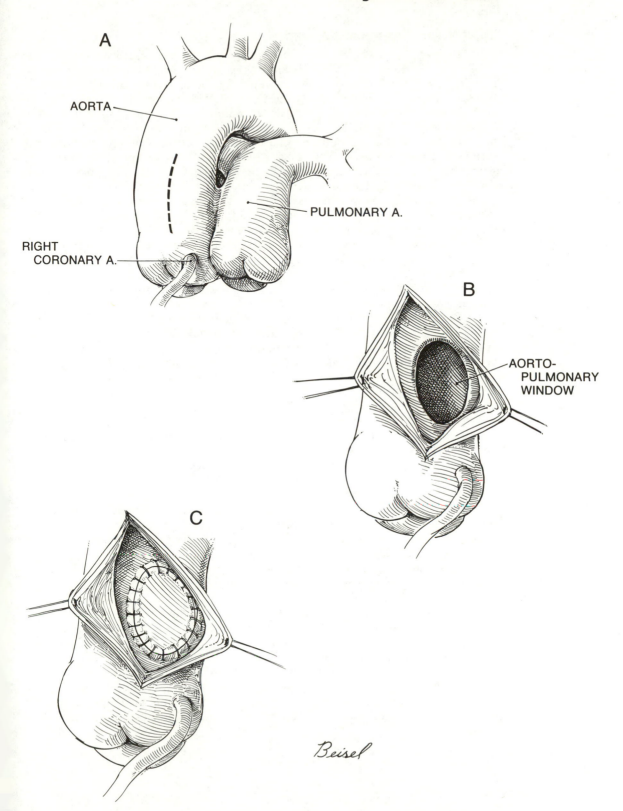

A

AORTA

PULMONARY A.

RIGHT
CORONARY A.

B

AORTO-
PULMONARY
WINDOW

C

Beisel

Resection with End-to-End Anastomosis

Fig 18–6, A.—The chest is entered through the left fourth interspace. The collateral circulation may have made the arteries in the muscles and intercostal space quite large, and careful hemostasis is essential. The lung is retracted anteriorly, and the area of coarctation is exposed by opening widely the mediastinal pleura over the aortic isthmus. Dissection of the tissue surrounding the aorta and the intercostal vessels must be done with the greatest care. Gentle, blunt dissection is preferable, for the most part, to sharp dissection. The highest intercostal vein crosses the aortic isthmus and must be divided in order to expose the coarctation. The intercostal arteries are often extremely thin-walled, and hemorrhage from them may be most troublesome. Bronchial arteries may originate from the posterior wall of the aorta just above or just below the constriction or from the posterior surface of the subclavian artery. A patent ductus arteriosus is not infrequently present and is usually near the point of maximum constriction (juxtaductal coarctation). It is divided and sutured as previously described. As the dissection proceeds, heavy silk ligatures are passed around the subclavian artery and the aorta to aid in controlling possible hemorrhage. A longer segment of the aorta than illustrated should be exposed when a longer segment is to be excised. The freeing of the aorta, almost to the diaphragm, will allow for its considerable upward displacement.

The length of aorta to be resected above and below the coarctation deserves the most careful consideration. When the aortic constriction is abrupt and there is a large lumen above and below it, reconstruction is simple. More often, however, above the constriction the aorta is small and below the constriction is quite large, requiring excision of a longer segment to achieve comparable lumina. Furthermore, the feasibility of an end-to-end anastomosis depends on the mobility and elasticity of both the aorta and the intercostal vessels. When excessive tension cannot be overcome by extensive freeing of the aorta, insertion of a graft may be necessary. In children it is usually possible to avoid using a graft by doing some type of plastic procedure instead, such as a subclavian flap procedure. If the upper end is narrow and cone-shaped, the lumen may be enlarged by incising the vessel longitudinally and inserting a diamond-shaped plastic prosthesis. This will allow growth of the remaining circumference of the vessel.

B.—When the dissection is complete, arterial clamps are applied above and below the constriction. It is important to obtain a large anastomosis, and several intercostal arteries may be occluded with Potts' ties, as shown. Rarely, an intercostal artery must be divided.

C and D.—A continuous everting mattress suture is illustrated. After the posterior suture is inserted and drawn taut, it is tied to an anchoring suture at each end.

E.—The anterior wall is completed with interrupted simple sutures. The lower clamp is removed first; then the upper clamp is removed slowly. By leaving the upper clamp on the aorta partially occluded, the aortic pulse is dampened, and less bleeding from the suture line is likely. The clamps are reapplied if additional sutures are required to control bleeding. Even when a large anastomosis is made, the lower part of the aorta is somewhat wider than the upper portion because of post-stenotic dilatation. The pleura is closed with a continuous synthetic absorbable suture. Utmost care should be taken to ensure hemostasis before the wound is closed.

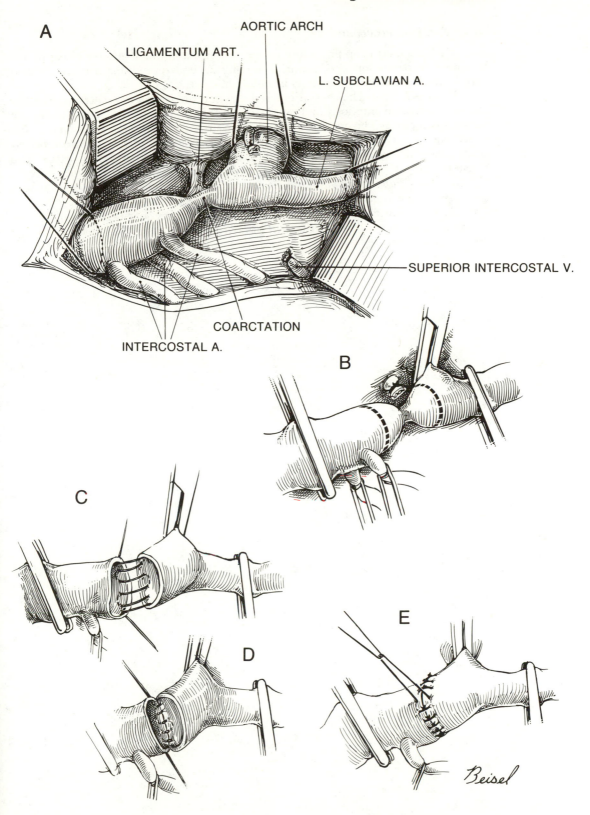

A

LIGAMENTUM ART.

AORTIC ARCH

L. SUBCLAVIAN A.

SUPERIOR INTERCOSTAL V.

COARCTATION

INTERCOSTAL A.

B

C

D

E

Beisel

Subclavian Flap Procedure

The subclavian flap procedure is primarily used in infants under 1 year of age in whom recoarctation is common following an end-to-end anastomosis. It also may be used for long coarctations in older children.

Fig 18–7, A.—The chest is entered through the fourth intercostal space. The lungs are retracted anteriorly and inferiorly, and the pleura over the aorta and aortic isthmus is incised. The aorta above and below the patent ductus arteriosus is dissected out, as is the subclavian artery. Heavy silk ligatures for retraction are placed around the transverse arch, the descending aorta, and the left subclavian artery. The patent ductus arteriosus is ligated with a heavy silk ligature. The subclavian artery is ligated at the origin of the vertebral artery, which is also ligated to prevent a subsequent steal syndrome.

B.—The aorta is incised distal to the area of narrowing. Staying laterally, the incision is carried up through the area of coarctation into the isthmus and the left subclavian artery.

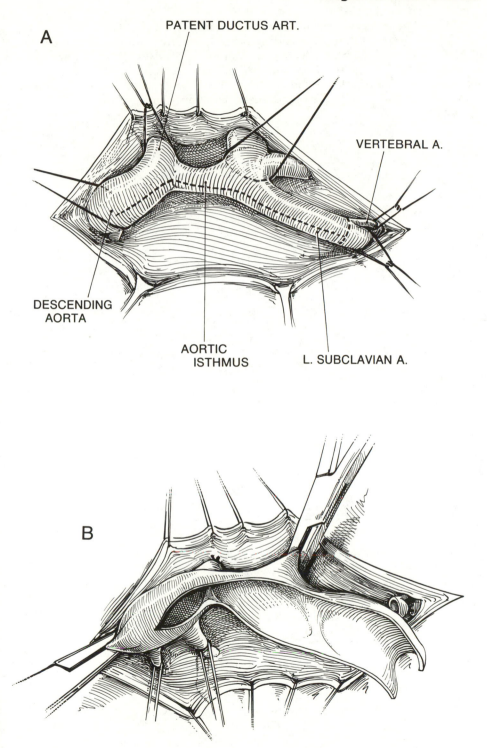

A

PATENT DUCTUS ART.

VERTEBRAL A.

DESCENDING
AORTA

AORTIC
ISTHMUS

L. SUBCLAVIAN A.

B

C.—The aorta is opened, and the coarctation shelf is excised.

D.—The tip of the subclavian flap is brought down into the aorta and sutured in place with 5–0 synthetic absorbable running sutures (PDS Suture; Ethicon). If nonabsorbable sutures are used, they should be interrupted. After hemostasis is achieved, the pleura is closed with a continuous 5–0 synthetic absorbable suture. A chest tube is placed for drainage, and the chest incision is closed in the routine manner.

C

D

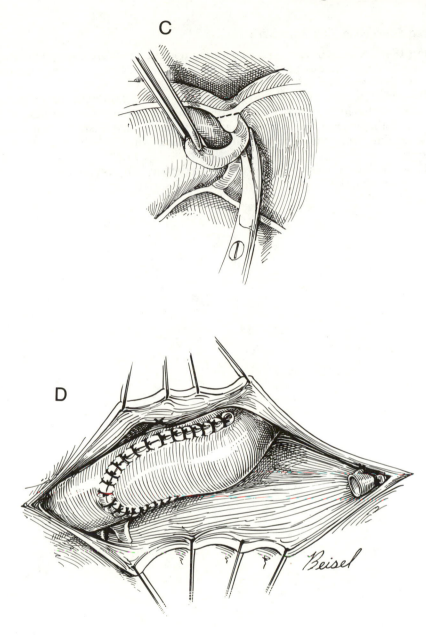

Beisel

Reversed Subclavian Flap Procedure

Fig 18–8, A.—In infants with a coarctation in the aortic arch, the narrowing is often between the left carotid artery and left subclavian artery. Here, a reversed subclavian flap can be of help.

B.—After ligation of the patent ductus arteriosus (not shown), the appropriate arteries are occluded with vascular clamps. The subclavian artery is ligated and transected at the origin of the vertebral artery, which is also ligated. An incision is made, extending from the aortic arch along the narrowing and into the left subclavian artery.

C.—The subclavian flap is then sewn into the incision, using either interrupted or running sutures, the latter being preferably of absorbable synthetic material (PDS Suture; Ethicon).

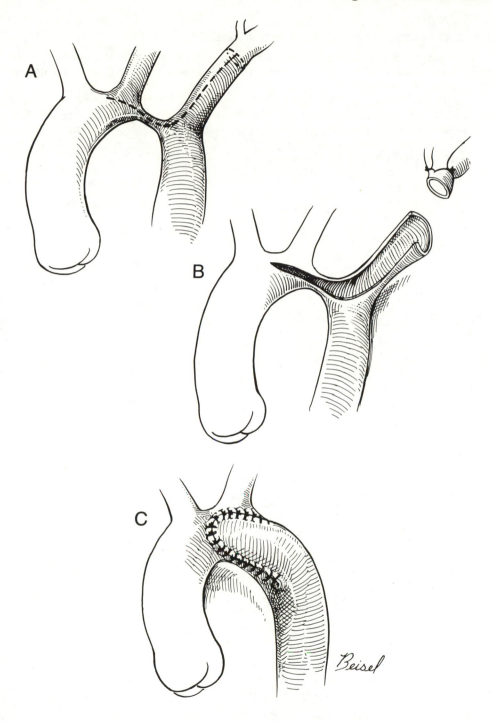

Repair of Coarctation of the Aorta with a Patch Graft

A patch graft of woven Dacron is used in patients with either sclerotic vessels or long coarctations. This kind of graft avoids excessive tension on the suture line of an end-to-end anastomosis.

Fig 18–9, A.—The chest is entered through the fourth intercostal space, and the area of coarctation including the transverse arch, the distal aorta, and the left subclavian artery, is dissected out as previously described. After placement of the vascular clamps, the aorta is incised anteriorly so that the incision extends from the distal aortic arch into the descending aorta.

B.—The coarctation shelf is excised.

A

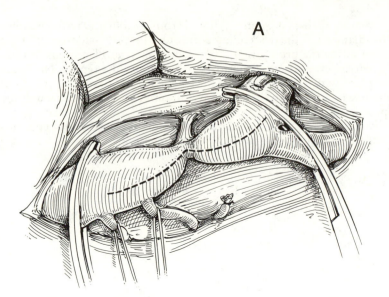

B

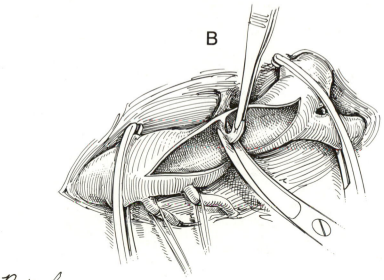

Beisel

C.—A large diamond-shaped patch is tailored from a tubular Dacron prosthesis having the same diameter as the descending aorta. Usually, the widest part of the patch will be three fourths the prosthetic graft's circumference. Placement of traction sutures at the narrowest portion of the aorta will simplify the repair. The patch is then sewn into place with continuous 4–0 Prolene sutures. Release of the distal clamp prior to the release of the proximal clamp will prevent bleeding through the woven Dacron prosthesis.

D.—After hemostasis is carefully obtained, the pleura is closed with a continuous absorbable suture, the chest is drained, and the chest incision is closed in a routine manner.

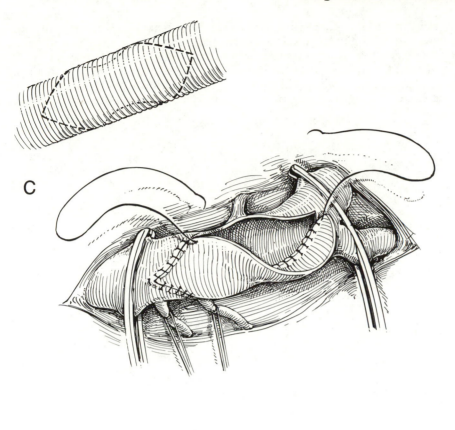

C

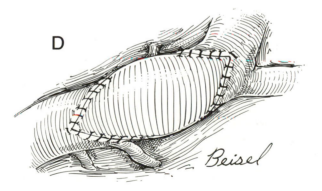

D

Beisel

Fig 18–10, A.—Repair of coarctation of the aorta with a tubular prosthesis. In patients with a long coarctation, and particularly in adults, a tubular prosthesis may be advisable in order to prevent excessive tension on the suture line.

B and C.—After the coarctation has been dissected out in the usual manner, clamps have been applied, and the area of coarctation excised, a woven tubular prosthesis of appropriate size is sutured into place using continuous 4–0 Prolene sutures.

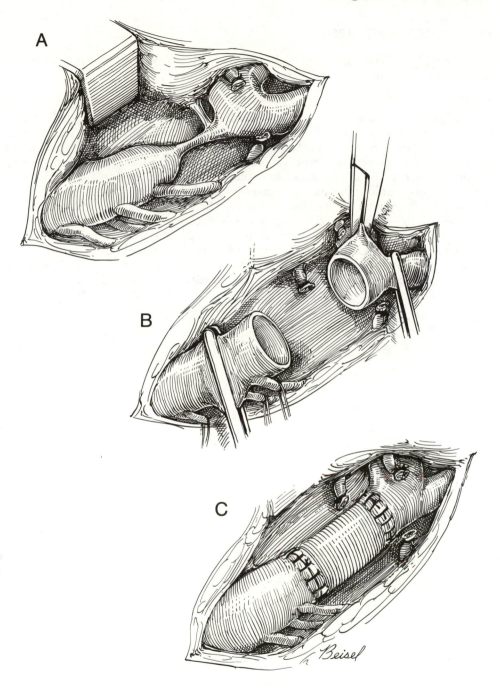

INTERRUPTED AORTIC ARCH

This highly lethal anomaly is characterized by absence of luminal continuity between the ascending and descending aorta.

Types

Figs 18–11, A to C.—It has been divided into types A, B, and C, depending on the location of the atresia. If it is beyond the left subclavian artery, it is called type A; if it is between the left carotid and left subclavian arteries, it is a type B; if it is between the innominate and left carotid artery, it is a type C. Type B is the most common. There is usually a ventricular septal defect and a patent ductus arteriosus. Left ventricular outflow tract obstruction is common. Prior to operations, maintaining ductal patency with prostaglandin E_1 is very helpful in ensuring distal perfusion of the body. Repair is achieved in either a one-stage or a two-stage procedure.

In a one-stage procedure advocated by some, the aorta is repaired by a direct anastomosis through a median sternotomy, using deep hypothermia and circulatory arrest. The ventricular septal defect is also closed. In a two-stage procedure, the aorta is repaired and the pulmonary aorta is banded. At a second operation, the ventricular septal defect is closed and the pulmonary artery band removed.

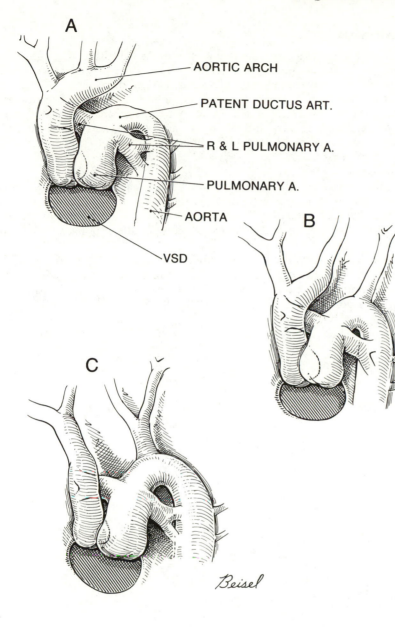

A

AORTIC ARCH

PATENT DUCTUS ART.

R & L PULMONARY A.

PULMONARY A.

AORTA

VSD

B

C

Beisel

Direct Anastomosis

Fig 18–12, A.—The aortic isthmus is approached either through a lateral thoracotomy in the fourth intercostal space for a two-stage procedure or through a median sternotomy in a single-stage procedure. After dissecting out the ductus arteriosus, the left carotid artery, the left subclavian artery, and the descending thoracic aorta, the ductus is ligated using a no. one silk ligature. Vascular clamps are placed on the descending aorta and obliquely across the transverse arch and left carotid artery. The ductal tissue beyond the ligature is excised to prevent subsequent narrowing of an anastomosis. The arch and left carotid artery are incised at the origin of the latter.

B.—The descending thoracic aorta, which has been well mobilized, is anastomosed end-to-side to the carotid artery, preferably using a monofilament absorbable suture (PDS Suture by Ethicon). The posterior row can be a continuous suture. Anteriorly, the suture line should be interrupted especially if nonabsorbable suture material is used.

If a single-stage procedure is being done, the ventricular septal defect is closed in the usual manner. In a two-stage procedure the pulmonary artery, which is huge, is banded. Care must be taken to avoid placing the band too far distally and partially obstructing the right pulmonary artery.

A

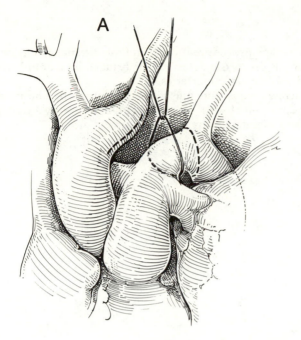

B

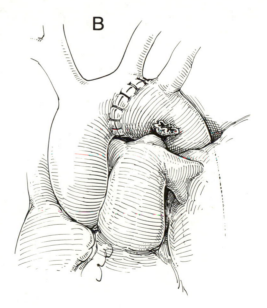

Beisel

Double-Flap Procedure

Fig 18–13, A.—If a two-stage procedure is done and the distance from transverse arch and descending aorta is great, the defect can be bridged by a double flap, using the divided left carotid and subclavian arteries.

B.—The two arteries each will constitute one half of the new arch. The anastomosis is made using a continuous 6–0 absorbable suture (PDS Suture by Ethicon). Adequate cerebral blood flow is maintained by the right carotid artery.

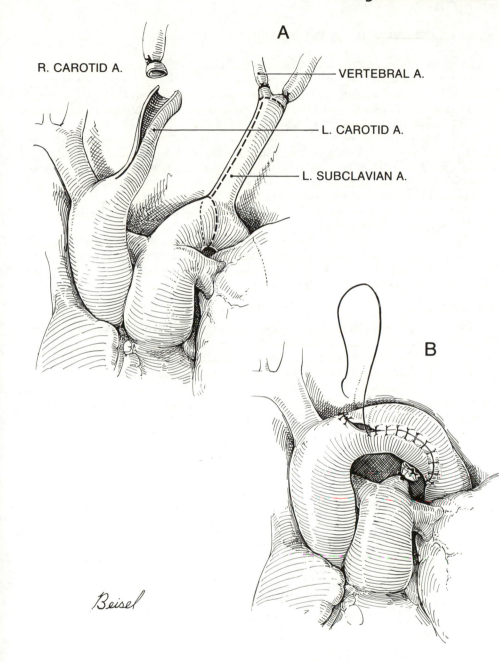

A

R. CAROTID A.

VERTEBRAL A.

L. CAROTID A.

L. SUBCLAVIAN A.

B

Beisel

VASCULAR COMPRESSION OF THE TRACHEA

Because of the softness and relative smallness of the tracheobronchial tree in infants, these structures, as well as the esophagus, can be compressed by aberrant arteries in the chest. Compression of these structures in infancy can produce dyspnea and "crowing" respirations and, less often, dysphagia. The diagnosis is confirmed by a roentgenographic study with a barium swallow.

The constricting band must be divided at a point that will not compromise normal blood flow to the arch vessels. Proximal division of the subclavian arteries, although not ideal, can be compensated for by collateral blood flow. The aim is not to reconstruct the normal anatomy but to release the constriction of the trachea and yet maintain adequate blood flow to tissues. There are several types of vascular compression, but the majority can be dealt with through a left-sided thoracotomy. A fourth interspace incision is used.

The right subclavian artery may arise from the left side of the descending aorta, below the origin of the left subclavian artery, and pass to the right behind the esophagus. Esophageal compression (dysphagia lusoria), although rare, can be relieved by division of the right subclavian artery at its origin.

Double Aortic Arch

Fig 18–14, A.—In this lesion, a smaller arch is usually situated to the left of the main one or anterior to it. The left arch must be freed widely to avoid continued pressure on the trachea and then divided at its narrowest point.

B.—The anterior arch is often divided between the left carotid and subclavian arteries. The ligamentum, or the patent ductus, must also be divided. If the smaller arch is situated posteriorly, it must be divided near its junction with the descending aorta. The larger anterior arch must be freed sufficiently to relieve pressure on the trachea.

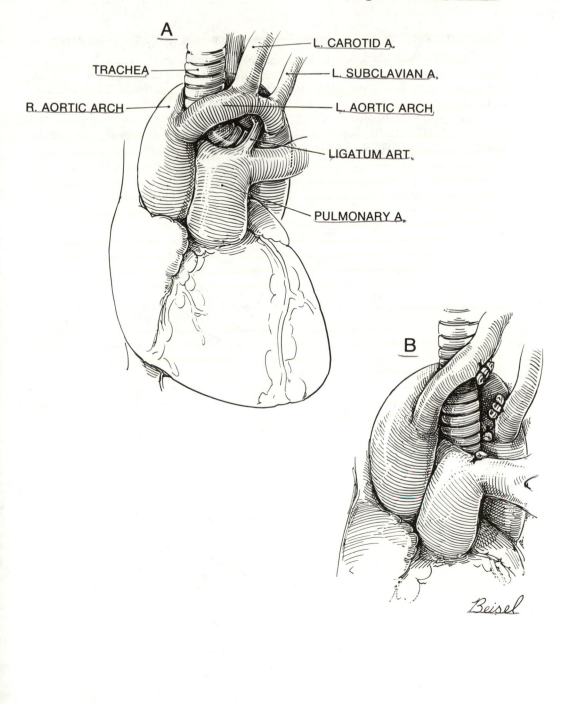

A

TRACHEA

R. AORTIC ARCH

L. CAROTID A.

L. SUBCLAVIAN A.

L. AORTIC ARCH

LIGATUM ART.

PULMONARY A.

B

Beisel

Right Aortic Arch, Retroesophageal Segment, Aberrant Left Subclavian Artery

Figs 18–15, A and B.—In the presence of a right aortic arch, a diverticulum may arise from the descending aorta. It protrudes behind the esophagus, with the left subclavian artery and ligamentum arising from it. This is seen from a posterior view in Fig 18–12, B.

C.—Usually, all that is required to relieve the constriction is to divide the ligamentum arteriosum. If the aberrant left subclavian artery contributes significantly to the constriction, it too should be divided.

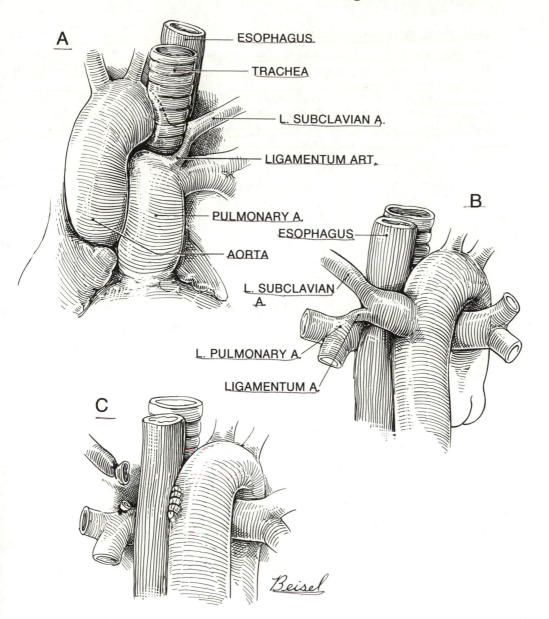

A
- ESOPHAGUS
- TRACHEA
- L. SUBCLAVIAN A.
- LIGAMENTUM ART.
- PULMONARY A.
- AORTA

B
- ESOPHAGUS
- L. SUBCLAVIAN A.
- L. PULMONARY A.
- LIGAMENTUM A.

C

Beisel

Innominate Artery Compression

Fig 18–16, A.—Anomalous innominate and carotid arteries may originate farther distally from the left-sided arch than normal and may cause compression as they cross the trachea.

B.—By suspending the aortic arch and anomalous innominate artery or the carotid artery from the anterior wall, using interrupted mattress sutures buttressed with Teflon pledgets, compression of the underlying trachea can be relieved.

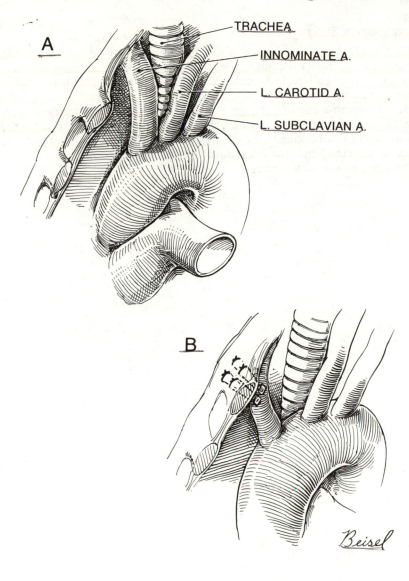

A

TRACHEA

INNOMINATE A.

L. CAROTID A.

L. SUBCLAVIAN A.

B

Beisel

Pulmonary Artery Sling

Fig 18–17, A.—Obstruction of the distal trachea by an aberrant left pulmonary artery arising from the right pulmonary artery and passing between the trachea and esophagus is often lethal. Associated anomalies of the tracheobronchial tree and heart are common.

B.—Through a median sternotomy, the left pulmonary artery is mobilized. The ligamentum arteriosum is divided. The left pulmonary artery is dissected from behind the trachea and divided near its origin from the right pulmonary artery. After suturing the proximal end, the left pulmonary artery is anastomosed to the partially occluded main pulmonary artery.

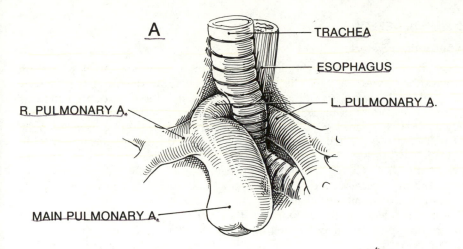

A

TRACHEA

ESOPHAGUS

L. PULMONARY A.

R. PULMONARY A.

MAIN PULMONARY A.

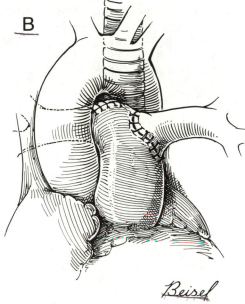

B

Beisel

ATRIAL SEPTAL DEFECT

Ostium Secundum Defect

Most atrial septal defects should be closed to prevent the development of pulmonary artery hypertension. The best time for such an operation is generally when the child is 5 to 6 years of age. These defects are closed through a median sternotomy. The patient is placed on cardiopulmonary bypass. The left ventricle may be vented with a catheter placed through the interatrial groove near the right superior pulmonary vein. The heart is stopped with cold cardioplegia solution injected into the aortic root.

Fig 18–18, A.—The right atrium is opened anterior to the sulcus terminalis. Ostium secundum defects are located in the fossa ovalis. Small defects may be closed directly using a continuous suture.

B.—Large defects should be closed with a patch. Autogenous pericardium is excellent for this purpose; it heals well and is resistant to infection. The patch is secured with a mattress suture of 4–0 Prolene. The suture is started at the superior margin, and each end is brought around the sides and tied at the inferior margin. If there is no inferior margin, the patch is sutured to the atrial wall at its junction with the inferior vena cava. The right atrium is then closed with a 4–0 or 5–0 Prolene suture. All air from the right atrium and the pulmonary artery is evacuated. Suction placed on the "cardioplegia" needle in the ascending aorta is helpful in removing any residual air which is ejected by the left ventricle after the heart has been restarted.

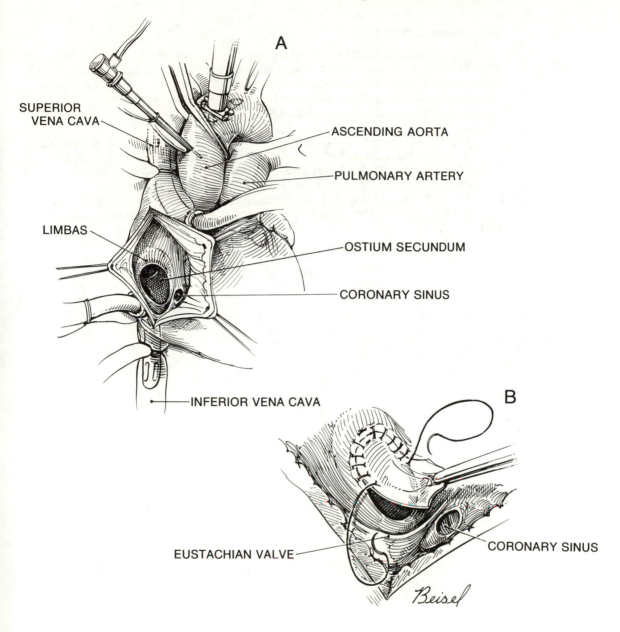

A

SUPERIOR
VENA CAVA

ASCENDING AORTA

PULMONARY ARTERY

LIMBAS

OSTIUM SECUNDUM

CORONARY SINUS

INFERIOR VENA CAVA

B

EUSTACHIAN VALVE

CORONARY SINUS

Beisel

Sinus Venosus Defect

Sinus venosus defects are located below the entrance of the superior vena cava into the right atrium. In these defects the right superior pulmonary vein usually enters into the superior vena cava at its junction with the right atrium. There may be additional pulmonary veins entering the superior vena cava. Blood from these anomalous pulmonary veins is routed into the left atrium through the sinus venosus defect.

Fig 18–19, A.—The right atrium is opened using the incision illustrated.

B.—The high defect and the orifice of the anomalous vein are exposed.

C.—Using a patch of autogenous pericardium, the defect is closed and the anomalous pulmonary vessels' returns are routed into the left atrium.

D.—The atrium is closed by advancing the flap from the atrial appendage (see Fig 18–19, A, 2) into the incision in the superior vena cava (1) thus avoiding caval narrowing.

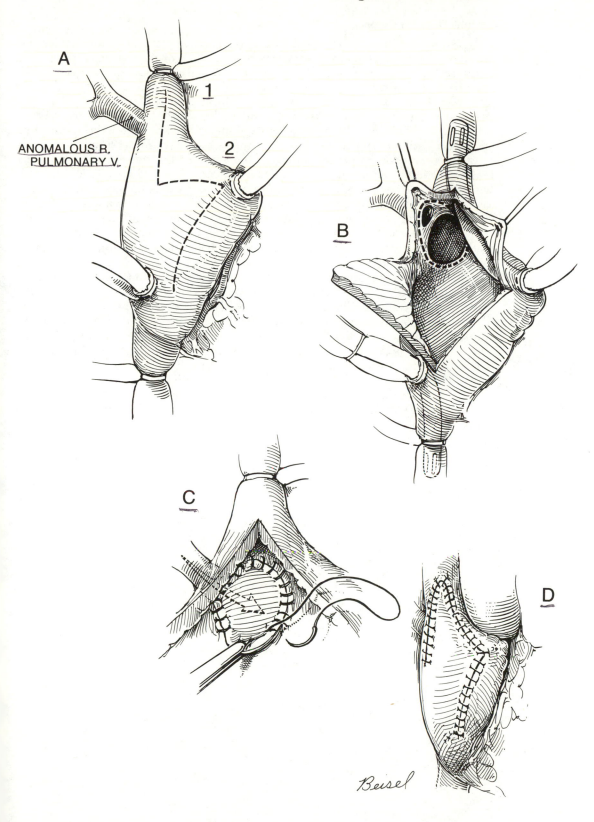

A

1

2

ANOMALOUS R.
PULMONARY V.

B

C

D

Beisel

Ostium Primum Defect

Ostium primum defects usually have an associated cleft in the mitral valve and are a partial form of an endocardial cushion defect. The mitral cleft may give rise to mitral regurgitation, in which case closure of the cleft is indicated. Its repair, in the absence of regurgitation, is controversial.

Fig 18–20, A.—The defect is exposed through a right atriotomy. It lies between the mitral and tricuspid valves and is due to the absence of the septum primum. There may also be an ostium secundum defect. The cleft in the mitral valve is repaired with interrupted 4–0 Dacron sutures. Where the initial suture is placed is most important for proper alignment of the edges of the two parts of the septal leaflet. The initial suture should approximate the thickened edge of each leaflet half without producing stenosis. After closure of the cleft valve, competence should be assessed by injecting saline solution into the left ventricle and allowing the leaflets to close. A regurgitant jet will be evident. Rarely, an annuloplasty may be required.

B.—The conduction system lies at the apex of the triangle of Koch and extends beneath the valve tissue on the left side of the ventricular septum and continues just beyond the cleft of the septal leaflet of the mitral valve. Here, the branching bundle extends along the inferior margin of the membranous septum and then divides into right and left bundles, which veer downward into the sinuses of the ventricles, the right bundle entering the anterolateral papillary muscle.

C.—To avoid damage to the conduction bundle, 4–0 Prolene interrupted sutures are placed superficially, staying more to the right side, between the two valves. The sutures are placed parallel to the conduction fibers to minimize any damage. At the coronary sinus, the sutures are placed to the left of the coronary sinus valve and continued to the left of the tendon of Todaro.

D.—Once the patch has been sutured into place along the lines of the conduction system, it can be attached to the free margin of the atrial septal defect using a continuous 4–0 Prolene suture. The atriotomy is then closed.

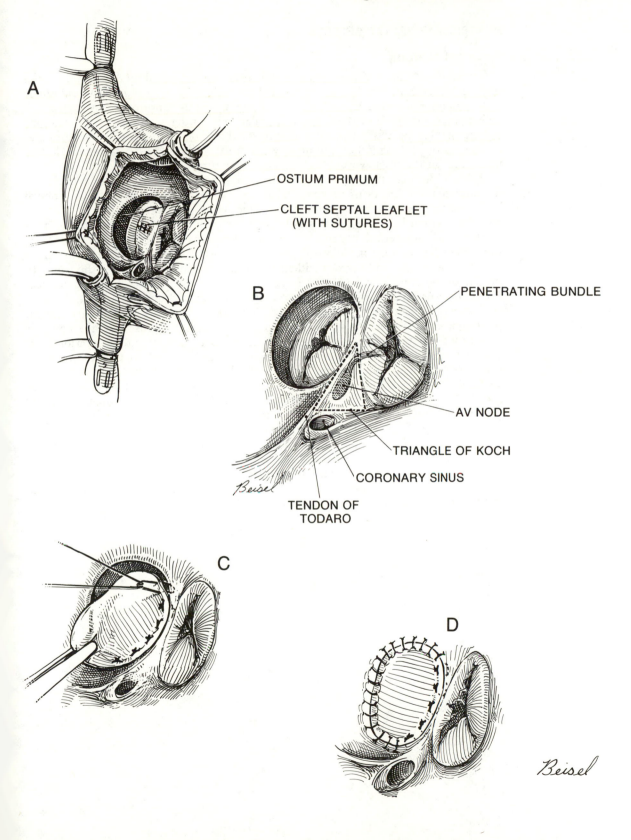

A

OSTIUM PRIMUM

CLEFT SEPTAL LEAFLET
(WITH SUTURES)

B

PENETRATING BUNDLE

AV NODE

TRIANGLE OF KOCH

CORONARY SINUS

TENDON OF
TODARO

C

D

Beisel

VENTRICULAR SEPTAL DEFECTS

Types and Anatomy

Fig 18–21, A.—Ventricular septal defects may be found in all portions of the ventricular septum. The septum is divided into inlet (*C*), trabecular (*B*), and outlet (*A*) components and is completed by the membranous septum. Perimembranous defects may extend into the inlet, trabecular, and outlet portions of the septum. Subarterial defects result from the absence of the outlet (infundibular) septum and are roofed by the conjoined pulmonary and aortic valves. Muscular septal defects may occur in the inlet septum and trabecular septum.

B.—The anatomic landmarks of surgical importance in the right ventricle and the characteristic locations of ventricular septal defects are illustrated. The medial border of the tricuspid valve ring is a key landmark. The outflow tract of the right ventricle, which lies between this point and the pulmonary valve, is another landmark and rises rather steeply in both anterior and cephalad directions. The third key site is the crista supraventricularis, a prominent muscular band which spans the floor of the outflow tract and is readily identified at operation. The fourth is the papillary muscle of the conus, which arises from the septum, and whose chordae tendineae insert adjacent borders of the septal and anterior tricuspid leaflets.

About 70% of all ventricular septal defects are in the membranous septum (perimembranous ventricular septal defect). The papillary muscle of the conus is usually inferior to defects in this area, but larger defects may extend inferior to it. The left ventricular outflow tract lies posterior and caudad to that of the right ventricle. Perimembranous septal defects, which extend above and below the papillary muscle of the conus, are in close relationship to the right and the noncoronary cusps of the aortic valve, which can be seen through the defect. A small number of ventricular septal defects lie between the crista supraventricularis and the pulmonary valve (subarterial ventricular septal defect). They are in proximity to the left cusp of the aortic valve and the pulmonary valve. Two less common sites are the posterior portion of the septum beneath the septal leaflet of the tricuspid valve, where it is an endocardial cushion defect and is part of the atrioventricularis communis defect, and the muscular portion of the septum, as shown. The two latter defects are not related to the outflow tract of either the right or the left ventricle.

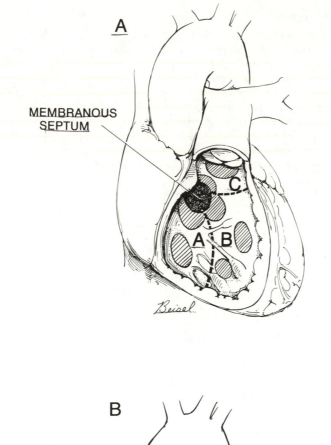

A

MEMBRANOUS
SEPTUM

C

A B

Beisel

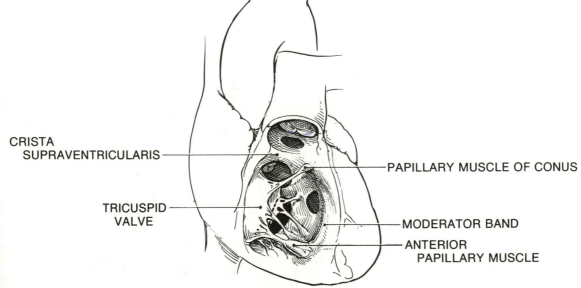

B

CRISTA
SUPRAVENTRICULARIS

PAPILLARY MUSCLE OF CONUS

TRICUSPID
VALVE

MODERATOR BAND

ANTERIOR
PAPILLARY MUSCLE

The Conduction System

C.—The atrioventricular node lies at the apex of the triangle of Koch, which is formed by the tendon of Todaro and the tricuspid valve anulus. The base of the triangle is the coronary sinus. The penetrating bundle of His passes through the central fibrous body into the septum, staying at the inferior border of the membranous septum on the left side. The branching portion gives off the fasciculi of the posterior radiation of the left bundle branch. At its bifurcation, it then divides into the right bundle and the anterior radiation of the left bundle branch. The right bundle branch passes to the right side of the septum and goes to the anterolateral papillary muscle (moderator band). Conduction tissue does not extend beyond the papillary muscle of the conus (medial papillary muscle).

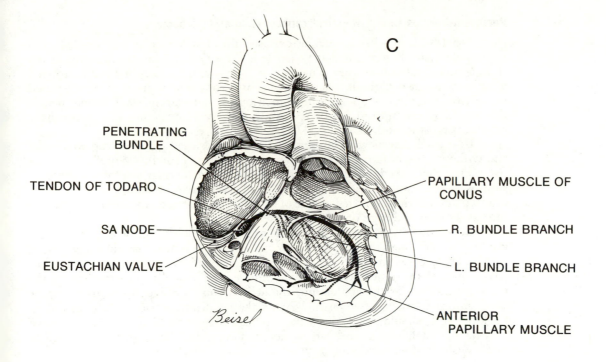

C

PENETRATING
BUNDLE

TENDON OF TODARO

SA NODE

EUSTACHIAN VALVE

PAPILLARY MUSCLE OF
CONUS

R. BUNDLE BRANCH

L. BUNDLE BRANCH

ANTERIOR
PAPILLARY MUSCLE

Beisel

Perimembranous Defect Repair: Transventricular Approach

Fig 18–22, A.—The heart is exposed through a median sternotomy. On cardiopulmonary bypass, the left ventricle is vented with a catheter inserted at the right superior pulmonary vein. The aorta is cross-clamped, and the heart is stopped with cardioplegia solution injected into the aortic root. The ventricle may be opened by either a transverse or a longitudinal incision. A transverse incision is said to split the muscle fibers and thus to be less injurious. Avoiding injury to the coronary arteries is most important.

B.—Small defects with fibrous margins can be closed with interrupted sutures and without a patch. However, most defects do require a patch. We prefer a Dacron felt *matrix*. Since the bundle of His lies on the left ventricular side of the septum, sutures in the septum, posterior to the papillary muscle of the conus, should be inserted into the right ventricular side of the septum. Mattress sutures are placed 2–3 mm away from the edge on the right side.

C.—When the tricuspid valve is the posterior border of the defect, the sutures can be placed through the base of the tricuspid valve. A transitional suture will close a possible gap between the tricuspid valve and the septal wall. One arm of the suture passes through the right side of the septal muscle. The second arm passes through the tricuspid leaflet near the anulus into the atrium and then back through the valve tissue into the ventricle (see *inset*). Beyond the papillary muscle of the conus, full-thickness bites should be taken. At the cephalad edge of the defect, the aortic valve may be injured unless extreme care is exercised in placing the sutures. The ventriculotomy is closed with a double row of continuous 4–0 Prolene suture.

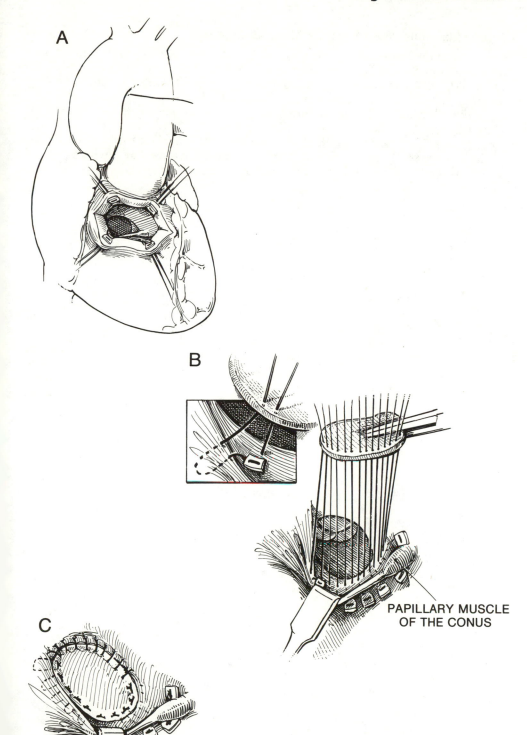

PAPILLARY MUSCLE
OF THE CONUS

Perimembranous Defect Repair: Transatrial Approach

This is our preferred approach, especially in infants. By avoiding a ventriculotomy, the function of the right ventricle is preserved. After establishing cardiopulmonary bypass and inserting a left ventricular vent, the heart is stopped using cardioplegia solution. The atrium is opened widely anterior to the sulcus terminalis.

Fig 18–23, A.—The perimembranous ventricular septal defect is exposed by retracting the septal leaflet of the tricuspid valve.

B and C.—The defect is then closed in a routine manner, using interrupted 4–0 Ticron sutures. As these are placed through muscle tissue, they are backed with Teflon pledgets; as the sutures pass through the fibrous base of the tricuspid leaflet, they may be unbacked.

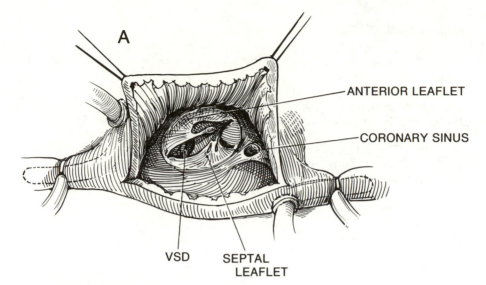

A

ANTERIOR LEAFLET

CORONARY SINUS

VSD SEPTAL
LEAFLET

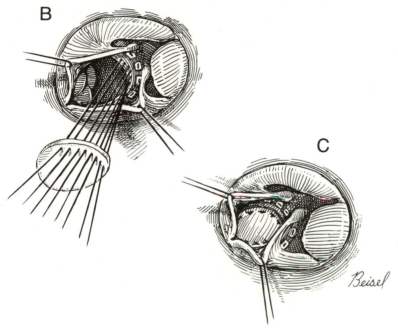

B

C

Beisel

Muscular Defect Repair

Muscular ventricular septal defects in the trabecular septum are often multiple and have a "Swiss cheese" appearance, especially when viewed on the right side. The closure from the right side is difficult due to the trabeculae.

Fig 18–24, A.—The apex of the left ventricle is incised parallel to the left anterior descending coronary artery. The defect is usually evident anteriorly. Although the defect has multiple exits on the right side, it has a single orifice on the left side.

B.—The defect is closed with a Dacron patch and a running suture of 4–0 Prolene. Conduction tissue is not present in the rim of the defect. The ventriculotomy is closed with a continuous suture of 4–0 Prolene.

A

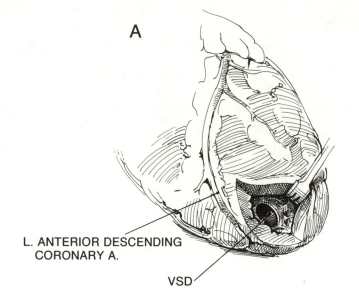

L. ANTERIOR DESCENDING
CORONARY A.

VSD

B

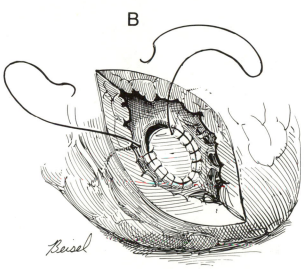

Beisel

Pulmonary Artery Banding

Although pulmonary artery banding has been superseded by complete repair of most lesions, there still remain occasions for its use.

Fig 18–25, A.—Through a left anterior thoracotomy in the third interspace, the pericardium is opened anterior to the phrenic nerve.

B.—The pulmonary artery is carefully dissected from the ascending aorta. The right pulmonary artery lies hidden as it passes behind the aorta and can be readily injured. A 5-mm wide, woven Teflon tape is passed around the aorta. It is essential that the tape be impervious to fibrous ingrowth so that it can be removed with ease at a later date.

C.—The tape is tightened until a fine thrill is palpable distal to the band. Usually there is an associated rise in systemic arterial pressure as more blood is forced into the ascending aorta.

D.—The band is secured with several interrupted sutures, incorporating some pulmonary artery tissue to prevent distal migration. At this time, pressures distal to the band are compared with systemic pressures. A mean pulmonary artery pressure equaling one half to one third of the mean systemic arterial pressure is usually an appropriate pressure reduction.

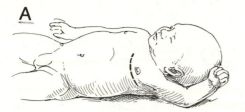

A

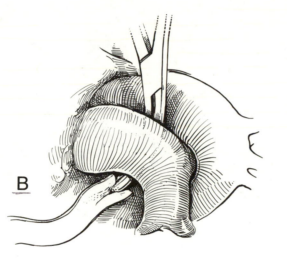

B

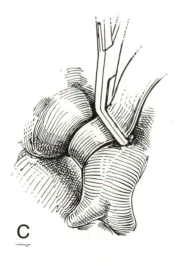

C

Beisel

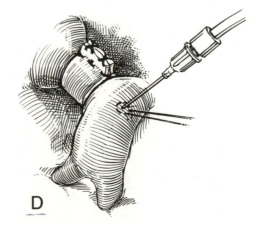

D

Removal of Pulmonary Artery Band

Removal of a pulmonary artery band is usually performed at the same time as total correction of the lesion. Both are approached through a median sternotomy.

Fig 18–26, A and B.—The tissue overlying the band is incised on each side of the area where the band is secured. The band is divided and removed (*arrow*).

C.—The piece of band with the incorporated pulmonary artery tissue is excised, and the defect in the pulmonary artery is closed with a patch of autologous pericardium.

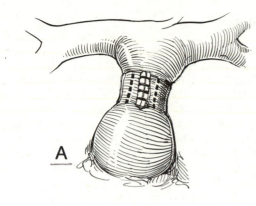

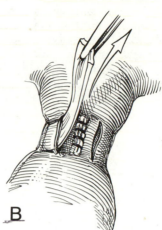

A

B

Beisel

C

COMPLETE ATRIOVENTRICULAR CANAL

In this lesion, the endocardial cushion defect involves the ventricular septum (inlet septum) as well as the septum primum. The conjoining mitral and tricuspid valves form a common atrioventricular orifice. Clefts in their septal leaflets often result in valve insufficiency. Pulmonary hypertension is common. The ventricular septal defect commonly extends anteriorly beneath the aortic valve and posteriorly to the atrioventricular junction and may vary significantly in breadth and length. When the anterior common bridging leaflet is not divided into mitral and tricuspid components, it is usually free-floating, without chordal attachments to the septum. The associated posterior cushion elements also may be bridging and are often partially divided, but have chordal attachments to the septal crest. In contrast, the anterior leaflet may be totally or partially separate with distinct mitral and tricuspid components. The edges of the anterior divided leaflet have chordal attachments to the septal crest. In this circumstance the posterior leaflet is almost always attached to the septal crest. These defects may be repaired by the one-patch technique or the two-patch technique. The latter has the major advantage in that the anterior and posterior leaflets are not cut and thus will not dehisce at their attachment to the patches.

Single-Patch Technique

Fig 18–27, A.—Through a median sternotomy the heart is exposed. Using cardiopulmonary bypass and cardioplegia solution, the right atrium is opened anterior to the sulcus terminalis.

B.—The anatomy of the defect and the valve leaflets are inspected. If not naturally divided, the anterior and posterior leaflets are incised, staying to the right atrial side on the plane of the ventricular septum. This ensures that the mitral side has adequate tissue to provide subsequent valve competence.

C.—The leading edges of the anterior and posterior leaflets are approximated, and the cleft of the septal leaflet of the mitral valve is repaired with interrupted 3–0 or 4–0 nonabsorbable suture.

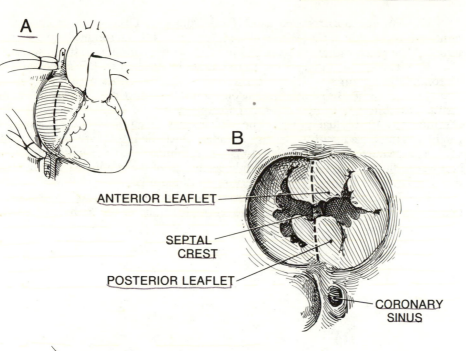

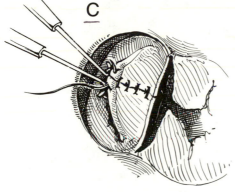

A

B

ANTERIOR LEAFLET

SEPTAL CREST

POSTERIOR LEAFLET

CORONARY SINUS

C

Beisel

D.—An appropriate-sized patch (pericardium or Dacron) is attached to the right ventricular side of the septum using interrupted 4–0 Ticron pledgeted mattress sutures. The patch can also be sutured in place with a running mattress suture.

E.—The septal leaflet of the mitral valve is attached to the patch with 4–0 Ticron mattress sutures which are backed with a strip of either pericardium or felt. The appropriate height of attachment on the patch is best determined by existing chordal attachments. In general, this corresponds to the level of the plane of the common atrioventricular orifice. The sutures pass through the mitral leaflet, the patch, and the cut edge of the tricuspid leaflet. Once the leaflets are attached, mitral valve competence is tested by injecting saline solution into the left ventricle. All necessary adjustments, including complete suturing of the residual cleft, shortening the chordae, and annuloplasty, are performed as required.

F.—The patch is then sutured into the atrial defect with a continuous suture, taking care to avoid damaging the atrioventricular node in the triangle of Koch.

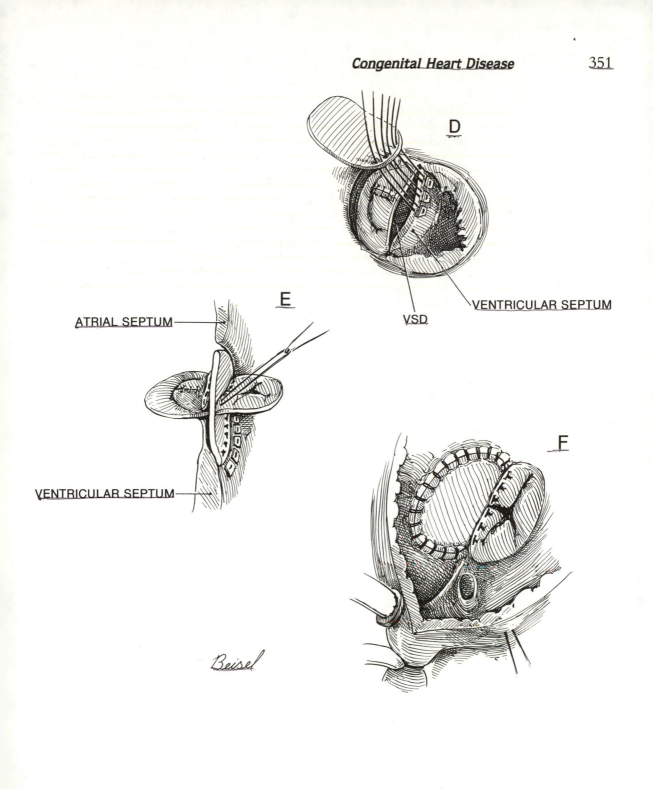

D

VENTRICULAR SEPTUM

VSD

E

ATRIAL SEPTUM

VENTRICULAR SEPTUM

F

Beisel

Two-Patch Technique

Fig 18–28, A.—The anterior and posterior leaflets are approximated at their midpoints above the septal crest. The ventricular septal defect is then carefully measured in length and height. A patch is cut using these measurements, adding 4 mm to the length and 2 mm to the height.

B.—The patch is sutured into the ventricular septal defect, staying well to the right side of the crest of the septum. The suture may be running or interrupted, and pledgets of Teflon felt are used.

C.—Mattress sutures of 4–0 Prolene are passed through the top of the Dacron prosthesis and the anterior and posterior leaflets. It is essential that these leaflets are sutured in the appropriate positions so that their margins are in apposition to their centers.

D.—The mattress sutures passing through the valve tissue are then passed through the edge of a pericardial patch and tied.

E.—The mattress sutures at the edge of the valve are used to suture the pericardial patch into the atrial defect.

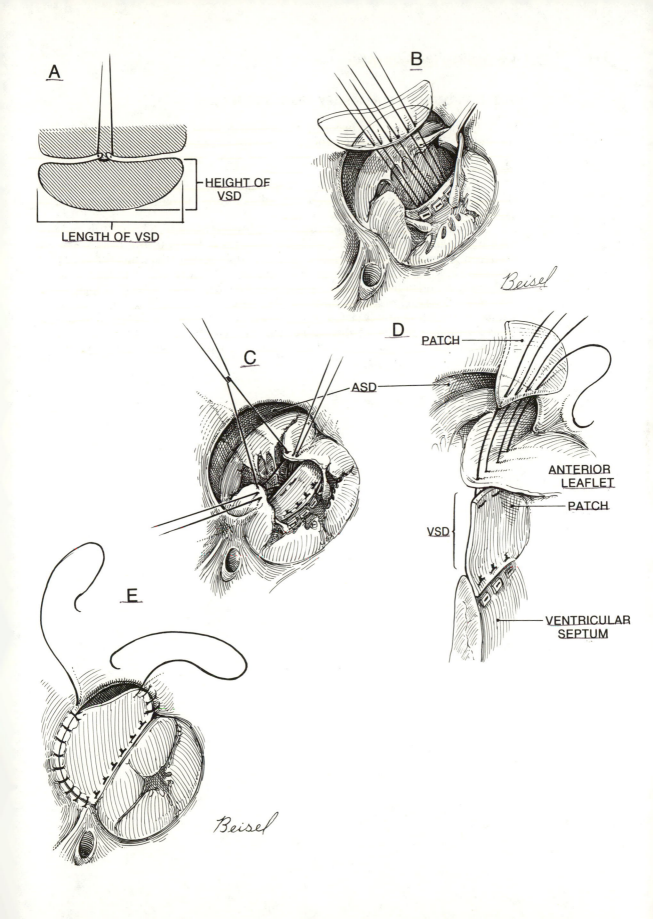

A

HEIGHT OF
VSD

LENGTH OF VSD

B

Beisel

C

ASD

D

PATCH

ASD

ANTERIOR
LEAFLET

PATCH

VSD

VENTRICULAR
SEPTUM

E

Beisel

TOTAL ANOMALOUS PULMONARY VENOUS DRAINAGE

This anomaly usually produces profound failure in infants in the first days of life and requires immediate operation, even in the presence of only mild symptoms.

Supracardiac Type

Fig 18–29, A.—The pulmonary veins join a transverse common trunk behind the left atrium and drain through a vertical vein into the left innominate vein. A patent foramen ovale is essential for life.

B.—The heart is exposed through a median sternotomy. Using cardiopulmonary bypass and deep hypothermia (20°C), the apex of the heart is lifted up, and the common pulmonary venous trunk is exposed. After incising the trunk for a distance of 2 cm, the vertical vein is ligated at its origin. The left atrium is incised, and the incision is extended from the atrial septum into the base of the left atrial appendage.

C.—To prevent future stenosis, the left atrium is anastomosed to the common trunk with either continuous 6–0 Prolene sutures, which are interrupted in several areas for future growth, or absorbable synthetic sutures (PDS Suture; Ethicon).

D.—The foramen ovale is closed through a separate right atriotomy.

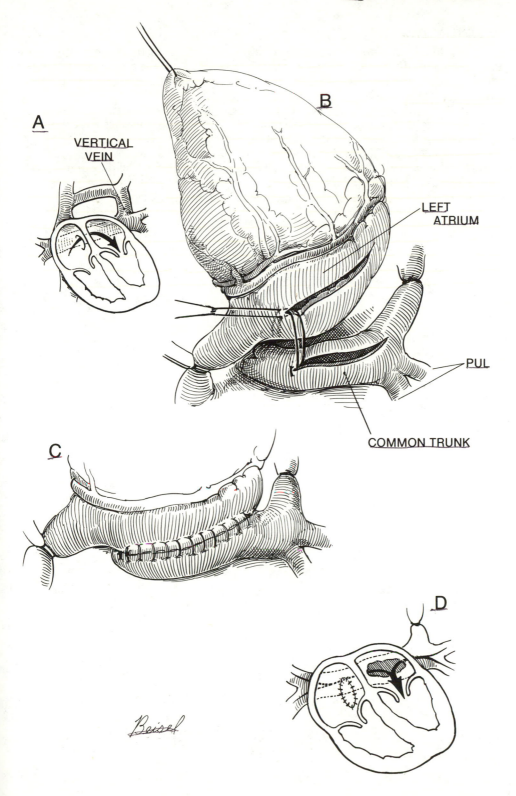

A

VERTICAL
VEIN

B

LEFT
ATRIUM

PUL

COMMON TRUNK

C

D

Beisel

Infracardiac Type

Fig 18–30, A.—In the uncommon infracardiac type of total anomalous pulmonary venous drainage, the common trunk drains through the esophageal hiatus of the diaphragm and joins the portal vein, the ductus venosus, or rarely, the inferior vena cava. There is a widely patent foramen ovale.

B.—A wide anastomosis between the left atrium and the common pulmonary venous tract is established. This may require a "T" incision in the tract and extension of the incision down into the draining vein.

C.—The anastomosis is completed with an absorbable synthetic suture (PDS Suture; Ethicon), and the descending vein is ligated. At times, the descending vein may require division to prevent kinking.

D.—The atrial septal defect is closed through a right atriotomy.

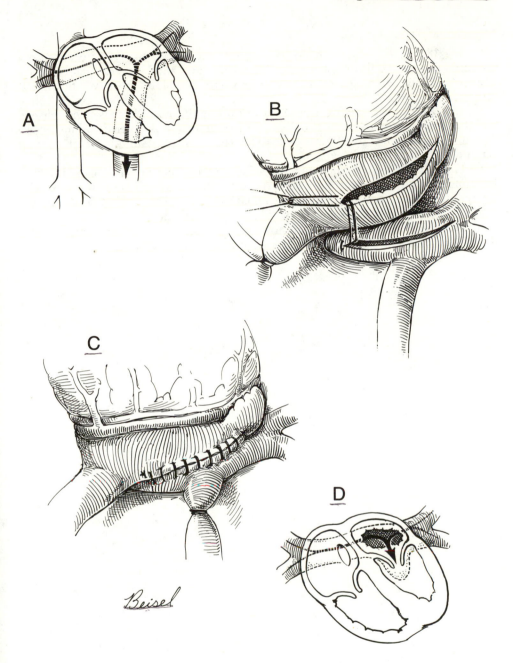

A

B

C

Beisel

D

Intracardiac Type

Fig 18–31, A.—In the majority of cases, the pulmonary veins drain into a common venous trunk which, in turn, drains through a greatly enlarged coronary sinus. A widely patent foramen ovale is necessary for blood to flow into the left atrium.

B.—Through a median sternotomy, cardiopulmonary bypass is established and the temperature is lowered to 20°C. The right atrium is opened and inspected. The atrial septal defect usually lies close to the large coronary sinus. The intervening septum (left atrial wall) is excised.

C.—The coronary sinus and the atrial septal defect are then closed with a ballooning patch of pericardium. The sutures at the coronary sinus must be relatively superficial to avoid damage to the nodal tissue. By placing them down into the coronary sinus, the nodal tissue is less likely to be damaged.

D.—Following repair, the pulmonary veins drain into the left atrium as does the coronary sinus. This produces an insignificant right-to-left shunt.

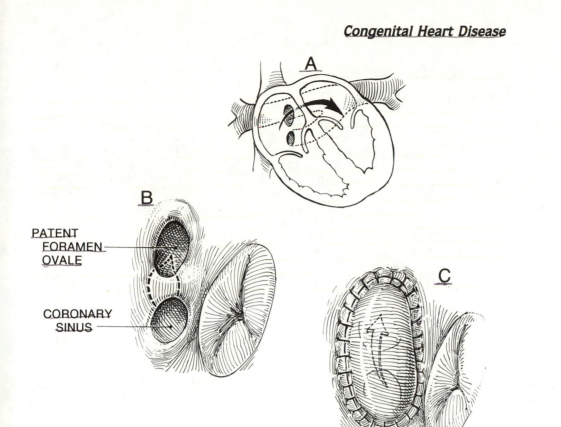

PATENT
FORAMEN
OVALE

CORONARY
SINUS

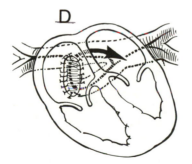

PULMONARY STENOSIS: VALVULAR TYPE

Transventricular Approach

Critical pulmonary stenosis in infants requires an emergency operation, which is best accomplished by a transventricular pulmonary valvotomy.

Fig 18–32, A.—The heart is exposed through a median sternotomy. A mattress suture of 4–0 Prolene, backed with Teflon felt, is placed in the outflow tract of the right ventricle, and a rubber keeper is applied. Through a stab wound between the sutures, a 5-mm Brock knife is advanced into the pulmonary artery. As the sharp edges of the knife cut through the stenotic valve, a distinct "give" can be felt. It is essential that the point of the knife can be felt far out in the pulmonary artery to ascertain that the valve has actually been cut, not merely pushed forward. A 7-mm or even 10-mm knife may then be passed into the pulmonary artery. The size of the knife will be determined by the size of the pulmonary anulus.

B.—A small, sharp Kerrison rongeur is then advanced through the same tract, and the valve tissue at the anulus is excised to further open the valve. This is done on both sides of the valvular incision. The rongeur is then removed, and the mattress suture tied.

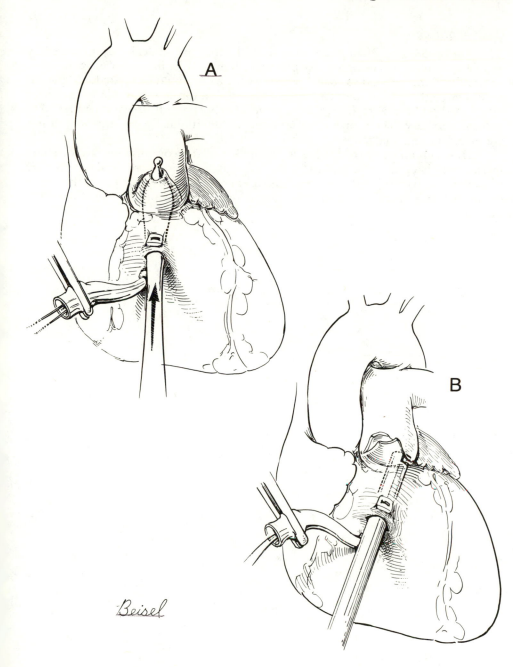

Beisel

Open Approach

Fig 18–33, A.—Pulmonary stenosis in children and adults is best managed by an open valvulotomy using cardiopulmonary bypass. It is important that the heart be fibrillating or arrested so that it cannot eject air that could be sucked into the left atrium through a patent foramen ovale. Direct vision through the pulmonary artery offers the best chance to open the valve accurately through its commissures. The pulmonary artery may be opened transversely or longitudinally, and traction sutures are placed along its edges.

B.—The dome-shaped valve is exposed, and the commissures are carefully incised well back into the anulus. If the valve is bicuspid, both commissures are incised; if it is tricuspid, all three commissures are opened. By staying in the center of the fused commissure when making the incision, subsequent valve insufficiency is minimized.

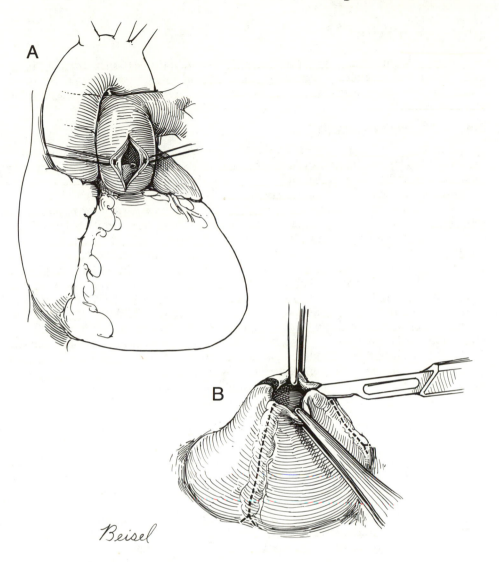

Beisel

TETRALOGY OF FALLOT

Systemic pulmonary artery anastomosis is still an important palliative operation for the management of tetralogy of Fallot in infants, as well as for other conditions that cause inadequate pulmonary blood flow and that are unsuitable for total correction.

Blalock-Taussig Anastomosis

The Blalock-Taussig operation remains the operation of choice because of the ease with which the shunt can be obliterated at the time of total correction, the minimal distortion of the pulmonary artery, and the almost ideal shunt flow, which is limited by the size of the subclavian artery.

Fig 18–34, A.—The subclavian artery to pulmonary artery anastomosis is most easily made on the opposite side of the aortic arch. Thus, with a left arch, a right-sided anastomosis is made. Through a right posterolateral thoracotomy in the fourth intercostal space, the lung is retracted inferiorly and posteriorly. The pleura over the right pulmonary artery is incised, and the artery is dissected out. Care is taken to expose not only the artery to the upper lobe but also the entire artery, including the middle and lower lobe branches. Potts ties are placed around these vessels. The pulmonary veins from the upper lobe lie anterior and slightly inferior to the pulmonary artery and can be mistaken for the artery, especially if the latter is small. The mediastinal pleura posterior to the superior vena cava is incised, and the azygos vein is ligated and divided. The subclavian artery is mobilized above as well as below the vagus nerve and its recurrent laryngeal branch. The innominate artery and right carotid artery are also widely mobilized, and Potts ties are placed around them. The subclavian artery may be brought closer to the pulmonary artery by freeing the common carotid artery high into the neck.

B.—The subclavian artery is ligated above the origin of the vertebral artery, which is also ligated to prevent a possible subclavian steal. The subclavian artery is occluded with a straight vascular clamp proximal to the recurrent nerve and then divided proximal to where it was ligated. It is then turned down after passing behind the recurrent laryngeal nerve. The adventitia is stripped off the distal subclavian artery to prevent subsequent constriction.

C.—The pulmonary artery is occluded with a vascular clamp as medially as possible while the Potts ties are tightened. A longitudinal incision, 3–4 mm, is made in the superior aspect of the pulmonary artery in its midportion.

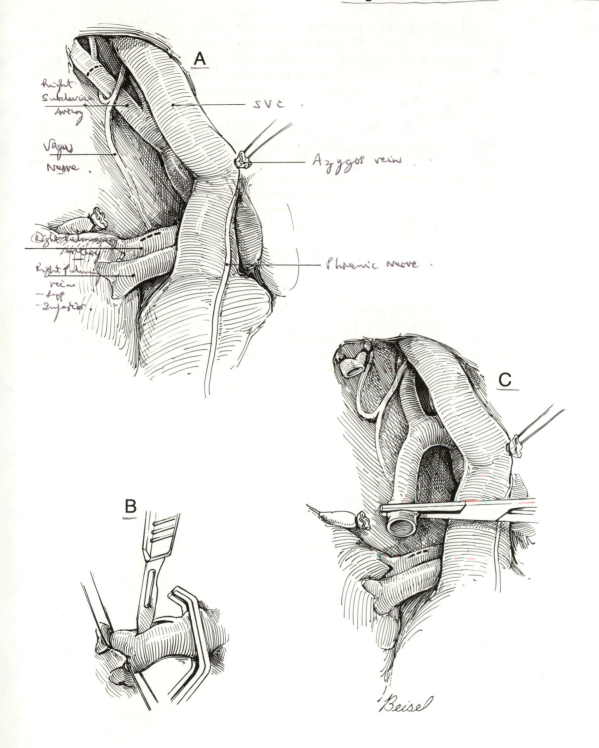

A

Right
Subclavian
Artery

Vagus
Nerve

Right Subclavian
Artery

Right Pulmonary
vein
— Sup
— Inferior

SVC.

Azygos vein

Phrenic Nerve

B

C

Beisel

D.—A posterior, continuous everting mattress suture of 6–0 Prolene is used to join the pulmonary and subclavian arteries. Each end of the suture is tied to an anchoring suture at either side of the anastomosis (*inset*). In small infants, the posterior wall is sewn with simple interrupted sutures of 6–0 Prolene, placing four or five sutures before tying them.

E.—The anterior line of the anastomosis is completed with 6–0 Prolene interrupted sutures.

F.—On completion of the anastomosis, the Potts ties are loosened, and the pulmonary artery clamp is released. This is followed by release of the subclavian artery clamp. A fine continuous thrill should be palpable in the pulmonary artery.

D

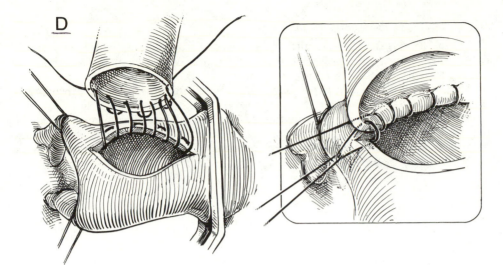

E

F

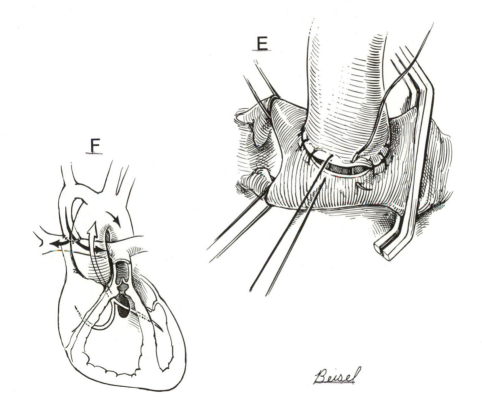

Beisel

Gortex or Impra Prosthetic Shunt

Figs 18–35, A to D.—A prosthetic shunt of either Gortex or Impra graft has an advantage over the classic Blalock-Taussig anastomosis in that the subclavian artery is not sacrificed. The major disadvantage of using artificial shunt material is a greater likelihood of shunt thrombosis. By placing the proximal anastomosis into the subclavian artery, the latter to a large extent will determine the shunt flow. The operation is performed in a manner similar to the Blalock-Taussig operation, although it is more readily performed on the left side. A 4- or 5-mm prosthesis is used in most infants. Intravenous heparin is given to the patient for the first 24 hours postoperatively to prevent shunt thrombosis.

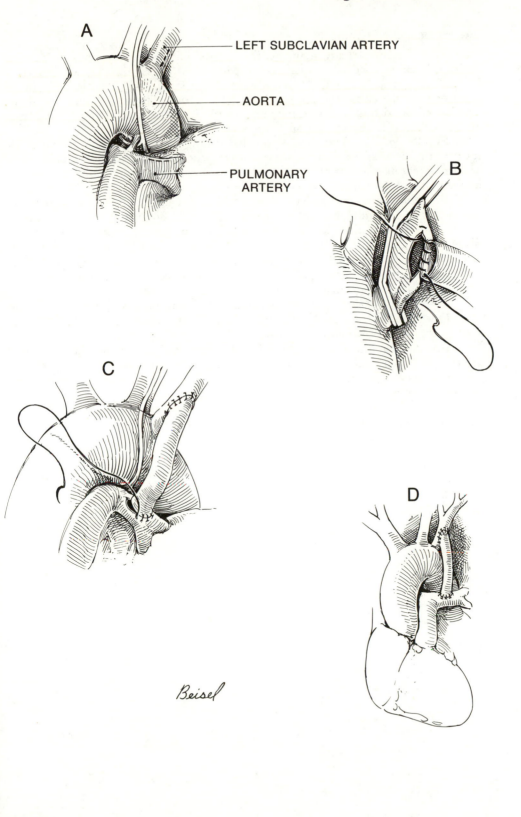

A

LEFT SUBCLAVIAN ARTERY

AORTA

PULMONARY ARTERY

B

C

D

Beisel

The Waterston Anastomosis

This operation is advantageous for infants who have very small pulmonary arteries. It can be used with equal ease in patients with a right or left aortic arch. It has two major disadvantages: (1) it can be made too large, and (2) if it is made too far anteriorly on the aorta, the pulmonary artery becomes kinked, forcing the major portion of blood flow to the right lung. In the latter case, the kinked pulmonary artery will require reconstruction at the time of takedown.

Fig 18–36, A.—The chest is opened through a right lateral incision in the fourth intercostal space. The pericardium is opened anterior to the phrenic nerve, and the ascending aorta is retracted to the left, exposing the right pulmonary artery between it and the superior vena cava.

B.—The pulmonary artery is dissected out, and heavy silk ligatures are placed around its upper and lower lobe branches. A small, angulated vascular clamp is placed with the posterior blade passing behind the pulmonary artery and the anterior blade occluding a posterolateral portion of the ascending aorta. The pulmonary artery is incised transversely, and a small incision, no greater than 3 mm (unless the operation is being performed on a larger child or an adult), is made into the occluded portion of the aorta parallel to the pulmonary artery incision.

C.—The posterior anastomosis is made with continuous 6–0 Prolene suture.

D.—The anterior row is completed with interrupted 6–0 or 7–0 Prolene sutures to prevent restriction of growth.

E.—After removal of the occluding ligatures and the clamp, the pulmonary artery is palpated. If the shunt appears excessive, as manifested by a rough thrill in the pulmonary artery, the anastomosis can be made smaller by placing a suture in the corner of the anastomosis, through both the pulmonary artery and the aorta, to occlude partially the opening between the vessels. Too large an anastomosis should be avoided, since severe postoperative cardiac failure may result.

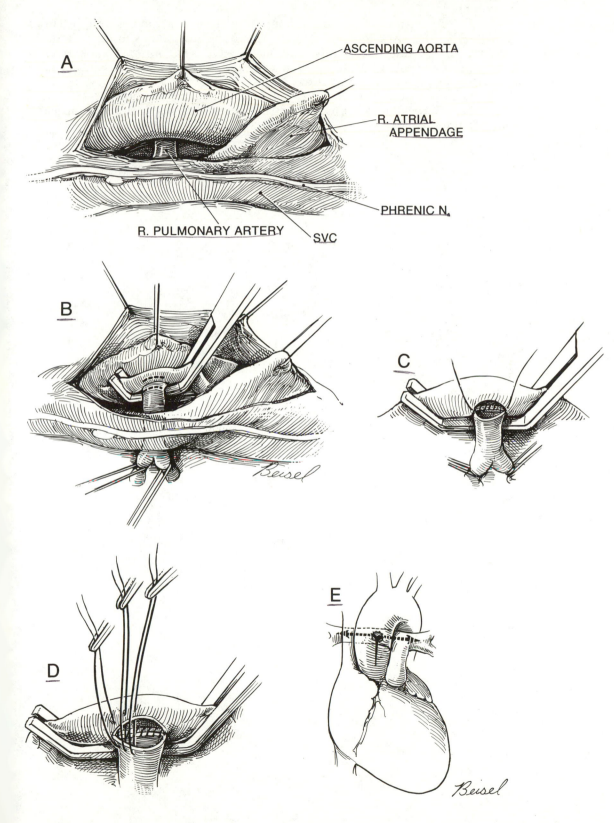

F.—At the time of total correction, the Waterston anastomosis can be closed by opening the aortic root and suturing closed the anastomosis to the pulmonary artery. This is only possible if the pulmonary artery is not distorted and kinked. In most cases, the pulmonary artery is cut away from the aorta, leaving a small cuff of aortic tissue on the pulmonary artery.

G.—The aorta is closed with a running 5–0 Prolene suture.

H.—The pulmonary artery is incised longitudinally and enlarged with a patch of pericardium.

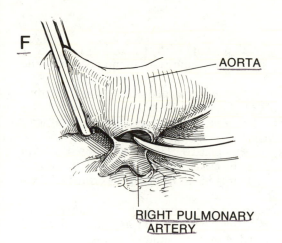

F

AORTA

RIGHT PULMONARY
ARTERY

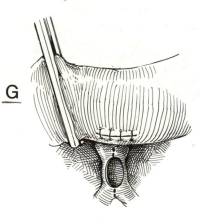

G

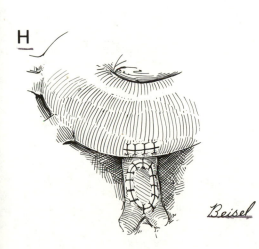

H

Beisel

Open Repair

Total correction is indicated in almost all patients with tetralogy of Fallot after the first year of life. Controversy still exists as to its indications in infants during the first year of life.

Fig 18–37, A.—The heart is exposed through a median sternotomy. Cardiopulmonary bypass with hypothermia (22–25°C) is established and the heart is arrested using cardioplegia solution. The left ventricle is vented with a catheter through the right superior pulmonary vein.

The outflow tract of the right ventricle is incised. The incision extends from the pulmonary anulus to the level just below the crista. It is essential that an anomalous left anterior descending coronary artery arising from the right coronary artery is not incised. Its transection is often fatal.

B.—Through the incision (here shown longer than actual to illustrate the anatomy), the perimembranous ventricular septal defect, the parietal and septal bands of the crista, and the pulmonary valve and its anulus are inspected. The parietal and, to a lesser extent, the septal bands are excised with care not to make the resection too extensive.

C.—The ventricular septal defect is then closed in a manner routine for a typical large perimembranous ventricular septal defect. Since the bundle of His lies on the left ventricular side of the septum, sutures in the septum, posterior to the papillary muscle of the conus, should be inserted into the right ventricular side of the septum. Mattress sutures are placed 2–3 mm away from the edge on the right side. Beyond the papillary muscle of the conus, full-thickness bites should be taken. When the tricuspid valve is attached to the posterior border of the defect, the sutures can be placed through the base of the tricuspid valve. At the cephalad edge of the defect, the aortic valve may be injured unless extreme care is exercised in placing the sutures.

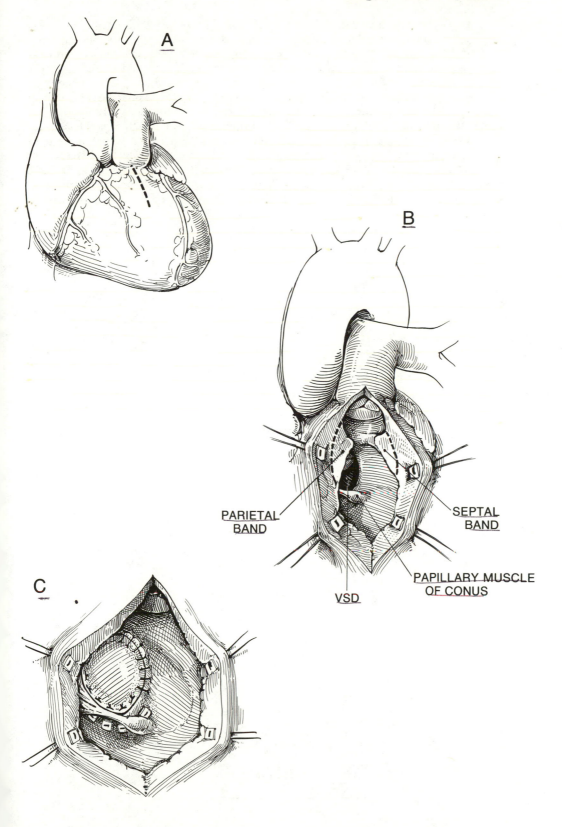

PARIETAL
BAND

SEPTAL
BAND

PAPILLARY MUSCLE
OF CONUS

VSD

D.—The pulmonary valve is inverted, and the fused commissures are incised. More commonly, the valve is opened through the pulmonary artery. The pulmonary artery is incised longitudinally. The dome-shaped valve is exposed, and the commissures are carefully incised well back into the anulus. If the valve is bicuspid, both commissures are incised; if it is tricuspid, all three commissures are opened. By staying in the center of the fused commissure when making the incision, subsequent valve insufficiency is minimized. After valvotomy, the anulus is calibrated with Hegar dilators. If it is of appropriate size (Tables 18–1 and 18–2), it is left alone.

E.—The outflow tract is closed with a pericardial patch. The patch must be wide enough (approximately two thirds of the normal circumference; see Table 18–1) to enlarge the inside diameter of the outflow tract to nearly normal. The patch is sutured into place using continuous 4–0 Prolene sutures. A concomitant atrial septal defect or patent foramen ovale should always be sought, and if present, closed.

TABLE 18–1.—INDICATIONS FOR PLACEMENT OF OUTFLOW PATCH IN TETRALOGY OF FALLOT*

WEIGHT (kg)	DIAMETER (mm)†	AREA (mm²)
3	6	28
4	7	38
5	7.5	45
6	8	50
7	9	63
8	9.5	72
9	10	81
10	11	90
12	12	113
14	13	126
16	13.5	144
18	14	162
20	15	177
25	17	225
30	18.5	270
35	20	314
40	20	314

* Assumes desired ratio of pulmonary valve area to weight = 9.
† If diameter is smaller than indicated, patch is placed across the valve anulus.
From Pacifico A.D., Kirklin, J.W., Blackstone, E.H.: Surgical management of pulmonary stenosis in tetralogy of Fallot. *J. Thorac. Cardiovasc. Surg.* 74:382, 1977.

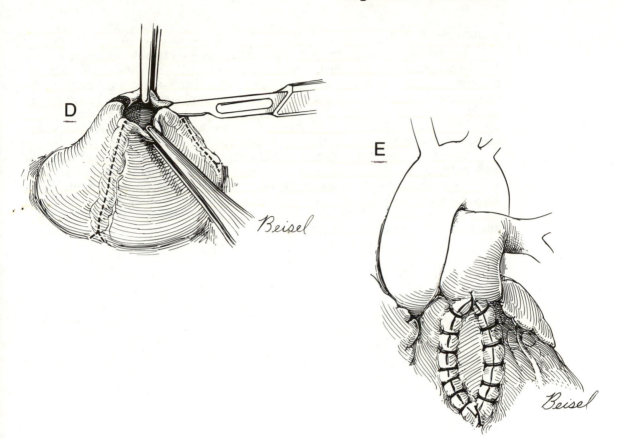

TABLE 18–2.—MEAN NORMAL VALVE DIAMETERS★

BSA (m²)	MITRAL (mm)	TRICUSPID (mm)	AORTIC (mm)	PULMONARY (mm)
0.25	11.2	13.4	7.2	8.4
0.30	12.6	14.9	8.1	9.3
0.35	13.6	16.2	8.9	10.1
0.40	14.4	17.3	9.5	10.7
0.45	15.2	18.2	10.1	11.3
0.50	15.8	19.2	10.7	11.9
0.60	16.9	20.7	11.5	12.8
0.70	17.9	21.9	12.3	13.5
0.80	18.8	23.0	13.0	14.2
0.90	19.7	24.0	13.4	14.8
1.0	20.2	24.9	14.0	15.3
1.2	21.4	26.2	14.8	16.2
1.4	22.3	27.7	15.5	17.0
1.6	23.1	28.9	16.1	17.6
1.8	23.8	29.1	16.5	18.2
2.0	24.2	30.0	17.2	28.0

Modified from Rowlatt et al: Surgical Clinics of North America (1963). The approximate standard deviations (±) are: mitral < 0.3 m² = 1.9 mm, > 0.3 m² = 1.6 mm; tricuspid < 1.0 m² = 1.7 mm, > 1.0 m² = 1.5 mm. BSA = body surface area.

★ Stark J., deLeval M.: *Surgery for Congenital Heart Disease* (eds.). London, Grune and Stratton, 1983, p. 460.

Transanular Repair

Fig 18–38, A.—If calibration of the anulus shows it to be too small (see Table 18–1) enlargement is indicated. An incision is carried across the anulus into the pulmonary artery. It is preferable to make the incision across the anulus in the commissure between two valve cusps. This will minimize subsequent valve regurgitation.

B.—The pulmonary valve commissures are widely incised, the crista is excised, and the ventricular septal defect is closed.

C.—The entire outflow tract, including the infundibulum, the anulus and the main pulmonary artery, is enlarged with a pericardial patch. The width of the patch at the infundibulum and the anulus should be sufficient to bring the outflow tract at these points to normal size, based on the figures in Table 18–1. Making the patch larger than necessary will contribute to pulmonary regurgitation, a condition poorly tolerated in the postoperative period.

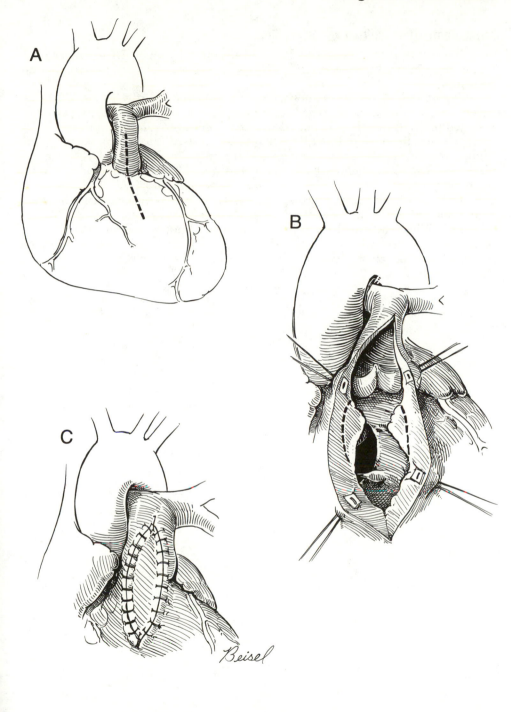

Beisel

Right Ventricular–Pulmonary Artery Conduit

In patients with pulmonary atresia and a ventricular septal defect, total correction is postponed until the age of 5 or 6 years, so that an adequate-sized conduit can be placed.

Fig 18–39, A.—The pulmonary artery is incised, usually to the left of the aortic arch. The ventricle is opened at its highest point. The ventricular septal defect is closed through this incision but can also be closed through the right atrium.

B.—Ideally, a 20- or 22-mm valved conduit is used. Preclotting the prosthesis using a mixture of the patient's blood and thrombin can be helpful. The valve is placed as close to the pulmonary artery as possible. The conduit is sutured to the pulmonary artery using continuous 4–0 or 5–0 Prolene sutures.

C.—The conduit is trimmed appropriately to fit into the ventriculotomy and then is sutured into place using 3–0 or 4–0 Prolene sutures.

D.—When the prosthesis is in place, it should not kink, especially where it inserts into the ventricle. To prevent the prosthesis from being compressed by the sternum, both pleural spaces may be opened to allow the heart to fall away from the anterior chest wall.

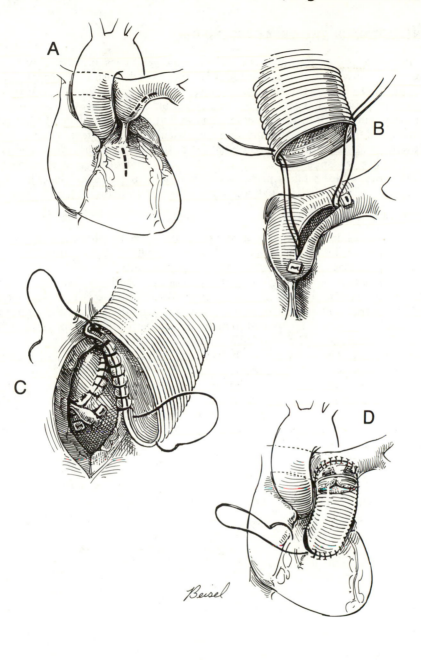

Beisel

TRANSPOSITION OF THE GREAT ARTERIES

In this common anomaly, the atria and the ventricles are normally related to one another. However, the great arteries are transposed, with the aorta arising from the right ventricle and the pulmonary artery arising from the left ventricle. The majority of patients have "simple" transposition in that, aside from the aorto-pulmonary transposition, there are no associated intracardiac defects. Other patients may have an associated perimembranous ventricular septal defect, a left ventricular outflow tract obstruction, or a combination of these two intracardiac lesions.

In simple transposition of the great arteries, vital mixing of pulmonary and systemic venous blood takes place through a patent foramen ovale. This opening must be enlarged by either a balloon septostomy or a Blalock-Hanlon procedure.

Blalock-Hanlon Septectomy

The Blalock-Hanlon operation as a palliative procedure for transposition of the great arteries is seldom used now. It has been replaced by balloon septostomy, which, in most instances, can be carried out successfully.

Fig 18–40, A.—Through a right thoracotomy the lungs are retracted posteriorly and the pericardium is incised anterior to the phrenic nerve. The interatrial groove is exposed. The right pulmonary artery is occluded, as are the right pulmonary veins. A clamp is then applied to include the anterior wall of the right atrium as well as the posterior wall of the left atrium.

B.—Portions of the walls of the two atria are excised along with as much of the septum as possible. A diagrammatic view of the operation is shown (*inset*). By loosening the vascular clamp, additional septum can be pulled into the opening and the resulting atrial septal defect enlarged.

C.—The edges of the walls are then approximated with a continuous 5–0 Prolene suture. The clamps are released as are the Potts ties. Finally, the pulmonary artery is released (*inset*).

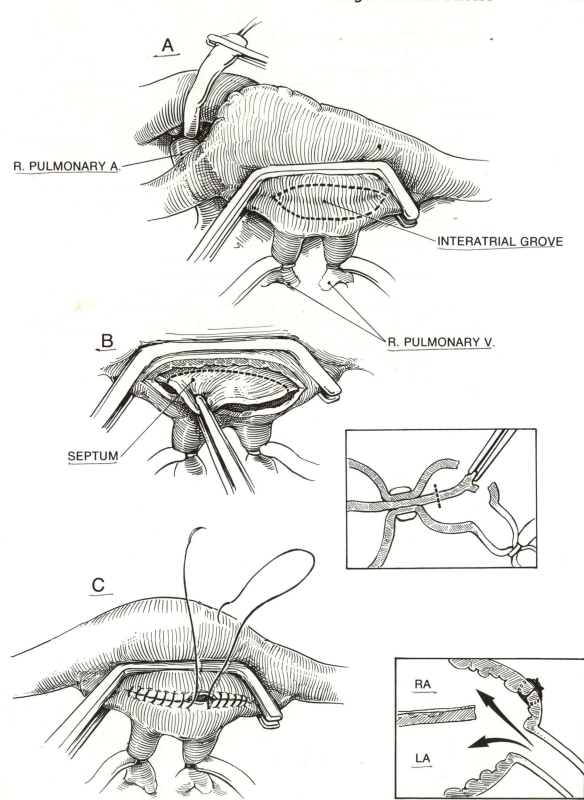

A

R. PULMONARY A.

INTERATRIAL GROVE

R. PULMONARY V.

B

SEPTUM

C

RA

LA

Atrial Switch Operation: The Mustard Operation

Patients with transposition of the great arteries and an intact ventricular septum are candidates for an atrial switch type of operation. This is usually done at 4 to 6 months of age but can be done earlier if the patient shows inadequate palliation or, more commonly, deterioration after balloon septostomy. The results of the Mustard and Senning operations are similar, and the choice depends on the surgeon's preference.

Fig 18–41, A,—The heart (*left*) is exposed through a median sternotomy. A large patch of pericardium is harvested and shaped according to the diagram shown (*right*):

$A \rightarrow B$: Distance between left upper and lower pulmonary veins.
$E \rightarrow D$: Flat diameter of superior vena cava.
$D \rightarrow F$: Flat diameter of inferior vena cava.
α: 30°.
R: 90°.

$$C \rightarrow D = \frac{ED + DF}{2}$$

B.—Venous cannulation is done by placing metal cannulas directly into the superior and inferior venae cavae. The arterial cannula is inserted into the ascending aorta. Cardiopulmonary bypass is established, using deep hypothermia (18–20°C) and cold potassium cardioplegia solution. The right atrium is opened vertically from the atrial appendage to just above the junction of the right superior and inferior pulmonary veins.

C.—The atrial septum is visualized and excised.

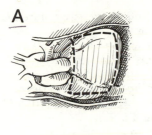

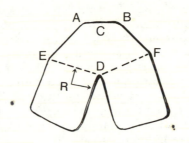

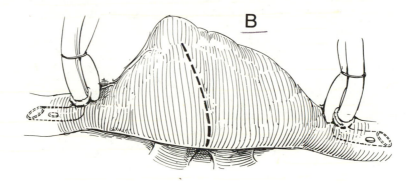

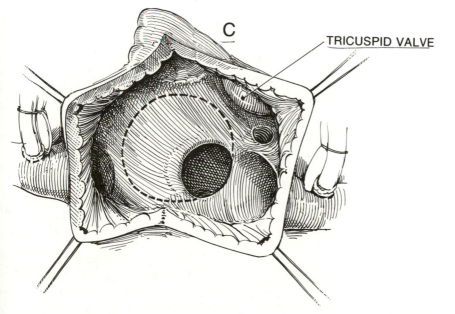

TRICUSPID VALVE

Beisel

D.—Starting to the left of the left pulmonary veins, the previously tailored patch is sutured into place using 5–0 synthetic absorbable suture.

E.—The suture line is carried around the pulmonary veins and the orifices of the venae cavae to the residual septum. Inferiorly, the patch is sutured to the eustachian valve. The coronary sinus is left behind in the new physiologic left atrium.

F.—The new left atrium is enlarged with a diamond-shaped patch of pericardium to prevent pulmonary venous obstruction. If there is an associated ventricular septal defect, it is closed through the tricuspid valve (see Fig 18–23).

In the patient who, in addition to transposition of the great arteries, has pulmonic stenosis, the pulmonary valve is exposed through the pulmonary artery. Fibrous subvalvular obstruction is excised after retracting the valve leaflets with a nasal speculum. Damage to the mitral valve and to the conduction system of the septum must be avoided. Subvalvular muscular obstruction is relieved by incising the muscle anterolaterally and excising part of the muscle.

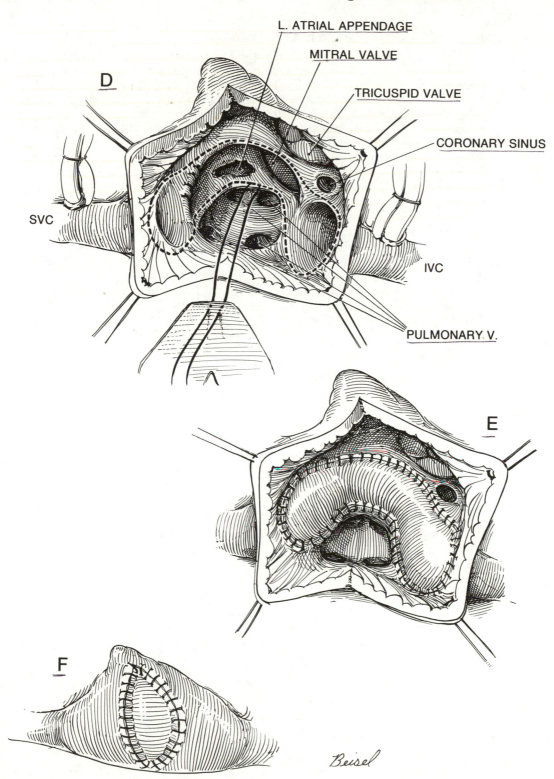

L. ATRIAL APPENDAGE

MITRAL VALVE

TRICUSPID VALVE

CORONARY SINUS

D

SVC

IVC

PULMONARY V.

E

F

Beisel

Atrial Switch Operation: The Senning Operation

This operation is an alternative to the Mustard operation. The results of both operations are similar. However, the Senning operation is preferred by many (including the author) because it is technically easier to perform.

Fig 18–42, A.—The heart is exposed through a median sternotomy. Cardiopulmonary bypass is initiated by direct cannulation of the superior and inferior venae cavae using metal cannulas. The aorta is cannulated in the usual way, and the heart is arrested using cardioplegia solution. The right atrium is incised 5 mm anterior to the sulcus terminalis, and the incision is extended down to the insertion of the eustachian valve at the orifice of the inferior vena cava.

B and C.—A septal flap is developed. Its base extends from the superior aspect of the right superior pulmonary vein to the inferior aspect of the right inferior pulmonary vein (approximately 3 cm). The tip of the flap is wide enough to extend across the orifice of the left pulmonary veins (usually 1.5 cm). The flap must be long enough to extend from the left atrial wall to the right atrial wall (usually 2 cm). This requires insertion of a piece of pericardium in the area of absent septum secundum. Accurate measurements using calipers are helpful.

D.—The tip of the flap is sutured around the left pulmonary vein orifices using 5–0 synthetic absorbable sutures (PDS suture; Ethicon). An initial mattress suture is placed between the orifices of the left pulmonary veins and the orifice of the left atrial appendage.

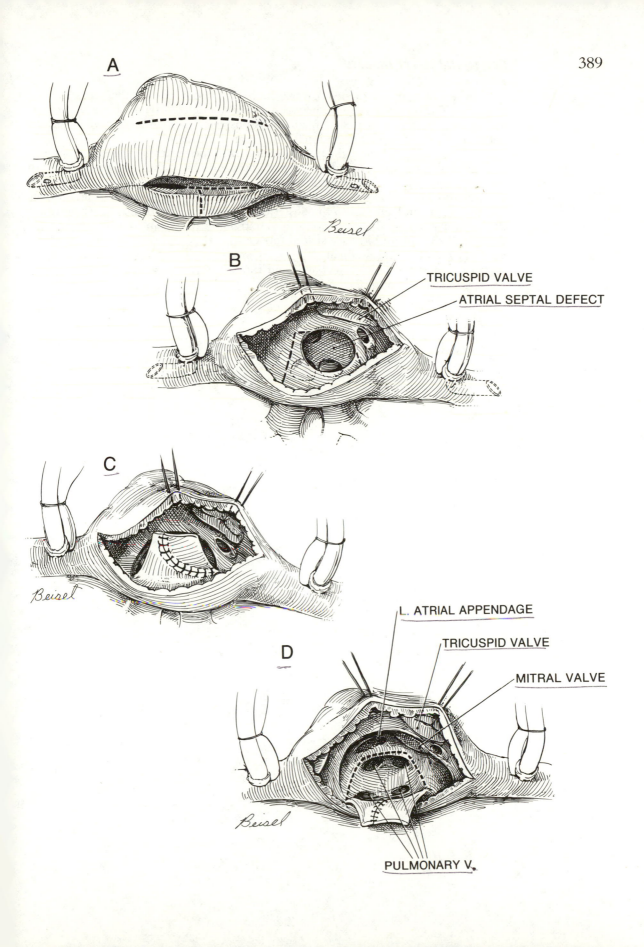

E.—The ends are carried toward the base on both sides of the flap.

F.—The interatrial groove between the right and left atria has been developed, and the left atrium is incised as medially as possible. The left atrial wall is incised between the right superior and inferior pulmonary veins.

The free edge of the right atrium is sutured to the remnant of the atrial septum and the eustachian valve. A catheter is placed through the right atrial appendage into the right ventricle to vent the latter.

G and H.—The anterior edge of the right atrium is not brought down over the vena cavae and sutured to the posterior edge of the left atrium. When suturing the atrial flap across the vena cavae, it is extremely important that it not be constricted. If the suture bites are spaced too widely, they can readily pursestring the vena cavae and compress them. By placing mattress sutures at the junction of the vena cavae and the pulmonary veins and running one arm across the vena cavae, using small bites, compression is less likely.

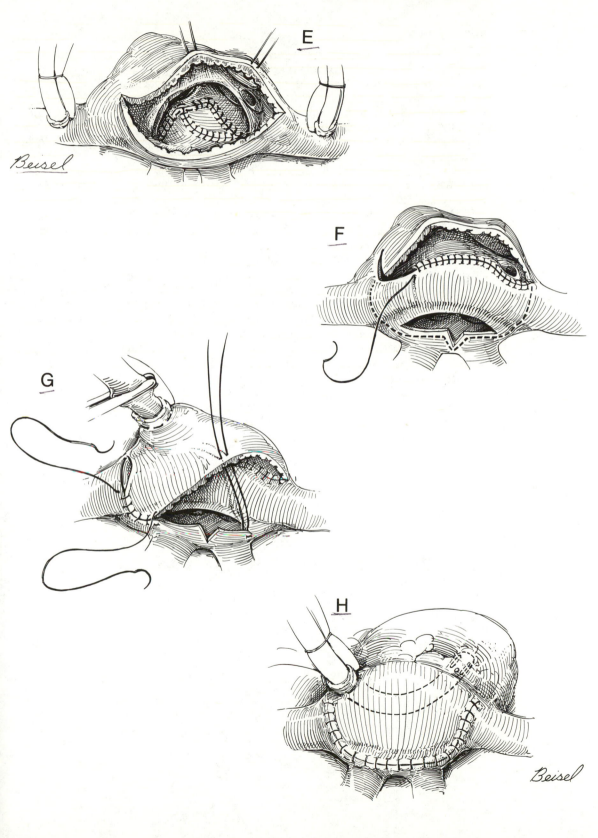

E

F

G

H

Beisel

Beisel

Rastelli Procedure

Although the combination transposition of the great arteries, a ventricular septal defect, and left ventricular outflow tract obstruction can be managed by an atrial switch operation, the results of closing the ventricular septal defect and correcting the subpulmonic stenosis have not been favorable. The Rastelli procedure, which has given good results and has the advantage of converting the left ventricle to the systemic pumping chamber, is preferred.

Fig 18–43, A.—The heart is exposed through a median sternotomy, and cardiopulmonary bypass is instituted in the standard manner.

The pulmonary artery is transected distal to the valve and the proximal end is oversewn. The right ventricle is incised high in the outflow tract, avoiding major coronary arteries.

B.—The ventricular septal defect and the aortic orifice are identified. If the ventricular septal defect is smaller than the aortic orifice, it is enlarged anteriorly to avoid damage to the conduction tissue.

C.—The orifice of the ventricular septal defect is then connected to the aortic orifice by an intraventricular tunnel of Dacron prosthetic material. The patch is cut from a tube graft of the same diameter as that of the aortic anulus. The length of the graft is determined by the distance from the anterior superior edge of the aortic anulus to the posteroinferior margin of the ventricular septal defect. The width is approximately two thirds the circumference of the graft.

D.—The patch is sutured into place with either continuous or interrupted sutures, taking care to avoid the conduction tissue near the posteroinferior margin of the ventricular septal defect.

E.—A conduit of appropriate size is sutured distally to the pulmonary artery. It is essential that the valve be as close to the pulmonary artery as possible to avoid future kinking. The conduit is then tailored to fit into the ventriculotomy and is sutured into place using 3–0 or 4–0 Prolene.

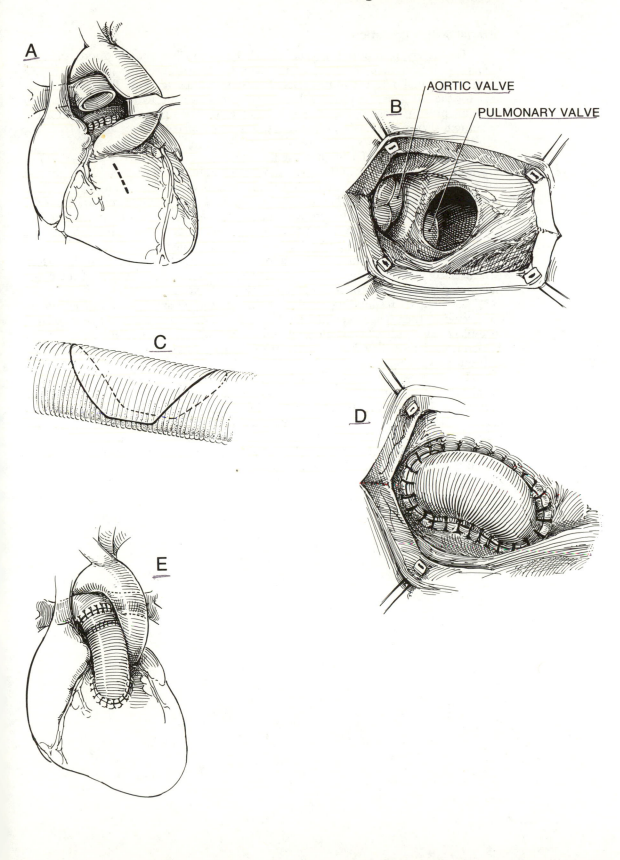

A

B   AORTIC VALVE   PULMONARY VALVE

C

D

E

Arterial Switch Operation

The newly introduced arterial switch operation has shown good promise. Generally, it is limited to those infants with transposition of the great arteries, a ventricular septal defect, and reversible pulmonary hypertension. The last is necessary for the left ventricle to have developed sufficient contractile force to maintain systemic pressure once the operation is completed. The operation should probably be limited also to patients with the left and right coronary arteries arising from the two posterior cusps.

Fig 18–44, A.—Through a median sternotomy, the heart is exposed. The aorta is dissected away from the main and branch pulmonary arteries. The right and left pulmonary arteries are mobilized to the hilum of the lung. The ligamentum arteriosum is divided. Cardiopulmonary bypass and deep hypothermia are initiated. The anatomy of the coronary arteries is inspected, and the site for their transfer into the pulmonary artery marked with fine stitches. The aorta is then cross-clamped and the heart protected with hypothermia and cold cardioplegia solution.

B.—The aorta is transected just above the sinuses, while the pulmonary artery is transected slightly more distally, just above its sinuses. The orifices of the coronary arteries with a rim of adjacent aortic wall are excised.

C.—The corresponding sinuses of the pulmonary arteries are incised where the previous stitches had been placed. The cuff and coronary artery are then sutured into place using either 6–0 Prolene or, preferably, absorbable vascular PDS suture, Ethicon. Care must be taken to rotate the coronary arteries into their new position without kinking them.

D and E.—The distal pulmonary artery is brought anterior to the aorta. The distal aorta is anastomosed to the proximal pulmonary artery using 5–0 Prolene or, preferably, PDS suture. Because of the discrepancy in their sizes, the aorta may require enlargement with a patch of glutaraldehyde-fixed bovine pericardium. Defects created by the excision of the coronary ostia are repaired with patches of bovine pericardium. A patch larger than the defect would enlarge the proximal aorta to match the size of the distal pulmonary artery.

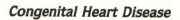

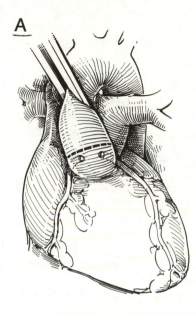

A

B

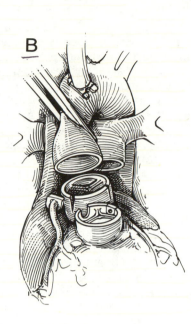

C

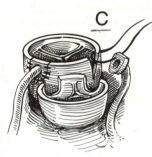

D

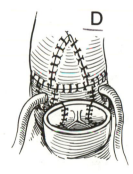

E

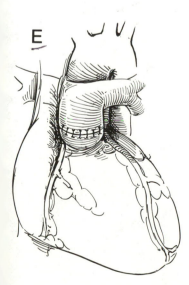

TRUNCUS ARTERIOSUS

Repair

Fig 18–45, A.—In this uncommon anomaly, the pulmonary arteries arise from the aorta either as a single trunk (type I), which occurs most often, or as individual branches (types II and III). A Type IV truncus is actually a pulmonary atresia with a ventricular septal defect (see Fig 18–39). A subvalvular ventricular septal defect is present. The common truncal valve may be tricuspid or have four leaflets and in some patients it is insufficient. Pulmonary hypertension develops early. The surgical management of types I, II, and III is similar. Although pulmonary artery banding has been used with limited success, total correction, even in infancy, is more likely to succeed, even though replacement of the conduit will be required two or three times as a child grows.

The heart is exposed through a median sternotomy. Cannulation for cardiopulmonary bypass is carried out putting the arterial cannula into the distal ascending aorta. Using hypothermia, perfusion is initiated. The pulmonary artery is occluded, and the heart is stopped with cold cardioplegia solution after the aorta has been cross-clamped. The left ventricle is vented with a catheter placed through the right superior pulmonary vein.

B.—The pulmonary trunk is dissected free and is separated from the aorta, leaving adequate tissue to close the aorta without deforming it. The right ventricle is incised high, just below the truncus, using a vertical incision.

C.—The ventricular septal defect is closed using a Dacron patch in such a manner that the truncus arises from the left ventricle. Since the ventricular septal defect is subarterial, full-thickness sutures can be placed without damaging the conduction system.

D.—The largest valved conduit that can be placed in the patient without compression (in an infant, a 12-mm prosthesis) is sutured to the pulmonary artery with 5–0 Prolene, keeping the valve as close to the pulmonary artery as possible. It is essential that this suture line is tight. Bleeding is particularly difficult to control from the posterior suture line.

E.—The proximal prosthesis is tailored to fit into the ventricular incision. It is sutured into place with 3–0 or 4–0 Prolene.

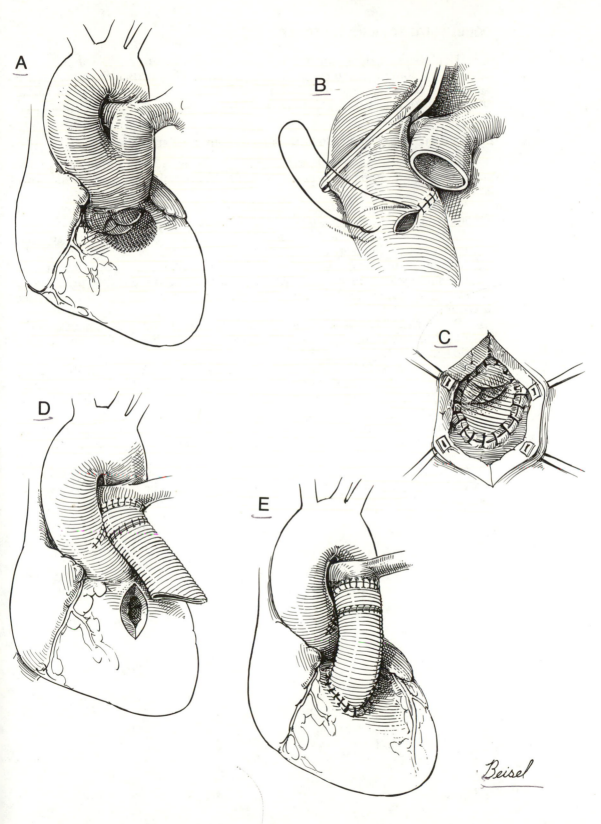

Beisel

DOUBLE-OUTLET RIGHT VENTRICLE

Double-outlet right ventricle is present when more than 50% of each great artery arises from the morphological right ventricle. The ventricular septal defect is categorized according to its relationship to the orifice of the great arteries and can be either a subaortic defect, a subpulmonic defect, a doubly committed defect, or a noncommitted defect.

Double Outlet Right Ventricle With Subaortic Ventricular Septal Defect

In the classic double-outlet right ventricle, the aorta arises to the right of and posterior to the pulmonary artery. The ventricular septal defect is a perimembranous defect.

Fig 18–46, A.—The heart is exposed through a median sternotomy. Using hypothermia and cardiopulmonary bypass, the heart is stopped with cold cardioplegia solution. The left ventricle is vented with a catheter through the right superior pulmonary vein. The ventricular septal defect is exposed, preferably through the right atrium and the tricuspid valve (see Fig 18–20) but may also be exposed through a right ventriculotomy in the infundibulum. The ventricular septal defect's size must be equal to or larger than the aortic anulus. If not, it is enlarged in an anterior direction.

B.—A patch of Dacron is tailored from a tube graft having the same size as the aortic anulus. The length of the graft is determined by the distance from the anterior superior edge of the aortic anulus to the posteroinferior margin of the ventricular septal defect. The width is approximately two thirds the circumference of the graft.

C.—The patch is sutured to the ventricular septal defect inferiorly, with interrupted mattress sutures backed with Teflon felt. The sutures are placed well to the right side of the septal crest to avoid the conduction system. Posteriorly, the defect is sutured to the septal leaflet of the tricuspid valve with unbacked interrupted sutures.

D.—Anteriorly and superiorly, the patch is secured with continuous 4–0 Prolene suture.

In patients with concomitant pulmonic stenosis, the outflow tract is enlarged in a manner similar to that used in tetralogy of Fallot. The insertion of a valved conduit may be required to correct the pulmonic obstruction adequately.

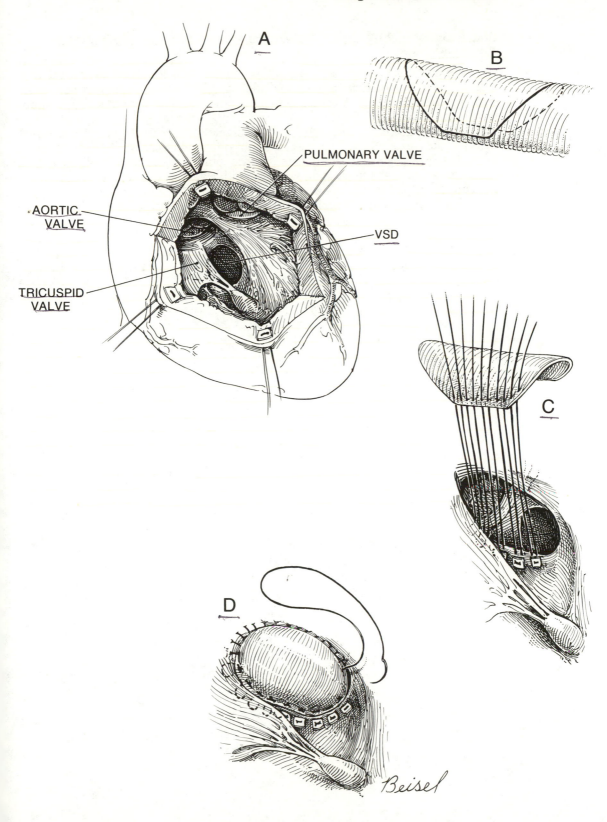

A

B

PULMONARY VALVE

AORTIC
VALVE

VSD

TRICUSPID
VALVE

C

D

Beisel

Double Outlet Right Ventricle With Subpulmonic Ventricular Septal Defect: Taussig-Bing Heart

Fig 18–47, A.—The intraventricular tunnel is usually placed so that the pulmonary artery is in continuity with the left ventricle, creating a complete transposition of the great arteries. An atrial switch operation, such as the Senning operation, is then performed.

B.—A variation is an intraventricular tunnel connecting the ventricular septal defect to the aortic anulus. This may encompass the pulmonary anulus if the latter is immediately adjacent to the aortic anulus. The pulmonary artery is divided and its distal end is connected to the right ventricle with a valved conduit. This technique is particularly helpful in patients with a doubly committed ventricular septal defect. It may also be applicable in patients with a noncommitted ventricular septal defect.

A

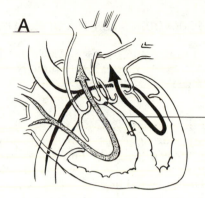

PATCH CLOSING
ANTERIOR
SUBPULMONIC VSD

B

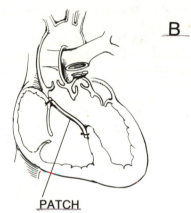

PATCH

RIGHT HEART BYPASS PROCEDURES FOR TRICUSPID ATRESIA

In some instances of cyanotic heart disease, such as tricuspid atresia, palliation has been achieved by diverting the venous return directly into the pulmonary artery. This requires low pulmonary vascular resistance.

Glenn Procedure

An anastomosis of the superior vena cava to the right pulmonary artery permits venous blood to bypass the right side of the heart and go directly into the right lung. It is now rarely performed, since the lung becomes subject to arteriovenous malformations and cyanotic returns.

Fig 18–48, A.—The right pulmonary artery is divided medial to the vena cava. When the superior vena cava is large enough, a clamp may be applied so that blood can go into the right atrium as the anastomosis is being made.

B.—In most instances, we prefer to heparinize the patient and insert a catheter as shown. With heavy ligatures around the superior vena cava above and below the site of the anastomosis, an oval part of the wall of the vena cava may be excised. This allows a good end-to-side anastomosis. We now commonly place a second catheter in the right atrium and connect the two.

C.—Since the blood flows through the tube from the vena cava to the right atrium, the anastomosis can be carefully made with interrupted mattress sutures, everting the edge of the anastomosis. After completion of the anastomosis, the tube is removed, and the vena cava is divided to allow a more direct flow. Because of the greater probability of clotting in a venous anastomosis, heparinization is continued if hemostasis can be adequately controlled. The patient is maintained in the upright position as soon as possible to aid blood flow through the anastomosis into the pulmonary artery. Intravenous therapy is avoided in the upper extremities.

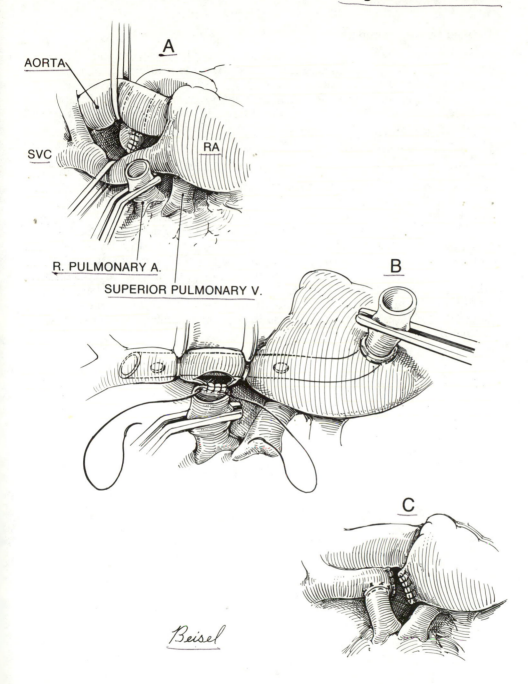

AORTA

SVC

RA

R. PULMONARY A.

SUPERIOR PULMONARY V.

A

B

C

Beisel

Modified Fontan Procedure

This procedure requires a low pulmonary vascular resistance and a large pulmonary artery. If there is no right ventricle, the atrium must be connected to the pulmonary artery with or without a conduit. If a right ventricle is present, even if it is too small, and if there is an adequate pulmonary anulus, the right atrium is connected to the right ventricle, since the latter will assist in expelling blood into the pulmonary artery.

Right atrium-to-right ventricle connection.

Fig 18–49, A.—In the presence of a small right ventricle and an adequate pulmonary anulus, the right ventricle is incised, and the ventricular septal defect is closed. Using flaps from the right atrium as well as from the right ventricle, the posterior wall of the anastomosis is established using 4–0 or 5–0 Prolene suture.

B.—The anterior portion of the connection between the right atrium and the right ventricle is accomplished by placement of either a pericardial or a Dacron patch. The conduit must be large enough to accommodate the entire venous return or, if a previous Glenn procedure had been performed, the inferior vena caval flow. If the conduit is completed with a Dacron tube, the prosthesis should be at least the size of the pulmonary artery. Its width will then be determined by using two thirds of its circumference. The length is determined by the distance between the atrial and ventricular incisions.

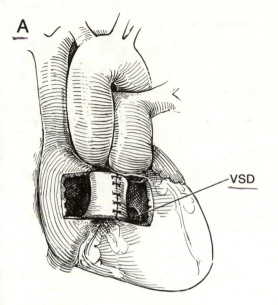

VSD

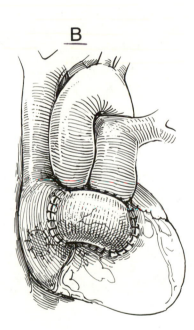

Beisel

Right atrium-to-pulmonary artery connection without conduit.

C and D.—In patients with tricuspid atresia and transposition of the great arteries, the pulmonary artery lies posteriorly and to the right of the aorta. The right atrial appendage is anastomosed to the pulmonary artery, making the anastomosis as large as possible. This may require an anterior patch of pericardium. We have used absorbable synthetic suture for the anastomosis (PDS Suture; Ethicon) to allow future growth. The atrial septal defect is closed through the incision in the atrial appendage.

Right atrium-to-pulmonary artery with conduit.

E and F.—In patients with normally related great arteries, the atrium is connected to the pulmonary artery with as large a Dacron conduit as can be placed. A valve in the conduit is not desirable, since it probably does not function but stays open at all times. The atrial septal defect is closed through the atrial appendage incision.

C

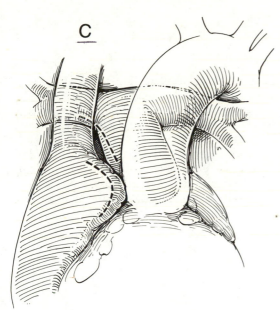

D

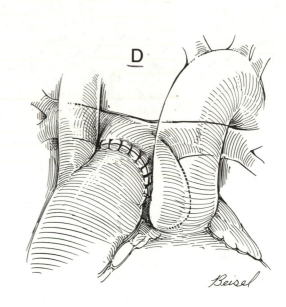

Beisel

E

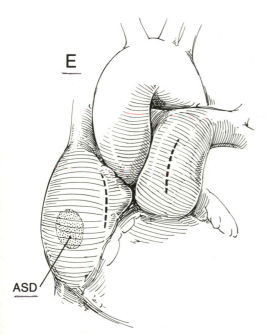

ASD

F

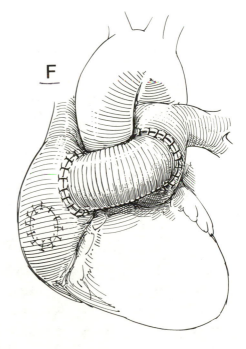

Beisel

EBSTEIN'S ANOMALY

Repair

In this anomaly there is a widely patent foramen ovale. The septal and posterior leaflets of the tricuspid valve are usually displaced down into the right ventricle. The leaflets are thickened, shortened, and adherent to the wall of the right ventricle. The anterior leaflet is large and billowy. The entire right ventricle is dilated and thinned, and the right atrium is greatly enlarged.

Fig 18–50, A.—The heart is exposed through a median sternotomy. Cardiopulmonary bypass is established, and the heart is stopped with cold cardioplegia solution. The right atrium is incised with a curving anterior incision.

B.—The anterior leaflet is reattached to its normal position at the anulus using interrupted plegeted mattress sutures.

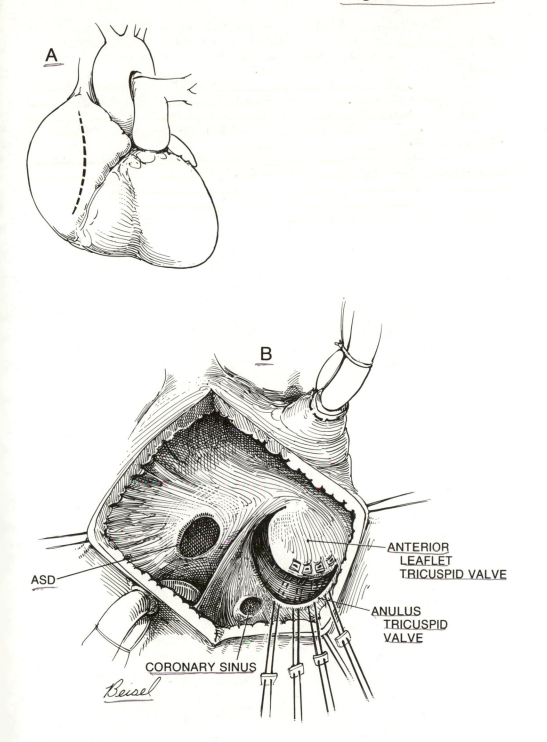

A

B

ASD

CORONARY SINUS

ANTERIOR
LEAFLET
TRICUSPID VALVE

ANULUS
TRICUSPID
VALVE

Beisel

C.—These sutures will imbricate the atrialized portion of the ventricle if they are passed through the myocardium, care having been taken to avoid damaging the coronary arteries externally. To avoid damage to the conduction system, the sutures should not pass beyond the coronary sinus.

D.—The anterior commissure may require an additional plication suture to make the valve competent. The valve is tested by injecting saline solution into the ventricle. The atrial septal defect is closed with a patch of pericardium.

E.—An ellipse is excised from the right atrium to reduce its size, and then the atrium is closed.

On occasion, if the tricuspid valve cannot be restored to reasonable competence, a bioprosthesis can be used to replace it.

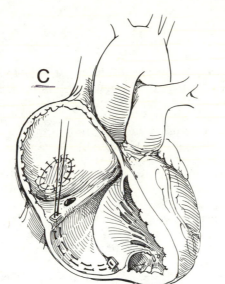

C

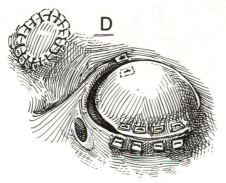

D

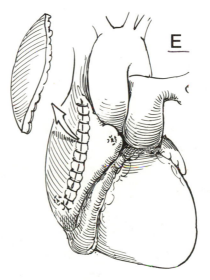

E

Beisel

AORTIC STENOSIS

Supravalvular Repair

Supravalvular aortic stenosis may be localized just distal to the aortic valve and have either a diaphragm-like narrowing, a figure-of-8 narrowing of the ascending aorta, or diffuse narrowing of the entire ascending aorta, extending even into the transverse arch.

The heart is exposed through a median sternotomy, and cardiopulmonary bypass is instituted. The left ventricle is vented. The aortic cannula is placed as distally as possible.

Fig 18–51, A.—The aorta is cross-clamped proximal to the aortic cannula, and the heart is stopped with cold cardioplegia solution. A vertical incision is made into the ascending aorta distal to the narrowing. The incision is brought into the noncoronary sinus across the narrowing and must be extended to the valve anulus. If this incision inadequately opens the aorta, a "Y" extension can be made into the right coronary cusp, taking care not to injure the right coronary artery. When a diaphragm is present, it is excised.

B.—The aorta is enlarged with a preclotted Dacron patch cut from a tube graft the size of the aortic anulus or slightly larger. Glutaraldehyde-fixed bovine pericardium has also been used. The patch should measure one half to two thirds the circumference of the tube graft. If a "Y" incision is made, the patch must be made to have an appropriate extension into both sinuses. The patch is sutured into place with 5–0 Prolene, starting with a pledgeted mattress suture in the noncoronary cusp. Small bites are taken to prevent leakage.

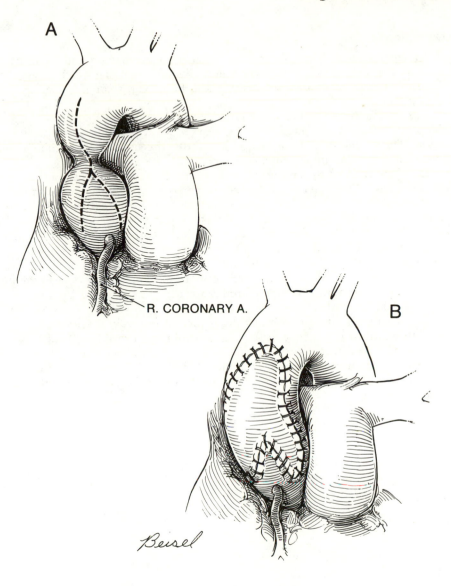

R. CORONARY A.

Valvular Repair

Valvular stenosis is usually seen as a bicuspid valve having both commissures fused and an eccentric orifice, with one leaflet divided by a raphe which appears to be the result of imperfect commissural formation. However, there is a wide spectrum of abnormalities.

Fig 18–52, A.—The heart is exposed through a median sternotomy. Cardiopulmonary bypass is instituted, and the heart is protected with cold cardioplegia solution. The ascending aorta is incised just above the sinus in an oblique manner, the incision extending into the noncoronary cusp.

B.—The aortic wall is retracted with sutures passed through the aortic adventitia. The extent of the valvotomy depends on the type of valvular stenosis found. In monocusp valves, only a single incision is made. As a rule, the extent of the commissurotomy should be related to the height of the developed commissures and the depth of the developed adjacent sinuses. Thus, if the commissural height is normal, the commissure is incised to the anulus. If the commissure and sinus development are only 50% of normal, the valve should be opened only halfway from the central orifice to the aortic valve anulus. If there is only rudimentary sinus development and no height of the commissure (the commissure being represented by a raphe), no incision should be made at all.

C.—Using a knife, the commissure is incised precisely in the midline. After the commissurotomy, the new orifice can be calibrated using Hegar dilators.

D.—The aortotomy is closed with 4–0 or 5–0 Prolene, starting with a pledgeted everting mattress suture at each end of the incision and approximating the edges with a running mattress suture. The initial suture is reinforced with a second over-and-over suture.

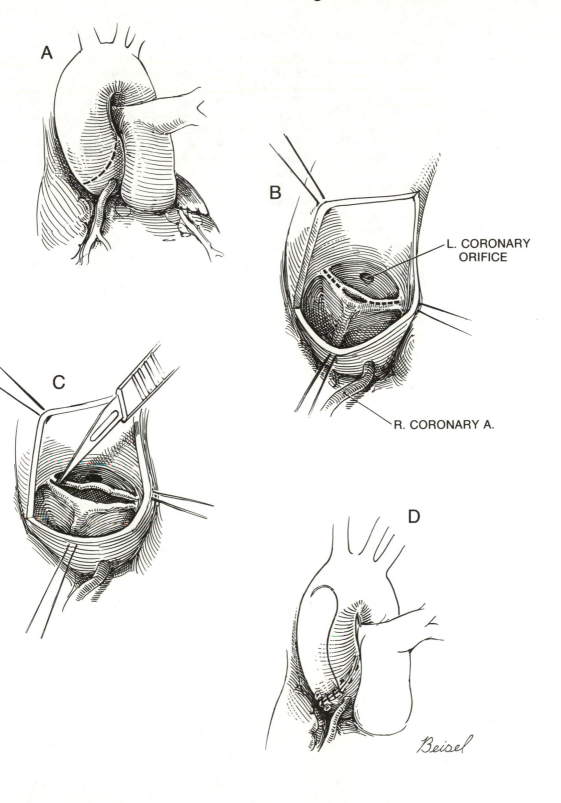

L. CORONARY
ORIFICE

R. CORONARY A.

Beisel

Subvalvular Resection of Membrane

Subvalvular aortic stenosis is often caused by a discrete subaortic membrane.

Fig 18–53, A.—Through a median sternotomy, the heart is exposed. Cardiopulmonary bypass is instituted, and the heart protected with cold cardioplegia solution. The aorta is incised, and the valve leaflet is retracted to expose the diaphragm. Traction sutures are at times placed in the diaphragm to bring it into better view. Fine skin hooks are also helpful in doing this.

B.—With great care, the diaphragm is dissected from the left ventricular outflow tract. The diaphragm is cut away from the ventricular septum and the mitral valve leaflet without injuring either the mitral leaflet or the conduction system. At times, the outflow tract is further enlarged by incising the myocardium to a depth of 5 mm just below the commissure between the right and left coronary cusps.

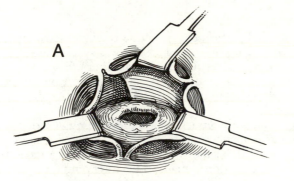

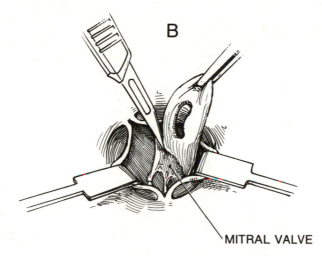

MITRAL VALVE

Morrow Operation

Idiopathic hypertrophic subaortic stenosis is due to asymmetric hypertrophy of the septum in the left ventricular outflow tract. There is systolic anterior motion of the anterior leaflet of the mitral valve. Although a number of surgical procedures have been proposed, the best results are obtained with the Morrow myectomy.

Fig 18–54, A.—Using cardiopulmonary bypass and cold cardioplegia solution, the aortic root is opened.

B.—The aortic valve leaflets are retracted, and the bulging ventricular septum is visualized. The muscle bar is incised just to the right of the center of the right coronary cusp. The incision extends 4 cm down into the ventricle. A second incision 10–12 mm to the left of the first incision is made. This intervening bar or wedge of muscle is then excised by making a transverse incision connecting the two previous incisions. The left ventricle is lavaged with saline solution to remove any debris, and the aorta is closed.

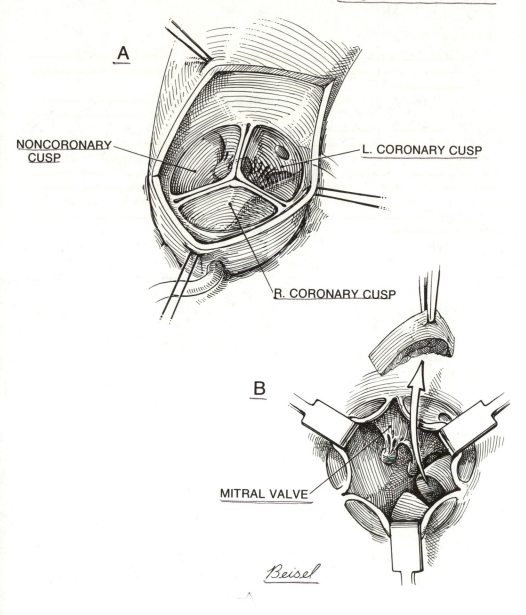

A

NONCORONARY
CUSP

L. CORONARY CUSP

R. CORONARY CUSP

B

MITRAL VALVE

Beisel

Nicks Operation

The Nicks operation is used to enlarge the diameter of the aortic anulus by 2–3 mm so that an adequate-sized valve prosthesis (usually 19 mm for a Björk-Shiley valve prosthesis) can be inserted.

Fig 18–55, A.—The aortic root is incised obliquely, and the incision is extended into the noncoronary cusp.

B.—The valve leaflets are excised, and the anulus is measured with a valve sizer. If the anulus is smaller than desired, the aortotomy incision is extended across the anulus into the right fibrous trigone for a distance of approximately 5 mm.

C.—A blunt wedge-shaped Dacron patch is cut. Its tip is sutured to the apex of the aortotomy with a 4–0 Prolene mattress suture backed with a Teflon pledget. The patch is sutured into place just beyond the anulus using both arms of the suture.

D.—The patch should enlarge the circumference of the anulus by 6–9 mm. It is measured with a valve sizer. An appropriate valve prosthesis is sutured into the natural anulus. In the areas where the patch extends up to the anulus, the valve sewing ring is sutured to the patch with two or three interrupted mattress sutures.

E.—The aortotomy is closed by sewing the remaining part of the patch into place, using both arms of the first suture.

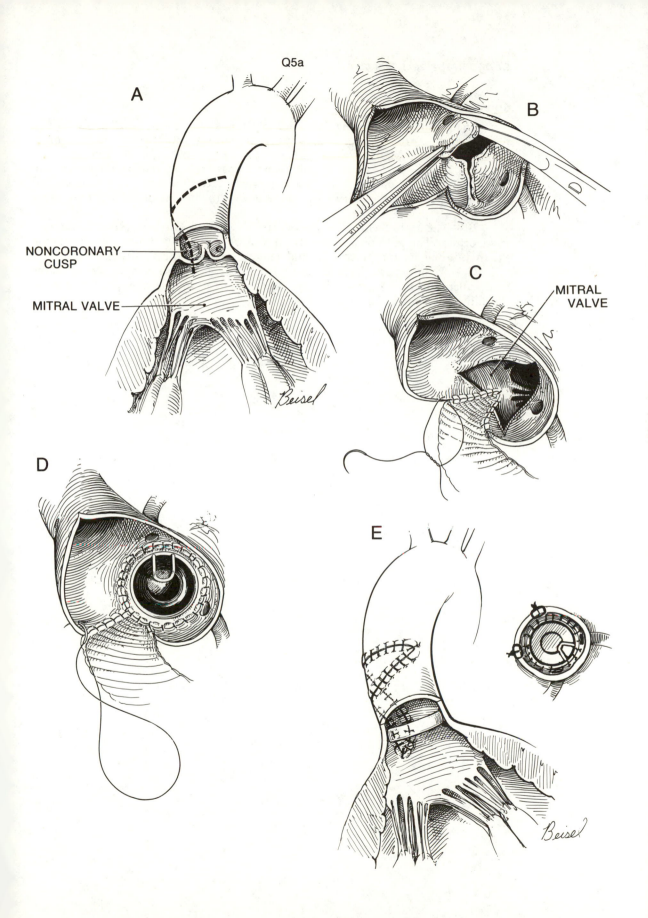

A

Q5a

NONCORONARY
CUSP

MITRAL VALVE

Beisel

B

C

MITRAL
VALVE

D

E

Beisel

Konno Operation

The Konno operation is used either in patients with a very small anulus which requires a valve prosthesis or in those patients with significant subanular fibromuscular obstruction. Many of these patients have a combination of the two lesions.

Fig 18–56, A.—On cardiopulmonary bypass and protecting the heart with cold cardioplegia solution, the aorta is incised vertically. The incision is carried down into the right coronary cusp, staying well to the left of the right coronary orifice.

B.—The right ventricle is incised transversely 1 cm below the pulmonary valve orifice. The pulmonary valve extends more proximally into the ventricle than the myocardial arterial junction would suggest, and it can be easily damaged.

C.—A high incision, staying away from the conduction system, is made in the ventricular septum. The septal incision and the aortotomy are then joined, opening the entire left ventricular outflow tract.

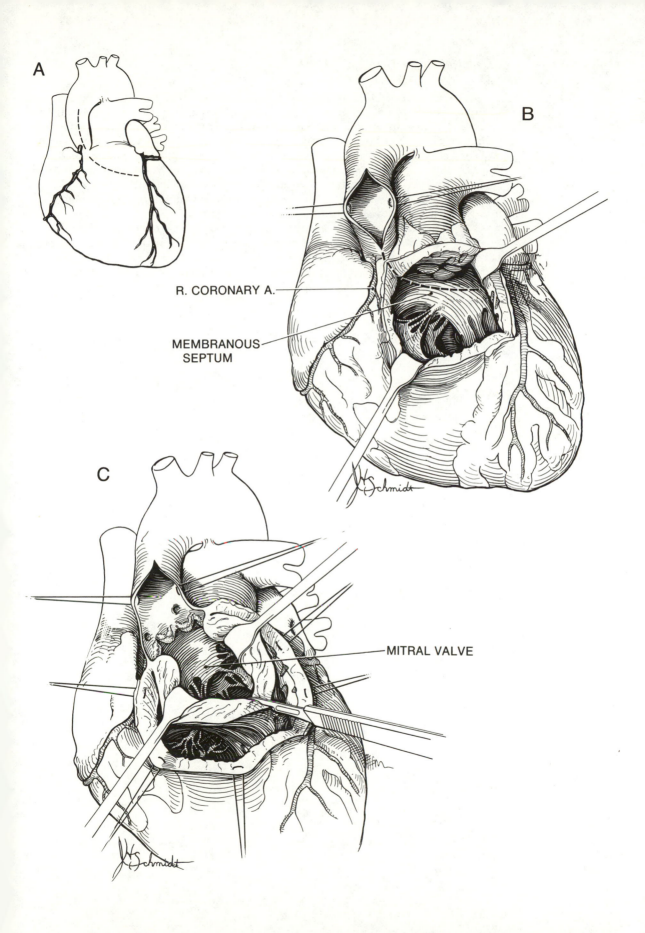

A

B

R. CORONARY A.

MEMBRANOUS
SEPTUM

C

MITRAL VALVE

D.—A patch of Dacron is tailored to fit the area from the septotomy, across the anulus, to the ascending aorta. At the anulus, the patch must be large enough to accommodate an appropriate valve prosthesis (approximately one third to one half of the new diameter). Mattress sutures of 3–0 Dacron backed with Teflon pledgets are passed through the full thickness of the septum and the patch and are tied.

E.—The cut anulus is sutured at each end to the patch, creating an enlarged "anulus." The valve prosthesis is then sutured to the natural anulus (the valve cusps have previously been excised) with mattress sutures. The valve sewing ring is sutured to the patch with a continuous 3–0 Dacron suture.

F.—The patch is sutured into the aortotomy using 4–0 Prolene.

G.—An inverted patch of pericardium, triangular in shape, is sutured at its base across the Dacron patch using 4–0 Prolene. It is then folded back into the ventriculotomy. The two arms of the suture are carried around the triangle to secure the pericardium into the right ventriculotomy.

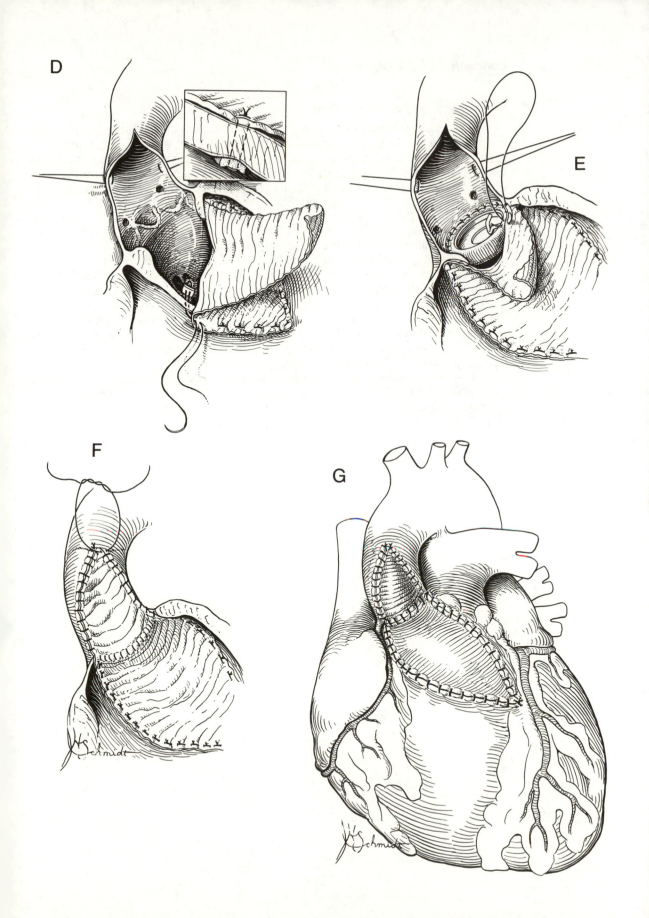

D

E

F

G

Left Ventricular Apicoaortic Conduit

This type of operation has been used in patients with tunnel stenosis of the left ventricle as well as other obstructive lesions. If the diagnosis is evident and if the aortic valve and subvalvar area do not require inspection, the operation can be done with left atrial-to-femoral bypass through a left sixth interspace thoracotomy. Otherwise, it is performed through a median sternotomy, using cardiopulmonary bypass.

Fig 18–57, A.—The apex of the left ventricle is exposed. A stab wound is made in the apex well to the left of the anterior descending coronary artery. A plug of myocardium is excised using a specially devised "cork borer." The hole that is created should be slightly smaller than the cannula to be fitted into it.

B.—A commercially available flanged cannula is inserted into the left ventricle and held in place with several closely spaced pledgeted mattress sutures of 2–0 Dacron. To obtain a leakproof anastomosis, the myocardial edge is sutured to the flange with a running Prolene suture (not shown). The rigid cannula tip must penetrate the entire myocardium to avoid occlusion of the outflow tract during systole. The cannula also must be large enough to readily accommodate the cardiac output (greater than 20 mm in diameter for an adult).

C.—A commercially available conduit with a valve bioprosthesis is sutured to the intracardiac tube. If the approach is made through a median sternotomy, the conduit is sutured distally to the infrarenal aorta. If a left thoracotomy is used, the conduit is anastomosed to the descending thoracic aorta.

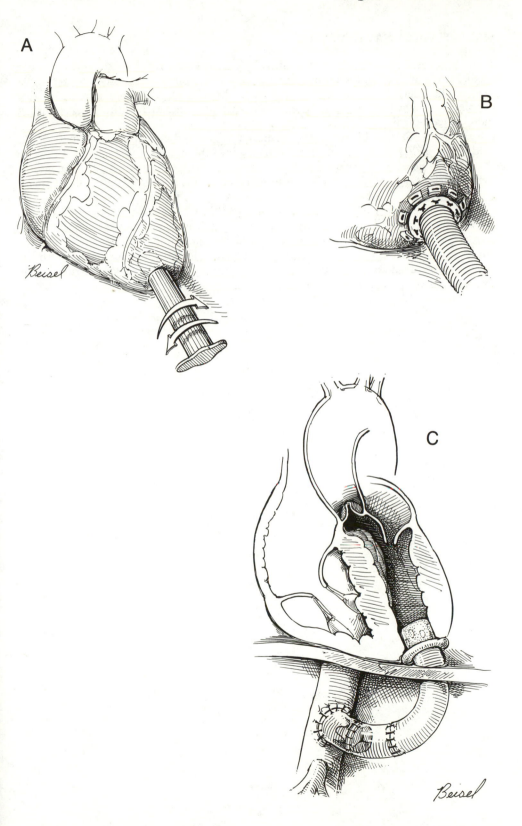

SINUS OF VALSALVA ANEURYSMS

Aneurysms and fistulas of the sinus of Valsalva are a result of separation of the medial aortic wall from the anulus fibrosis. The aneurysms eventually rupture into a cardiac chamber. There is controversy as to the best surgical management of this problem. However, the author prefers a transaortic approach rather than opening the involved cardiac chamber, directly.

Fig 18–58, A.—Using cardiopulmonary bypass, the aortic root is opened and cold cardioplegia solution is infused directly into the coronary ostia.

B.—The aneurysm and fistula are exposed and carefully probed. At times, a "wind sock" can be withdrawn into the aortic root. It is excised, leaving an adequate sewing margin.

C.—The defect is then closed with a patch of Dacron sewn into place with interrupted sutures. Direct closure without a patch is not advisable, since it may distort the aortic valve. On occasion, there is concomitant aortic valve disease, which requires the insertion of a valve prosthesis. Closing the sinus defect with the same sutures used to attach the valve prosthesis has given excellent results. The sewing ring of the prosthesis functions as a buttress for the repair.

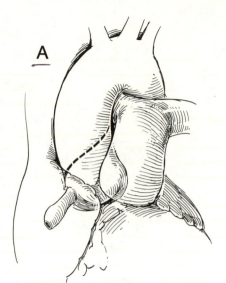

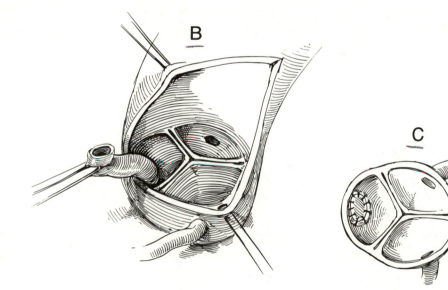

Part IV

Acquired Heart Disease

CHAPTER 19

Repair of Valvular Heart Disease

CLOSED MITRAL COMMISSUROTOMY

LEFT ventricular angiography and ultrasound examination are helpful in determining whether valvulotomy by the closed commissurotomy technique is feasible. More than a trace of mitral incompetence or immobility of the leaflets due to significant calcification indicate that an open technique should be employed. While it is clear that satisfactory, long-term results can be achieved using the closed technique, many surgeons, including ourselves, prefer the open technique.

Fig 19–1, A.—Closed operations on the mitral valve are performed through a left anterolateral thoracotomy performed at the level of the ventricular apex, which is usually the fifth intercostal space. This approach allows use of the transventricular dilator. The pericardium is opened widely.

B.—A generous pursestring suture of 2–0 polypropylene is placed in the atrial appendage and brought through a Rummel tourniquet.

C.—The appendage is then incised and about 200 ml of blood is allowed to spill onto the operative field. This allows any loosely attached atrial thrombus to be expelled from the heart rather than be forced into the circulation either by application of a vascular clamp to the appendage or by advancement of the index finger.

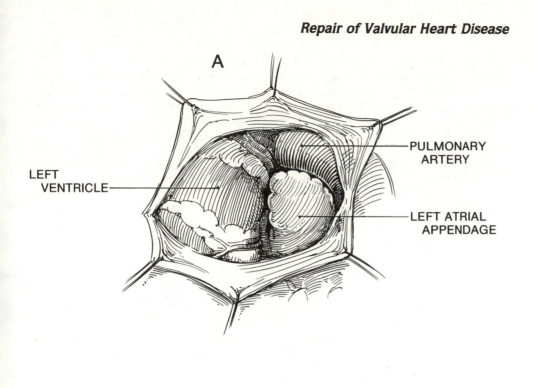

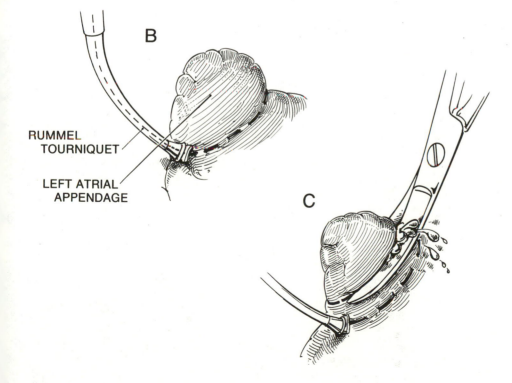

D.—The valve is first explored with the index finger.

E.—A normal valve is shown diagrammatically (*left*). The commissures occupy an anterolateral and posteromedial position and are open nearly to the valve ring (**1**). The least problematic type of defect is shown in the *middle* drawing (**2**). The edges of the valve leaflets are thickened and fused except for the irregular opening, which is slightly posterior to the center of the valve. The drawing on the *right* (**3**) depicts the narrowed opening in a more anterior position. The presence or absence of regurgitation and the general character of the leaflets regarding thickness or calcification or both are assessed during the preliminary exploration.

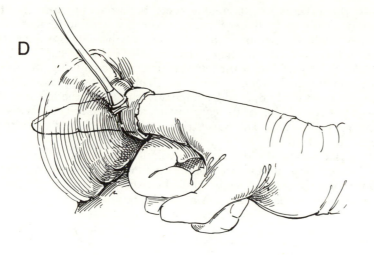

D

ANTEROLATERAL
COMMISSURE

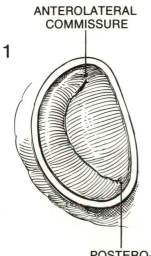

1

POSTERO-
LATERAL
COMMISSURE

E

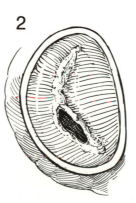

2

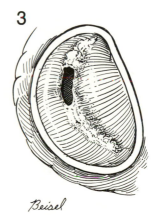

3

Beisel

F.—If the valve is of a favorable type, both commissures may be opened completely or nearly so by finger fracture. Experience and judgment indicate how long to persist with efforts to open the valve digitally before resorting to the dilator. If too great a force is used with finger fracture, there is great danger of tearing the atrial appendage or perforating the left ventricle as the commissure opens. Rather than using too much force, it is wiser to change to the dilator. The posterior commissure is most easily opened by finger fracture from the left side.

G.—After completion of the commissurotomy, the finger is withdrawn, and the appendage is clamped. The pursestring suture is tied, and the incision in the appendage is oversewn.

If the atrial wall is torn during the manipulation of finger fracture, the finger should be kept in the atrium to occlude the opening until the tear can be visualized. A curved vascular clamp can often be applied satisfactorily. If not, the tear should be sutured by an assistant as the finger is gradually removed.

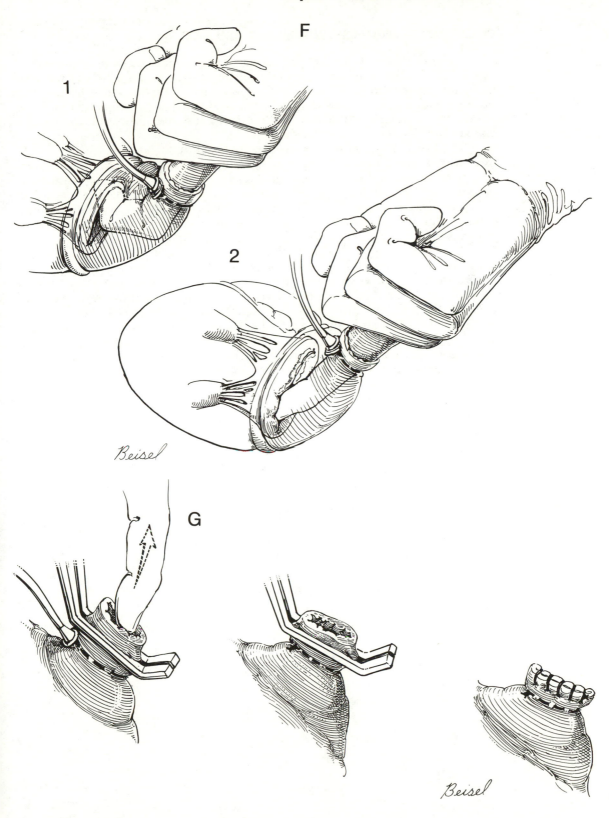

CLOSED MITRAL COMMISSUROTOMY WITH DILATOR

The mechanical dilator has provided a significant advance in the technique of closed mitral commissurotomy. With the dilator, greater pressure can be applied to the commissures and to the valve leaflets than can be applied safely by exerting pressure with a finger. Some surgeons have been so favorably impressed with the advantages of using a dilator that they use it for almost every patient in whom a closed commissurotomy is performed.

Fig 19–2, A.—A heavy synthetic mattress suture, backed with Teflon felt, is inserted in a bare area near the apex of the left ventricle. A Rummel tourniquet is used to prevent blood loss. An oblique tunnel is made through the left ventricular myocardium by passing progressively larger Hegar dilators into the left ventricular cavity so that the muscle fibers are gradually separated rather than cut. The mitral valve dilator is then inserted and passed through the orifice of the mitral valve, where it is readily palpated with the tip of the index finger.

B.—The dilator is usually opened by squeezing together its handles with the left hand. Most dilators have a guard which can be set to limit the opening of the blades and which prevents an uncontrolled rupture of the valve and anulus. It is probably wise to use the dilator only to start the tear in the commissures and then to complete the opening by finger fracture. If this is not possible, further release of the valve may be accomplished by a gradual opening of the blades.

In spite of the greatest care, the valve may be torn by the dilator, resulting in significant regurgitation. Then the surgeon should be prepared to place the patient on cardiopulmonary bypass and either repair the valve or replace it under direct vision.

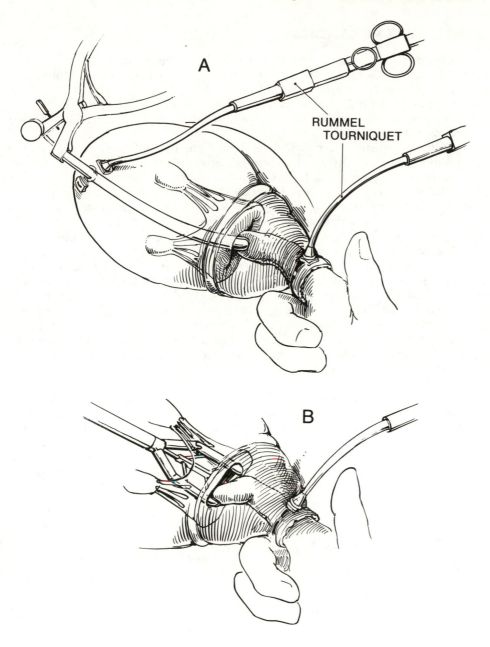

A

RUMMEL
TOURNIQUET

B

OPEN MITRAL COMMISSUROTOMY

Exposure of the mitral valve through the right chest wall has become a standard procedure. This approach can be used in patients in whom a mitral commissurotomy, annuloplasty, or valve replacement is to be performed. It provides excellent valve exposure but the approach limits access to other cardiac structures, such as the coronary arterial tree. In general, we now prefer to perform most mitral valve procedures through a median sternotomy.

With the patient in the right lateral position, the right side of the chest is opened through a standard fourth intercostal space incision. The lung is retracted posteriorly, and the pericardial sac is opened anterior to the phrenic nerve. The pericardial incision extends downward to the diaphragm and upward to the point of reflection on the superior vena cava. An additional incision is made in the pericardium anteriorly and at a right angle to the previous incision, at the level of the right atrial appendage. Traction sutures are inserted in the edges of the pericardium.

Fig 19–3, A.—Heparin (3 mg/kg) is administered, and the arterial perfusion cannula is inserted into the ascending aorta. Cannulas are then introduced into the superior and inferior venae cavae for drainage of venous blood into the heart-lung machine. Large cannulas are used to prevent difficulty with venous return. The inferior vena caval catheter is inserted through an incision in the right atrial appendage. Just before inserting this cannula, it is advisable to introduce the index finger and palpate the tricuspid valve. Unsuspected tricuspid stenosis is occasionally present. The superior vena caval cannula is inserted through an incision in the wall of the right atrium at approximately the position illustrated.

After the institution of cardiopulmonary bypass, the patient's temperature is cooled to 25°C. While cooling proceeds, the cardioplegia cannula is inserted into the ascending aorta, proximal to the aortic perfusion cannula. The aorta is cross-clamped between the aortic perfusion cannula and the cardioplegia solution cannula. Cold cardioplegia solution is infused, and the left atrium is opened.

B.—Exposure of the valve is facilitated with a Cooley-type retractor. The valve can be seen clearly when the blood level has been lowered below the valve.

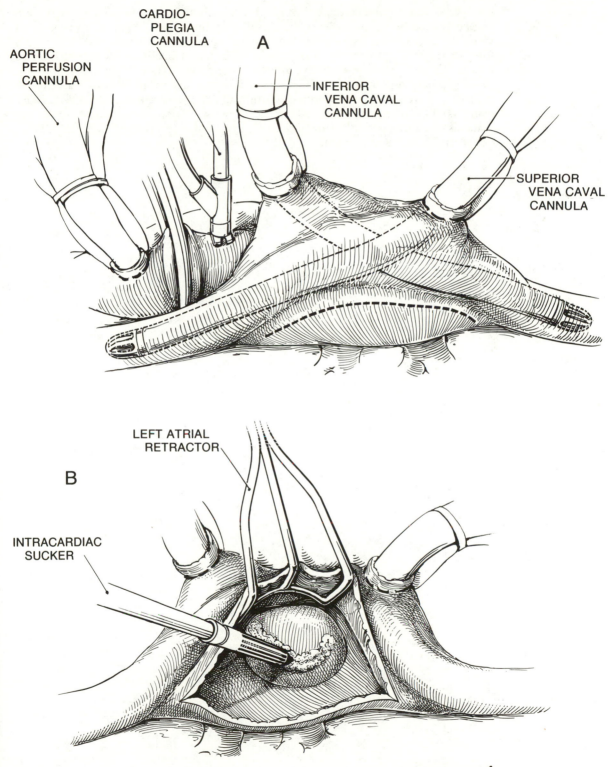

CARDIO-
PLEGIA
CANNULA

A

AORTIC
PERFUSION
CANNULA

INFERIOR
VENA CAVAL
CANNULA

SUPERIOR
VENA CAVAL
CANNULA

B

LEFT ATRIAL
RETRACTOR

INTRACARDIAC
SUCKER

Beisel

C.—The valve is carefully inspected. Elevation of the valve leaflets with right-angled Blanco retractors exposes the chordae tendineae and enables the operator to visualize the exact location of the commissural plane. Both a bistoury blade and a long clamp are helpful in separating the fused leaflets. Usually, with care, the fusion can be relieved almost to the valve anulus. In certain instances, careful incision of a fused papillary muscle head will provide added mobility to the leaflets. Valve competence is tested by injecting saline solution under pressure into the left ventricle, using a bulb syringe and visually checking for regurgitation. After completion of the commissurotomy, atrial closure and air removal are accomplished as described under Mitral Valve Replacement.

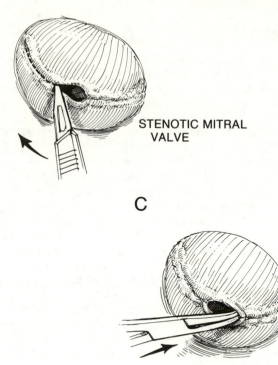

STENOTIC MITRAL
VALVE

C

MITRAL ANNULOPLASTY

Often some degree of mitral insufficiency occurs in conjunction with mitral stenosis. As the valve leaflets become thickened and scarred, there is an increasing tendency for the valve orifice to become fixed. The valve leaflets cannot come together during systole; thus, there is regurgitation. Contraction of the papillary muscles and the chordae tendineae also decreases the effective length of the leaflets. In patients with severe mitral insufficiency, the pathologic process may be as described below.

Fig 19–4, A.—Mitral insufficiency may be present even when the leaflets are relatively normal because of dilatation of the anulus. Often there is an associated lengthening of the chordae tendineae of the septal leaflet which causes it to prolapse above the mural leaflet even though the anulus has been shortened. In this case, the valve must be replaced. If the chordae tendineae are not lengthened too severely, however, regurgitation may be overcome by shortening the anulus. A heavy, nonabsorbable mattress suture is placed deeply in and around the anulus, adjacent to the posterior part of the mural leaflet. The suture is backed with a pledget of Teflon fabric to decrease the likelihood of its pulling through. More than one suture may be necessary.

When there is a deformity of the leaflets in addition to the dilatation of the anulus, it is most often in the posterior portion of the mural leaflet as shown; thus, the mattress suture is placed in this location. An "annuloplasty" at the anterior commissure is used less often. The chief limitations of annuloplasty are its tendency to produce stenosis, the difficulty of ascertaining whether or not the regurgitation has been completely corrected while the heart is still open, and the tendency toward recurrence of regurgitation due to either a partial pulling through of the sutures or a further enlargement of the anulus. Valve competence is tested by injecting saline solution under pressure into the left ventricle with a bulb syringe.

B.—If the mitral insufficiency is a result of generalized anular dilatation, use of the D-shaped ring, as described by Carpentier, has been helpful. A ring that is similar in size to the septal leaflet of the mitral valve is selected.

C.—Interrupted sutures, placed just beyond the base of the leaflet, are then passed through the ring.

D.—The ring is positioned and the sutures are tied.

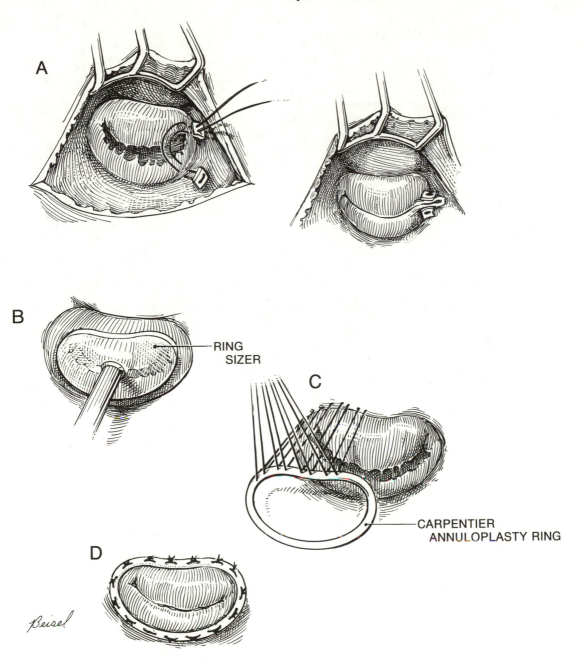

RING
SIZER

CARPENTIER
ANNULOPLASTY RING

Beisel

MITRAL VALVE REPLACEMENT

Thickening, distortion, and calcification are often present to such an extent that adequate valve function cannot be achieved with any procedure utilizing the patient's own tissues. Under such circumstances, total replacement of the valve offers the best chance for a favorable long-term result. Many types of artificial valves have been used. The Starr-Edwards ball valve, the Bjork-Shiley tilting disk valve, the stent-mounted porcine valve, and the stent-mounted bovine pericardial valve have all provided excellent results. The technique employed with the ball valve is illustrated, and a similar technique is employed with the other prosthetic valves.

Replacement of the mitral valve is generally performed through a median sternotomy.

Fig 19–5, A.—In preparation for mitral valve replacement, the pericardium is opened widely. Heparin is administered, and the aortic cannula is inserted through a stab wound high in the ascending aorta. Vena caval cannulas are inserted, and bypass is initiated. The patient is cooled, and a cannula is inserted into the ascending aorta for the administration of cardioplegia solution. When the body temperature has dropped to 25°C or when ventricular fibrillation occurs, the aorta is cross-clamped, and cold cardioplegia solution is given.

B.—The left atrium is opened widely through an incision beginning at the junction of the right superior pulmonary vein and the left atrium. The valve is exposed by use of a Cooley-type mitral valve retractor and by tilting the operating table away from the surgeon. The vulnerable position of the main circumflex artery, which is located in the posterior atrioventricular groove, is shown (*inset*). A suture placed too deeply in the posterior or mural leaflet edge can encircle this artery. There is also the possibility of encircling a portion of the atrioventricular node, which is located above the junction of the anterior (septal) leaflet and the posterior commissure. Accordingly, complete heart block may occur following mitral valve replacement.

A

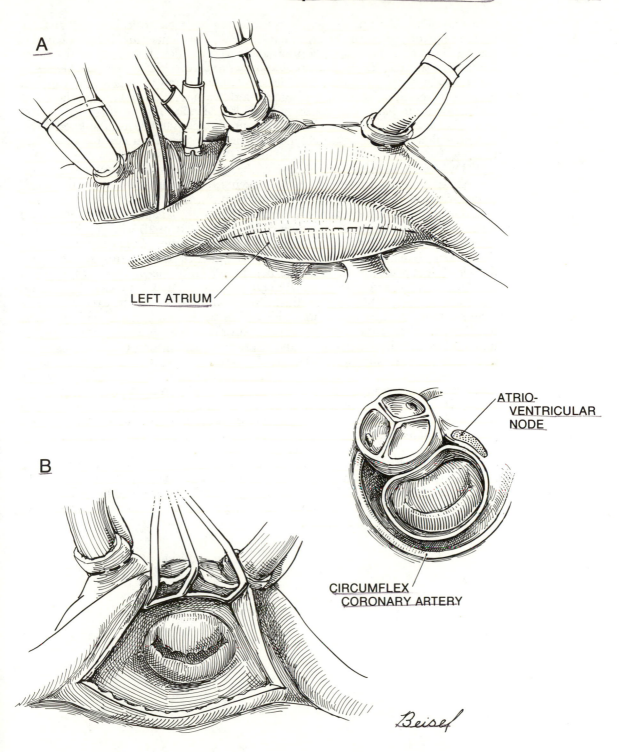

LEFT ATRIUM

B

ATRIO-
VENTRICULAR
NODE

CIRCUMFLEX
CORONARY ARTERY

Beisel

C.—When the mitral valve is excised, it is desirable to leave a rim of valve tissue rather than to excise the valve in its entirety. This remaining tissue is helpful in placing sutures in the proper position and gives additional strength to the tissue holding the sutures. It is particularly important to leave a cuff of the mitral leaflet in the region of the aortic valve. The chordae tendineae and the tips of the papillary muscles are removed sufficiently to avoid interference with the function of the valve. It is important to have adequate room in the left ventricle for the prosthesis, so it is probably better to use a valve that is "too small" than one that is "too large." In a patient with a small left ventricle, a disk-type valve may be preferable to the ball type.

D.—Many different techniques have been used to suture the valve into place. The objective is to distribute the tension evenly to the circumference of the mitral orifice. Suturing is begun at the anterior commissure and continued clockwise. Exposure of the anulus is improved as successive sutures are placed. If the valve rim is fibrous in nature, figure-of-8 sutures of 2–0 Dacron are used, with two bites being taken in the tissue with the same needle. If the anulus tissue is flimsy or calcified, the risk of perivalvular leak can be reduced by using felt-backed mattress sutures, with the felt pledget placed in the subanular position. With this technique, each needle of the double-armed suture is passed through the tissue anulus and then through the valve sewing cuff. When using a disk valve, we prefer to use a pledgeted mattress suture with the pledget on the atrial side to prevent any interference with the valve mechanism. In the patient with a large left atrium and an anulus of fibrous tissue, time may be saved by inserting a simple suture in each quadrant and then using an over-and-over running suture to secure the valve.

E.—The valve is in place with all the sutures tied. The valve holder which keeps the valve incompetent has been replaced with a small catheter through the valve. When using a Björk–Shiley valve, the surgeon should insert the catheter through the lesser orifice to ensure subsequent easy removal. As the heart is filled with blood, the left ventricle should be massaged to evacuate any residual air before the left atrium is closed and the catheter is removed.

F.—The atrial incision is closed with a 3–0 polypropylene suture using a mattress technique, which is then reinforced with an over-and-over suture. The suturing is done from either end of the incision and the sutures tied in the middle of the incision. For clarity of illustration, the catheter used to maintain incompetence of the prosthetic valve is not shown.

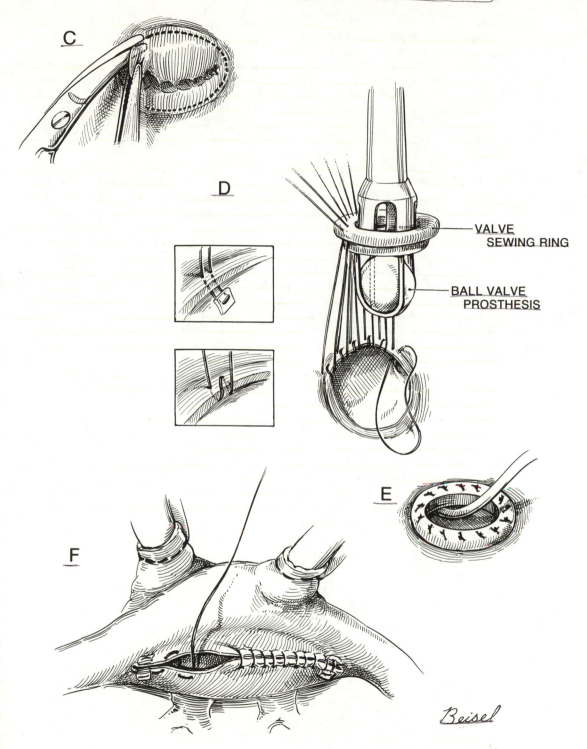

C

D

VALVE
SEWING RING

BALL VALVE
PROSTHESIS

E

F

Beisel

AORTIC VALVE REPLACEMENT

Patients with hemodynamically significant acquired aortic valve disease, which may be a result of rheumatic or atherosclerotic heart disease, almost always require valve replacement. Moreover, many patients with bicuspid aortic valves ultimately will develop stenosis due to degenerative changes and calcification of the valve. Tissue, ball-in-cage, and tilting disk valves are in common usage. The Bjork–Shiley tilting disk valve has a large orifice-to-anulus ratio and provides considerable advantage in the patient with a small aortic root.

Fig 19–6, A.—A median sternotomy provides excellent exposure of the aortic valve. After cannulation has been completed, cardiopulmonary bypass is begun, and the patient's temperature is cooled to 22°C. A small cooling pad is wrapped around the ventricles to provide external myocardial cooling. A vent is inserted through the junction of the right superior pulmonary vein and left atrium and is passed across the mitral valve into the left ventricle. When the heart fibrillates or when the myocardial temperature is below 30°C, the aorta is cross-clamped. The valve is exposed through a curved aortic incision that extends into the midportion of the noncoronary cusp.

B.—The cardioplegia solution cannula (12–14 F) is purged of air, and about 500 ml of solution (7 ml/kg) is infused into the left coronary orifice. About half of that amount (3 ml/kg) is then infused into the right coronary orifice. The goal is to stop all electrical activity and to bring the septal temperature (thermistor needle) to 12°C or lower. Lesser amounts of cardioplegia solution are infused every 20–30 minutes during the procedure to maintain an acceptable myocardial temperature.

C.—It is usually advisable to remove the major portion of the diseased aortic leaflets, leaving only a rim of tissue at the base of the cusp. This tissue is often thick in patients with aortic stenosis, but may be quite thin in patients with aortic regurgitation due to a dilated aortic root with attenuated leaflets. When the leaflets are calcified, care should be taken to prevent bits of calcific debris from falling into the left ventricle. A gauze sponge in the left ventricle collects some of the debris, and forceful irrigation of the left ventricle with 500 ml of fluid helps in the removal of any remaining particles.

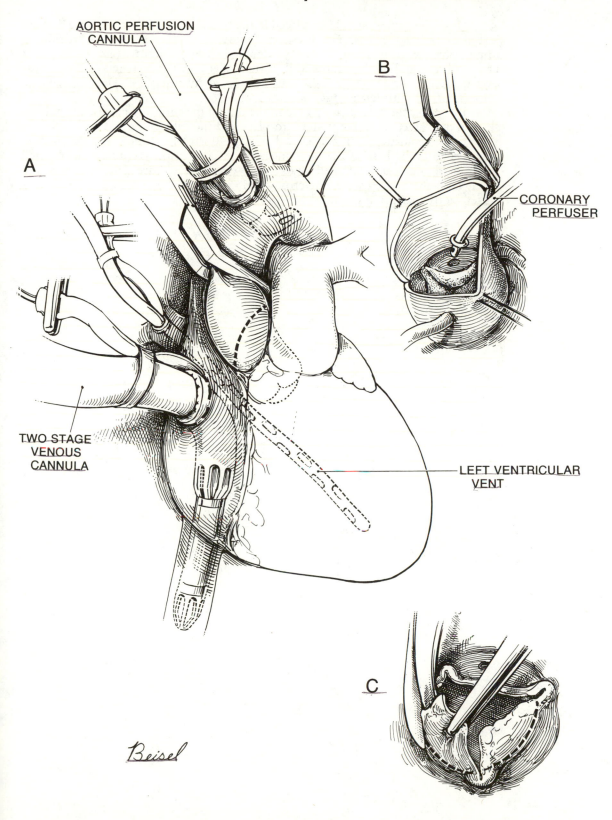

AORTIC PERFUSION
CANNULA

A

B

CORONARY
PERFUSER

TWO STAGE
VENOUS
CANNULA

LEFT VENTRICULAR
VENT

C

Beisel

D.—The sutures should be placed in the tissue of the root of the aorta and not just in the residual leaflets. This is especially important when the leaflets are thin, as in pure aortic regurgitation. We take a double bite in the anular tissue if the leaflet base is fibrous and holds sutures well. If the leaflet base is attenuated or if calcification is present, perivalvular leaks can be avoided by using 2–0 Dacron mattress sutures backed with felt pledget (shown).

E.—After the sutures are placed in the root of the aorta and passed through the skirt of the valve, the valve is slid into place and the sutures are tied.

F.—The aortic incision is closed using 4–0 Prolene suture. The first suture row, begun at the base of the incision, is placed as a mattress suture. The everted aortic incision is then reinforced by over-and-over suture. Care is taken to evacuate all air from the aortic root as the cross-clamp is removed and the aortic incision is closed (aortic perfusion cannula not shown).

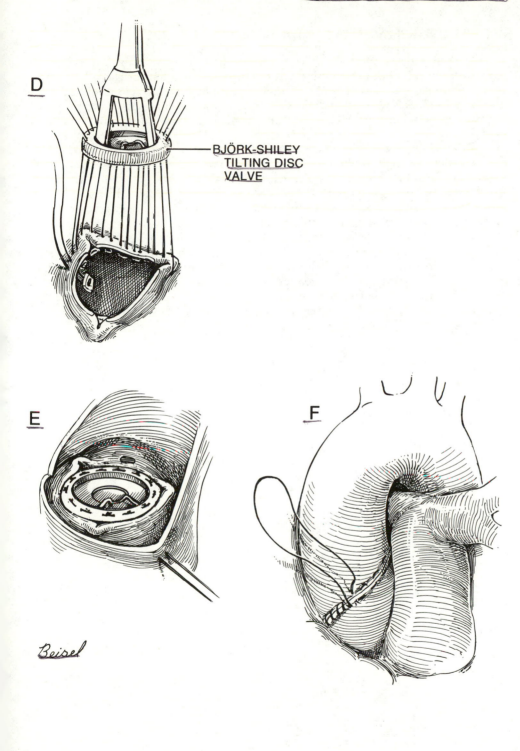

BJÖRK-SHILEY
TILTING DISC
VALVE

Beisel

AORTIC VALVE REPLACEMENT IN THE NARROW AORTIC ROOT

Certain patients with aortic valve disease have a narrow aortic root. If the narrowing includes both the anulus and the proximal segment of ascending aorta, aorto annuloplasty using the Nicks or Konno procedure is indicated (see page 422).

Fig 19–7, A.—In certain patients, the narrowing is confined to the proximal segment of ascending aorta. The aortotomy is made and extended into the noncoronary cusp.

B.—While a standard size Bjork-Shiley valve can be inserted, the aorta above the anulus is too small to allow the disk of the valve to open properly (inadequate tertiary orifice). In a similar manner, should a ball valve be inserted, inadequate space would exist between the ball and the aortic wall. This would result in improper valve function and an unacceptable systolic pressure gradient across the left ventricular outflow tract even during resting cardiac output.

C.—The aortic root is enlarged with a diamond-shaped patch of glutaraldehyde-preserved bovine pericardium or preclotted Dacron graft. Adequate enlargement of the aortic diameter requires the width of the patch to be greater than might be thought. For example, to enlarge the aortic diameter from 20 to 30 mm, the patch must be 30 mm at its widest point (new circumference = 30 π or 90 mm, original circumference = 20 π or 60 mm; width of patch needed to obtain new diameter = 90 mm − 60 mm = 30 mm).

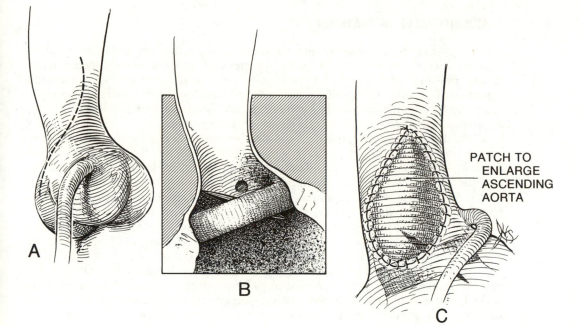

PATCH TO
ENLARGE
ASCENDING
AORTA

TRICUSPID VALVE OPERATIONS

Tricuspid regurgitation frequently accompanies mitral valve disease, particularly in patients with pulmonary artery hypertension. In such patients, competency of the tricuspid valve should be restored to provide the best chance for a good postoperative result. If tricuspid regurgitation is a result of anular dilatation, competency can be restored frequently by annuloplasty. We have found that the DeVega technique is effective and adds little to the operating time.

Fig 19–8.—The tricuspid valve is clearly visualized during cardiopulmonary bypass after the occluding tapes have been tightened to isolate the vena caval return. A double-armed, felt-pledgeted '0' polypropylene suture is placed, beginning at the anteroseptal commissure and continued around to the level of the coronary sinus orifice. It is put in the valve anulus, 1–2 mm beyond the base of the leaflet. The remaining arm of the suture is similarly placed but with the suture bites taken alternately to those in the first row. The suture is tied over a pledget with sufficient tension to reduce the anular area by about one third. Testing for competence by injecting saline solution into the ventricle is quite helpful.

In the patient with tricuspid regurgitation or stenosis that is a result of leaflet fibrosis or fusion, valve replacement using a bioprosthesis is usually necessary. Felt-backed mattress sutures are placed relatively superficial in the leaflet tissue along the septum. This prevents injury to the atrioventricular node and subsequent heart block.

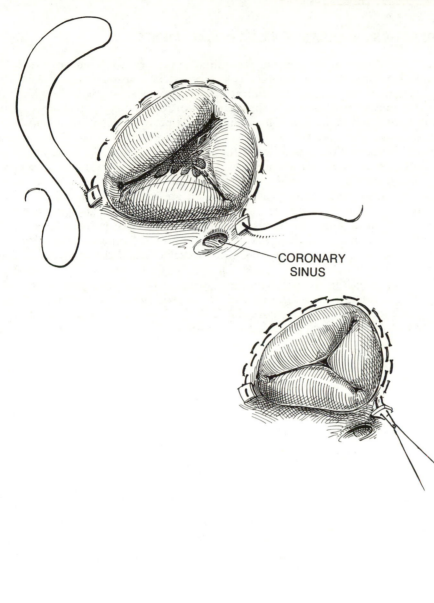

CORONARY
SINUS

CONSIDERATIONS IN MULTIPLE VALVE REPLACEMENTS

Not uncommonly, the surgeon is required to perform multiple valve replacement with or without accompanying coronary artery bypass grafts. It must be remembered that exposure of the mitral anulus may be extremely difficult in a patient with a prosthetic aortic valve because the aortic prosthesis prevents the aortic root from completely collapsing. Thus, our typical operative plan in a patient who is to have an aortic and mitral valve replacement for aortic regurgitation and mitral stenosis and regurgitation is as follows: Initiate cardiopulmonary bypass, cool patient to 20°C, cross–clamp aorta when heart fibrillates, open aorta, infuse cardioplegia solution to obtain myocardial septal temperature of 12°C, excise aortic valve, determine proper aortic prosthesis size, open left atrium, replace mitral valve, replace aortic valve, close left atrium, close aorta, and de–air aorta and left ventricle. Cardioplegia solution must be administered periodically. Tricuspid valve operations do not require the retraction required for exposure of the mitral anulus. Accordingly, tricuspid valve surgery is best performed after mitral and aortic valve procedures.

Aortic cross–clamp times for multiple valve and combined procedures may exceed 2½ hours. The risks associated with these procedures can be minimized by ensuring absence of electrical activity and a myocardial septal temperature at or below 12°C by the periodic (every 20–30 minute) infusion of cold cardioplegia solution.

CHAPTER 20

Coronary Artery Surgery

S CORONARY ARTERY BYPASS USING THE SAPHENOUS VEIN

URGERY for coronary artery disease has evolved over the past 15 years to become the most commonly performed cardiac procedure. Although there remains considerable debate as to the indications for coronary bypass surgery, it is generally agreed that a patient with left main coronary obstruction should have a bypass operation. Other patients with obstruction of one or more coronary artery branches should have an operation if they are refractory to medical management (class III or IV angina). Age and lifestyle must also be considered, since the operation does give far better relief of symptoms when compared to medical treatment.

Fig 20–1, A.—In preparation for coronary artery revascularization, a median sternotomy is made, and the ascending aorta is cannulated as far distally as possible. Ordinarily, the cannulation site is on the inner aspect of the aorta next to the pulmonary artery. This position avoids the origin of the innominate artery and provides more space for applying a partial occlusion clamp for the proximal anastomosis of the bypass grafts. We use a two-stage cannula,* with the larger proximal portion positioned in the right atrium and the extension, of smaller diameter, placed into the inferior vena cava. If the right coronary artery is occluded proximally, two vena caval cannulas with snares are employed to prevent the warmer venous return blood (25°C) from entering the right atrium and ventricle. After bypass has been established, the patient is cooled to 25°C, and the aorta is cross-clamped. Cold potassium cardioplegia solution (approximately 10 ml/kg at 3–5°C) is perfused through a small catheter,† and the line pressure is monitored. The perfusion pressure should be maintained between 60 and 80 mm Hg. The myocardial temperature is lowered to 10°C and is measured in several locations in the myocardium distal to the coronary occlusions, to be certain that distribution of the cardioplegia solution is adequate. The myocardium is maintained cold also by placing a plastic jacket,‡ with cold (4°C) water circulating through it, around the left ventricle posteriorly. Following infusion of the cardioplegia solution, the cannula is clamped and the proximal aorta is vented through the sidearm. A flaccid heart provides greatly improved exposure of the obstructed coronary arteries, particularly on the posterior wall of the ventricle. Occasionally, the aortic root vent is not adequate to handle the blood return from the right side of the heart, in which case the left ventricle must be vented by a left ventricular vent inserted through the anterior aspect of the junction of the right superior pulmonary vein and the left atrium.

---

* Two Stage Venous Return Catheter, Sarns Inc.
† Aortic Root Cannula with Attached Vent Line, DLP Inc.
‡ Cobe Temperature Cooling Device, Cobe Laboratories, Inc.

A

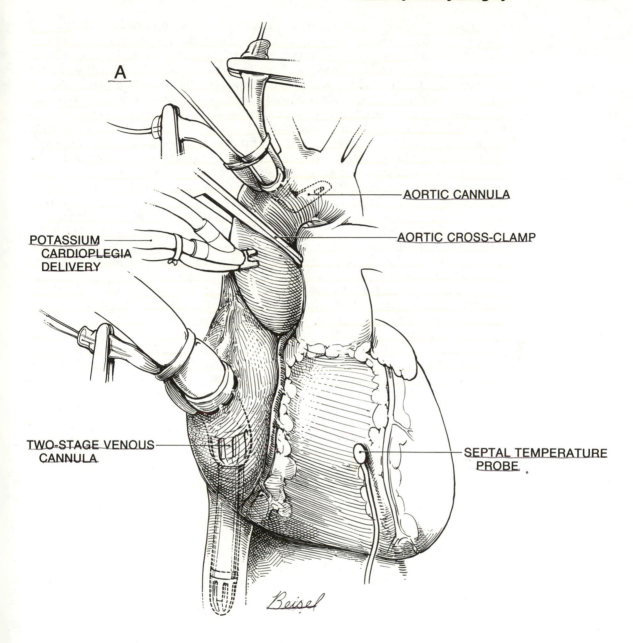

AORTIC CANNULA

AORTIC CROSS-CLAMP

POTASSIUM
CARDIOPLEGIA
DELIVERY

TWO-STAGE VENOUS
CANNULA

SEPTAL TEMPERATURE
PROBE

Beisel

B.—While one team exposes the heart, a second team harvests the vein. The patient's lower extremities are prepared circumferentially from foot to groin and placed on sterile drapes to permit access to both the greater and the lesser saphenous veins. The initial incision is made over the saphenous vein at the medial malleolus and extended proximally. In small women, however, the incision is made over the saphenous bulb and extended distally. If the lesser saphenous vein is to be removed, the incision is made posterior to the lateral malleolus and extended up over the calf. In most instances, a continuous skin incision is made to reduce the risk of injuring the vessel. After the overlying tissue has been incised, gauze sponges soaked in solution containing papaverine (30 mg/500 ml) are placed on the exposed vein. Then, it is dissected from the surrounding tissue. Side branches are tied off with 4–0 silk, with care not to place the ties close to the saphenous vein and thereby cause a drawing up of the adventitia and a constriction of the lumen of the conduit. A marking pen is used to scribe a line on the anterior surface of the vein prior to removal. This line is helpful in avoiding subsequent twisting of the vein graft. When the segment of saphenous vein is removed, a cannula is inserted into its proximal end, and the vein is gently distended with saline solution and placed into cold (3–5°C) saline solution until it is used.

Adequate exposure to permit an anastomosis to either the left anterior descending coronary artery or the diagonal branch of this vessel is obtained by elevating the heart on laparotomy pads. The site of the anastomosis is exposed by incising the overlying fat. Occasionally, the midsegment of the left anterior descending coronary artery is intramyocardial and can be difficult to find if its distal portion is small. Usually, it is found beneath a crease in the fat overlying the interventricular septum. The vessel is incised for 8–10 mm in an area which is free of atherosclerosis. Identification of a site suitable for anastomosis is usually not a problem with the left anterior descending coronary artery. Endarterectomy generally is not recommended for this vessel, but on occasion may be required if the vessel is extensively diseased. If an anterior descending diagonal vessel also requires grafting, the graft from it to the left anterior descending coronary artery should be placed at an angle to avoid kinking between the two.

B

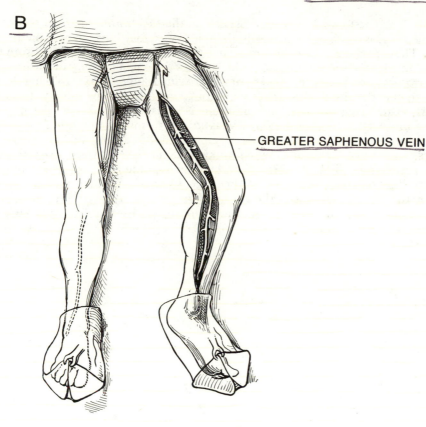

GREATER SAPHENOUS VEIN

C.—The anastomosis is begun distally (at the toe) with a mattress suture of 6–0 Prolene and is continued proximally about halfway along both edges of the arteriotomy. The saphenous vein is then retracted distally, which improves exposure for the proximal half of the anastomosis. This enables accurate matching of the graft to the arteriotomy and precise placement of the proximal sutures. Prior to tying down the suture line, the vessel is de-aired by injecting cold cardioplegia solution through the graft. After tying the knot, the anastomosis is tested for leaks and patency by injecting more cardioplegia solution. Bypass grafts to the left anterior descending diagonal coronary artery are usually done sequentially, as parallel side-to-side anastomoses. Care must be taken to avoid kinking of the vein between anastomoses. This is particularly difficult when the sites for anastomosis of sequential bypass grafts are close together. Usually it is advantageous to select a distal site for anastomosis on the left anterior descending coronary artery if the diagonal branch is to be grafted sequentially. The lie of the graft is improved so that the chances of kinking and axial torsion are reduced.

C

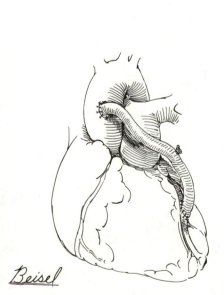

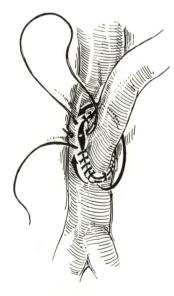

Beisel

D.—The circumflex coronary artery is the most difficult vessel to expose for coronary artery bypass grafting, but exposure is facilitated when the heart is arrested. The apex of the heart must be retracted anteriorly and to the patient's right side. The main circumflex artery is rarely grafted because of its position in the posterior atrioventricular groove and its proximity to the coronary sinus. Occasionally, the circumflex marginal branches will tunnel beneath the epicardial surface close to the atrioventricular ring. Locating these vessels can be troublesome unless an overlying epicardial ridge is present. Sometimes an adjacent vein that is on the epicardial surface will aid in locating an intramyocardial circumflex marginal vessel. Precise knowledge of the preoperative coronary arteriograms is essential in finding an obscure vessel. In many patients, more than one circumflex marginal artery is occluded, and several techniques have been used for revascularization, depending on the location and the size of the vessels. When a sequential graft is used, we prefer to make the distal anastomosis to the largest coronary artery. If just one vessel in the circumflex system is to be grafted and there are no occlusions of the right coronary artery, the anastomosis is started with a mattress suture at the proximal end of the arteriotomy. The proximal vein graft then drops away from the surgeon toward the base of the heart and allows him to sew toward himself along both edges of the arteriotomy. This technique can be used for the distal end of a sequential graft if there is sufficient distance between the two arteriotomy sites to prevent kinking of the graft between anastomoses. More commonly, the anastomosis of a sequential graft is brought off the arteriotomy either tangentially or directly perpendicular to the artery. This improves the lie of the graft and preserves the length of the conduit. In a perpendicular anastomosis, suture of the graft to the appropriate side of the arteriotomy is started at the apex of the vein graft and run toward both ends of the arteriotomy. This anastomosis can be facilitated by retracting the vein graft to the side and suturing from the luminal aspect.

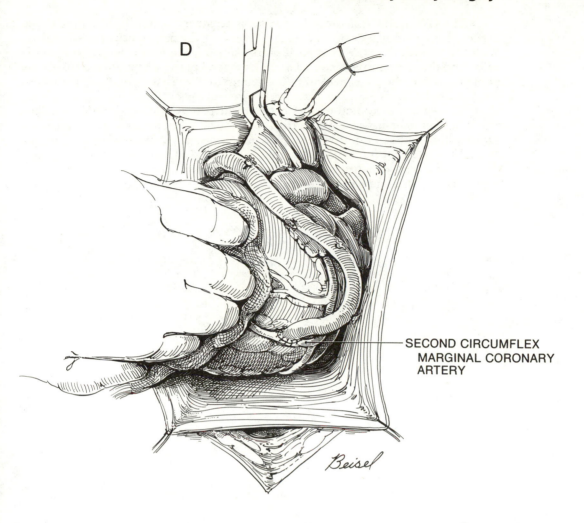

D

SECOND CIRCUMFLEX
MARGINAL CORONARY
ARTERY

Beisel

E1.—A sequential anastomosis can be done either as a parallel one, as with the left anterior descending diagonal coronary artery, or as a perpendicular anastomosis. With the most commonly used parallel anastomosis, the vein is incised longitudinally, and the anastomosis is started at the distal end of the vein graft and run to the midpoint. Here, the proximal end of the vein graft is retracted distally as the suture line is completed.

E2.—When the venotomy lies perpendicular to the long axis of the coronary artery, a diamond-shaped anastomosis can be done. The anastomosis is started by suturing the midpoint of the venotomy to either the apex or the base of the arteriotomy. The suture line is first completed along the distal edge of the arteriotomy from the luminal aspect, and then extended along the proximal edge. If the vein is large, a horizontal incision can be made and a parallel anastomosis performed.

E₁

E₂

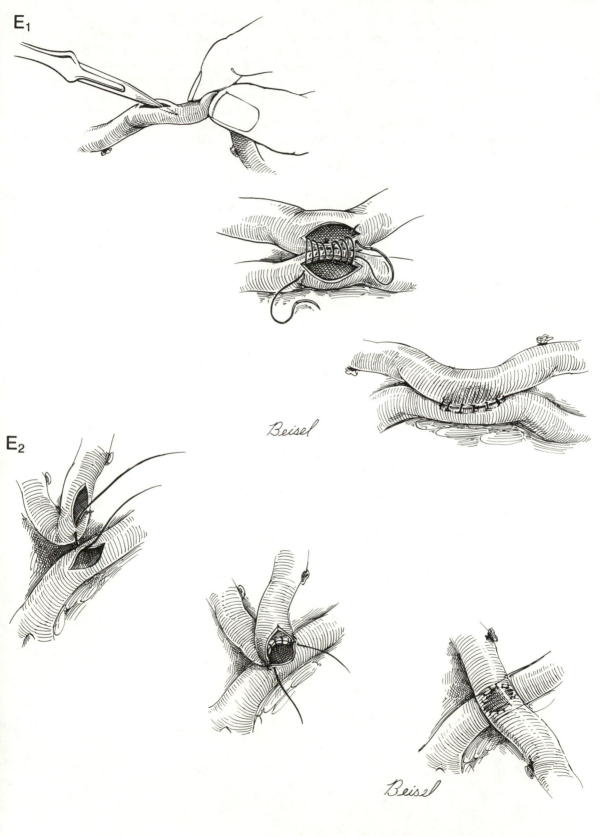

Beisel

Beisel

F.—Exposure of the posterior descending branch of the coronary artery is obtained by placing traction sutures of 0 silk deep into the crux of the right ventricle and elevating the posterior portion cephalad. A precise arteriotomy is then made in the posterior descending coronary artery. The anastomosis is begun distally (at the toe) with a mattress suture of 6–0 Prolene and continued proximally along both edges of the arteriotomy. The saphenous vein is then retracted distally, which improves exposure for the proximal half of the anastomosis. Prior to tying down the suture line, the vessel is de-aired by injecting cold cardioplegia solution through the graft. After tying the knot, the anastomosis is tested for leaks and patency by injecting more solution.

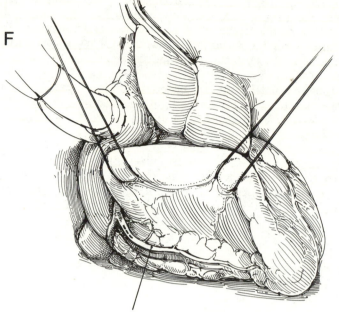

POSTERIOR DESCENDING CORONARY ARTERY

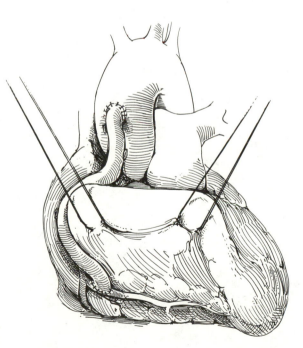

Beisel

G.—For a proximal right coronary artery occlusion, the arteriotomy is usually made in the atrioventricular groove. In this area, the arterial diameter is larger than it is distal to the bifurcation, and the course of the graft to the aorta is more suitable. If occlusive disease is found at the bifurcation of the right coronary artery, sequential anastomoses may be done to the posterolateral branches as well as to the posterior descending coronary artery.

Endarterectomy of the distal right coronary artery can be performed in selected patients when diffuse disease is present and the posterior descending coronary artery is too small for grafting. An arteriotomy is made just above the bifurcation of the distal right coronary artery through the adventitia and media to the intima of the vessel. With blunt dissection, using an endarterectomy spatula, the atheromatous intima core can be separated easily from the medial-adventitial wall. The atheroma is freed circumferentially as far as possible into each separate branch of the distal right coronary artery. The core is then removed by gentle traction with a small clamp. The coronary arteriotomy site is then used for anastomosing a vein graft.

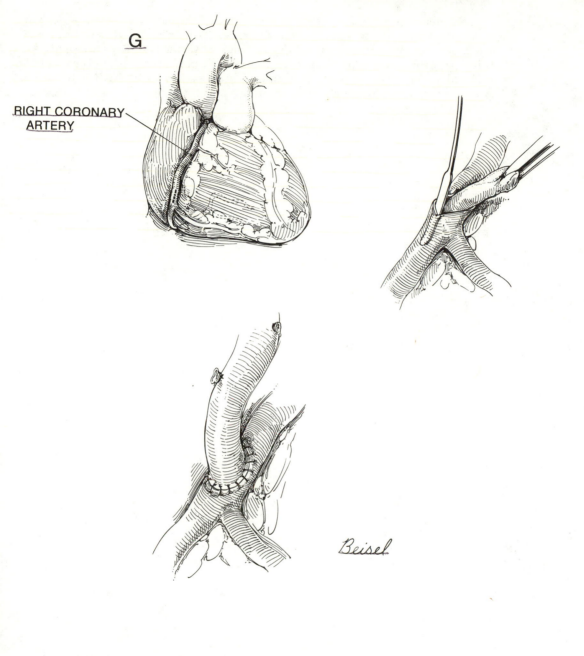

G

<u>RIGHT CORONARY ARTERY</u>

Beisel

H.—The proximal anastomoses are done after the distal anastomoses have been completed and after the removal of the aortic cross–clamp, but while the patient is still on cardiopulmonary bypass. The patient is rewarmed as these anastomoses are being performed. Prior to placing the partial occlusion clamp, the aorta should be palpated to detect the areas of calcification that must be avoided by the aortotomy. After the partial occlusion clamp is applied, a punch (4–5 mm) is used to form the site of anastomosis.

H

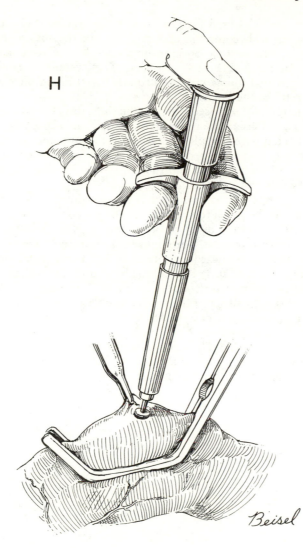

Beisel

I.—If suitable, the site used for perfusion of the cardioplegia solution is enlarged with the punch to become the proximal site for the anastomosis. With the vein graft coming off the aorta at an appropriate angle, the anastomoses are performed with continuous 5–0 Prolene sutures. The completed anastomoses are checked for both proximal filling and distal runoff by stripping the conduit distally and checking the refill of the vessel.

At the completion of the procedure, metallic rings can be used to mark the sites of aortic anastomoses. This facilitates subsequent coronary arteriography if it becomes necessary. Pacing wires are placed in the right atrium and the right ventricle. When the patient is rewarmed, cardiopulmonary bypass is stopped. Mediastinal drainage tubes are positioned away from the bypass grafts. The pericardium is left open so that the bypass grafts are not compressed.

In patients who undergo combined valve replacement and coronary bypass grafting, attention must be given to the order of the procedures. In general, there is an advantage to performing the distal coronary artery grafts prior to replacing the valve(s). This permits cardioplegia solution to be administered directly through the vein grafts, thus enhancing myocardial protection. It is unsafe to retract the heart to perform circumflex system grafting after a prosthetic mitral valve has been inserted. Disruption of the atrioventricular groove may result. We prefer to expose the valve anulus, remove the valve, and select the proper size valve. While the valve is being obtained (or, if a tissue valve, properly washed), the distal coronary anastomoses are performed. After the completion of the distal coronary artery anastomoses, the valve(s) are sutured into place. The left atrium or aorta is closed, and the aortic cross-clamp is removed. The proximal anastomoses are performed after the heart is de-aired, while the patient is being rewarmed.

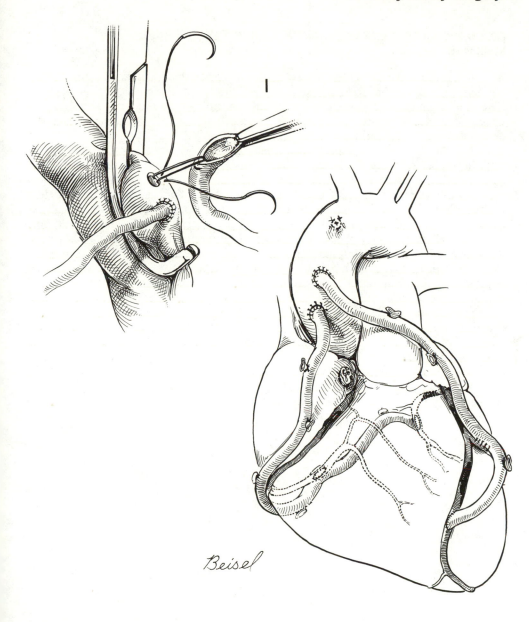

Beisel

CORONARY ARTERY BYPASS GRAFTING USING THE INTERNAL MAMMARY ARTERY

Internal mammay artery bypass grafts to either the left anterior descending coronary artery or the diagonal coronary arteries are performed on patients who require a single graft or patients who require multiple grafts but have a shortage of venous conduit. The internal mammary artery is not usually used to replace the circumflex and distal right coronary arteries.

Fig 20–2, A.—The internal mammary artery and its surrounding tissue are carefully dissected from the left chest wall. Small metallic clips are used to occlude side branches. A Favalaro retractor helps to obtain exposure. No attempt is made to separate the vein and adjacent tissue from the artery. The artery is dissected free proximally to the subclavian artery and distally to the costal margin. The pericardium is not opened until after the internal mammary artery has been dissected out. The internal mammary artery is transected distally only after the patient has been heparinized and cardiopulmonary bypass has been initiated. It is then cannulated carefully, gently dilated with papaverine solution (60 mg/1,000 ml), and wrapped in papaverine-soaked sponges to prevent spasm. The distal aspect of the artery is dissected free of tissue after it has been trimmed to length. Flow through the internal mammary artery is checked by allowing the blood to flow into a graduated vial. If the flow is less than 100 ml/min, the artery should be dilated again and checked for twisting and kinking. The coronary artery arteriotomy should be limited to between 0.5 cm and 1 cm.

B.—The anastomosis is then performed with interrupted 7–0 Prolene suture.

C.—The completed anastomosis is shown. The pericardial edge and anterior mediastinal fat are incised to prevent kinking and traction on the anastomosis.

A

INTERNAL MAMMARY
ARTERY

B

C

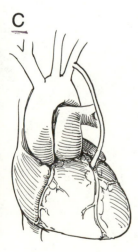

Beisel

CHAPTER **21**

Repair of Ventricular Aneurysms and Ventricular Septal Defects After Myocardial Infarction

REPAIR OF VENTRICULAR ANEURYSM

THE DEVELOPMENT of a left ventricular aneurysm following myocardial infarction occurs in approximately 8%–15% of patients. Approximately 90% of these aneurysms develop in the anterior apical area of the left ventricle. Aneurysms of the diaphragmatic portion of the left ventricle occur in only 3%–5% of patients. Indications for operation include congestive heart failure, embolization, and severe arrhythmias.

Surgical excision of the ventricular aneurysm using cardiopulmonary bypass is effective in relieving symptoms. Preoperative assessment of the functioning ventricular muscle as well as of the associated conditions, including mitral regurgitation, ventricular septal defect, and coronary artery disease, is necessary to correct the associated defects and to ensure survival.

Fig 21–1, A.—Operation for ventricular aneurysm is carried out through a median sternotomy and with the use of cardiopulmonary bypass. Venous cannulation is bicaval, and the arterial cannula is placed in the ascending aorta. Cold cardioplegia solution is delivered into the aortic root. To diminish the possibility of dislodging a mural thrombus, the area of the aneurysm is not dissected from the pericardial sac until the aorta has been cross-clamped, cold cardioplegia solution has been infused, and the heart is arrested. Pericardial adhesions over the surface of the aneurysm are then divided with scissors. The heart is elevated from the pericardial sac, and the center of the collapsed wall of the aneurysm is identified.

B.—The central portion of the aneurysm is incised, and any intramural clot is carefully removed. Clamps are placed on the edges of the aneurysm, and the lateral walls are excised. The interior of the left ventricle and the mitral valve apparatus are inspected. The presence of severe mitral valve insufficiency should be recognized from the catheterization study; the mitral valve can be replaced through a subanular approach. Fibrous tissue along the rim of the aneurysm must be retained intact to close the aneurysm securely without sacrificing healthy muscle. The right ventricle may be entered by mistake if too much aneurysmal wall is removed.

C.—Repair of the aneurysm is initiated by placing a wide strip of Teflon felt along each side of the aneurysm. The edge of each strip is sutured to the fibrous edge of the aneurysm with heavy horizontal mattress sutures of no. 1 Ethibond. The left ventricle is vented at the apex of the repair. After completion of the primary suture line, a secondary suture line joins the free edge of each strip with a continuous no. 2 Prolene suture along the entire length of the repair. The apex of the heart is elevated following removal of the aortic cross-clamp, the heart is defibrillated, and the vent is removed after the air has been evacuated. A previously placed horizontal mattress suture over the vent site is tied. The suture line is inspected for complete hemostasis.

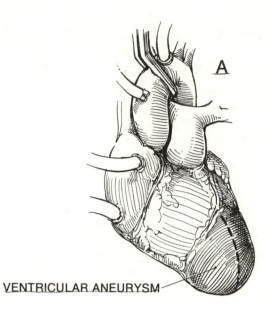

VENTRICULAR ANEURYSM

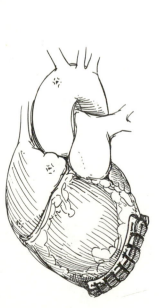

REPAIR OF VENTRICULAR SEPTAL DEFECT AFTER MYOCARDIAL INFARCTION

Nonoperative management of acute myocardial infarction complicated by a ventricular septal defect results in a survival of 15% at the end of two months. Moreover, 50% of the patients die within the first week following a rupture of the septum. Approximately 2% of the patients who sustain a transmural myocardial infarction will also sustain a septal rupture. Approximately 80% of ventricular ruptures will occur in the anterior portion of the septum near the apex. Hemodynamic instability and patient deterioration are commonly seen and are indications for early surgical intervention. Therefore, every patient with a ventricular septal rupture following myocardial infarction should be considered a candidate for surgical repair. As soon as a ventricular septal defect is diagnosed, left ventriculography and coronary arteriography should be performed. Also, hemoglobin saturations should be obtained from the right atrium and the pulmonary artery, following the insertion of a balloon-tipped Swan-Ganz catheter. A saturation increase of more than 5% between the right atrium and the pulmonary artery confirms the diagnosis of a ventricular septal defect. Any evidence of hemodynamic deterioration should be promptly treated with the insertion of an intra-aortic balloon for circulatory assistance, followed by an emergency operative repair.

Fig 21–2, A.—Operation for a ventricular septal defect is performed through a median sternotomy. Two venous cannulas with vena caval tapes are inserted for venous return, and an arterial cannula is placed in the ascending aorta. Myocardial preservation is achieved with systemic cooling to 20–24°C, and cold cardioplegia solution is injected into the aortic root to lower the left ventricular myocardial temperature below 15°C. Cold saline solution is infused into the pericardial well. The heart is elevated from the pericardial well, and the area of myocardial infarction is identified by the distinct discoloration of the epicardium. In an anterior infarction, the necrotic area is incised parallel to the anterior descending coronary artery. The defect is invariably associated with a large transmural infarction surrounding the distribution of the anterior descending coronary artery. The right free wall of the ventricle, next to the left anterior descending coronary artery, is usually involved also. Aortocoronary bypass grafting is performed on the diseased arteries including, when possible, the occluded left anterior descending coronary artery. Cold cardioplegia solution is infused into the ascending aorta every 20 minutes, while the aorta is cross-clamped, to ensure good myocardial preservation.

B.—The left ventricular margin of the infarction is trimmed of damaged tissue, and the papillary muscles to the mitral valve are inspected. The necrotic edges of the septum and the anterior right ventricle are also removed to expose normal myocardium. All necrotic muscle must be removed. In most cases, a Dacron patch will be required to close the defect. Mattress sutures of 2–0 Prolene are placed circumferentially, and buttressed with Teflon felt pledgets on the right side of the ventricular septum. Sutures placed on the edge of the anterior wall of the right ventricle are passed from outside into the right ventricle, with pledgets on the epicardial side. After the sutures have been placed, they are inserted into the edges of an elastic Dacron fabric patch, which is then slipped into place. The patch then lies on the left ventricular side of the septum and on the endocardial side of the free right ventricular wall (B_2).

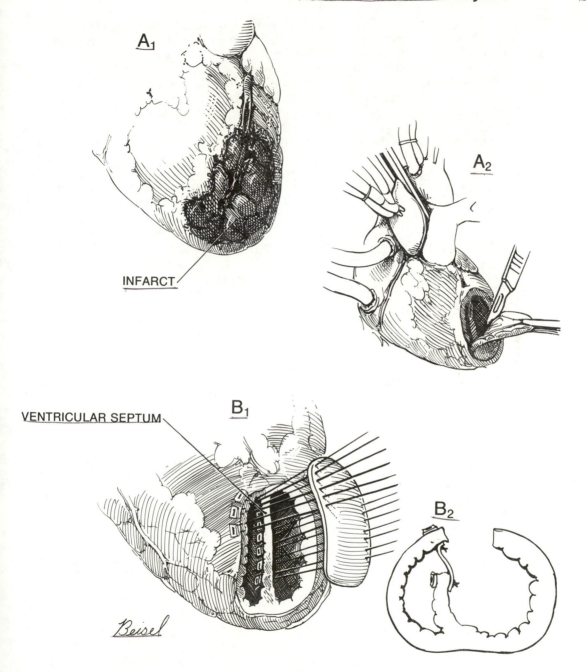

A₁

INFARCT

A₂

VENTRICULAR SEPTUM

B₁

B₂

Beisel

C.—When the septal defect has been repaired, the anterior infarctectomy site is closed with a patch of low-porosity woven Dacron to avoid a delayed rupture of the ventriculotomy. Mattress sutures of 0 Prolene with pledgets are placed circumferentially around the free wall margins of the left ventricular defect. The sutures are brought through the left ventricular wall from endocardium to epicardium. Sutures placed along the septal margin of the left ventricle pass through the edges of the septal patch and emerge through the epicardium of the anterior right ventricle.

D.—After all the sutures are placed, they are inserted into the edge of an oversized oval patch of low-porosity woven Dacron graft material, which has been prepared with autologous clot and autoclaved to further decrease porosity. The sutures are then tied, the heart is de-aired, the aortic cross-clamp is removed, the heart is defibrillated, and further de-airing maneuvers are carried out. Before bypass is discontinued, it is important to examine the ventricular wall repair for hemostasis and to place additional sutures with pledgets as needed. This technique of double-patch application was developed by Willard M. Daggett, M.D. The repair is also applicable to posterior ventricular septal rupture.

C₁

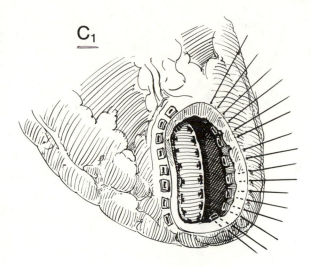

C₂

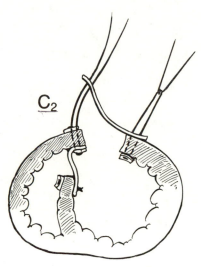

D

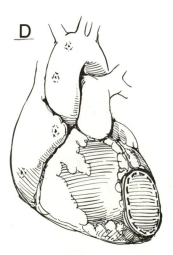

Beisel

CHAPTER 22

Aortic Aneurysms and Dissections

REPAIR OF ASCENDING AORTIC ANEURYSMS

RESECTION of the aneurysm and graft replacement is currently the treatment of choice for aneurysms of the ascending aorta. Fusiform aneurysms and, more commonly, saccular aneurysms caused by syphilis are virtually nonexistent in the United States because of effective medical therapy for syphilis. The fusiform aneurysms that do occur are secondary to cystic medial necrosis. Dilatation frequently extends to the aortic valve and causes aortic valve insufficiency. The aortic lesions seen in Marfan's syndrome are indistinguishable from Erdheim cystic medial necrosis. The most serious complication of Marfan's syndrome, and the one that accounts for more than one half of the deaths, is dissection and separation of the layers of the aorta within the fusiform aneurysm. Atherosclerotic aneurysms of the ascending aorta are increasing in frequency. The large size of the aneurysm and the presence of symptoms presage rupture and, if untreated, result in a five-year survival of less than 50%. Unfortunately, the majority of these patients have severe coronary artery disease, which increases the risk of operative correction of the aneurysm.

We believe that if the aortic valve is incompetent, the valve should be replaced. If there is no evidence that either the aortic valve with its anulus or the coronary ostia is involved, we replace the aneurysm with a woven Dacron graft of appropriate size. Replacement of the ascending aortic aneurysm with a composite valve and graft is almost always indicated in patients with Marfan's syndrome. This eliminates the late complication of aortic valve regurgitation if only the ascending aorta is replaced.

Fig 22–1, A.—Two techniques can be utilized for replacing the ascending aorta. The first technique shown retains the aneurysm for wrapping around the woven Dacron graft to achieve optimal hemostasis following the repair.

A₁.—The operation is carried out through a median sternotomy utilizing bicaval venous cannulation and ascending aortic cannulation if the aneurysm ends proximal to the innominate artery. Common femoral artery cannulation may be helpful if the aneurysm extends to the aortic arch. The aneurysm is incised longitudinally, and cold cardioplegia solution is delivered directly into the coronary ostia until the temperature of the myocardium (septum) reaches 12°C or lower.

A₂.—A woven Dacron graft of appropriate size is chosen and preclotted with blood obtained prior to the administration of systemic heparin. The proximal and distal anastomoses are reinforced circumferentially with external felt strips. The proximal and distal suture lines are completed using a simple continuous suture of 3–0 Prolene. Thus, the aorta is enclosed between the woven Dacron graft internally and the felt strip externally.

A₃.—Excess tissue is then trimmed from the edges of the aneurysmal wall, and the residual aorta is wrapped around the graft and secured with a running suture of 3–0 Prolene to aid in obtaining hemostasis. On completion of the aneurysm repair, air is removed from both the left side of the heart and the ascending aorta.

<u>A</u>₁

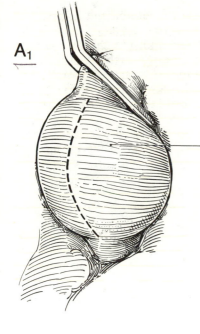

ASCENDING AORTIC ANEURYSM

<u>A</u>₂

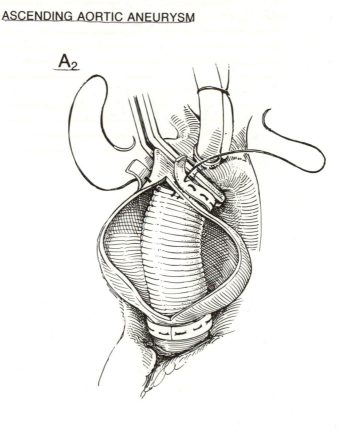

<u>A</u>₃

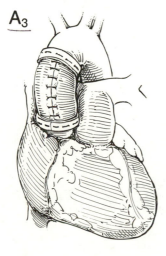

Beisel

B.—The second technique can be utilized with or without the necessity of replacing the aortic valve. A median sternotomy is performed. Venous cannulation is bicaval, and, if the aneurysm ends proximal to the innominate artery, the arterial cannula is inserted in the ascending aorta. Following exposure of the aneurysm, the ascending aorta is cross-clamped as close to the innominate artery as possible. The aneurysm is incised longitudinally, and cold cardioplegia solution is delivered directly into the coronary ostia until the septal temperature of the myocardium reaches 12°C or lower.

C₁.—In this drawing, the aortic valve has been replaced by standard technique, using double-armed, pledgeted 2–0 Ethibond sutures with the pledgets on the ventricular side of the anulus.

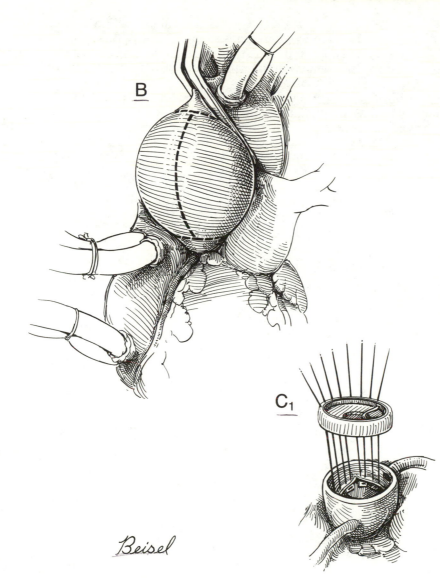

B

C₁

Beisel

C_2.—If the aortic tissue appears to be substantial, the preclotted Dacron tube is sutured in place using a simple continuous suture of 3–0 Prolene.

C_3, C_4.—If the aortic wall is thin, a strip of felt is incorporated into both the proximal and distal anastomoses, using parallel mattress sutures to evert the lip of the graft within the lumen of the aorta.

C_5.—When complete, the aortic wall is interposed between the external felt strip and the internal lip of Dacron graft.

The distal anastomosis is started posteriorly and performed in a similar manner. On completion of the aneurysm replacement, air is removed from both the left side of the heart and the ascending aorta. The aortic cross-clamp is then removed.

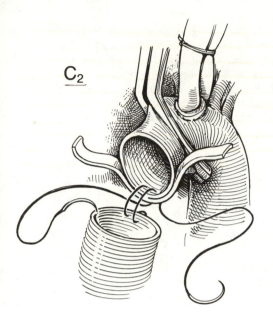

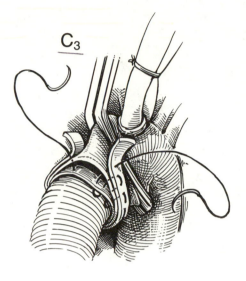

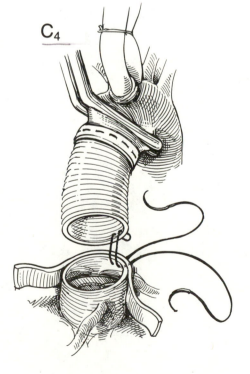

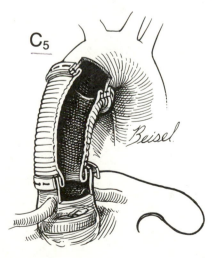

D.—In the case of Marfan's syndrome, the ascending aorta is incised and preserved to wrap around the graft. The composite valve and graft technique is employed in all patients with this disease. After the aneurysm is opened and cardioplegia solution has been delivered directly into the coronary ostia for myocardial protection, the valve is excised. A composite valve and graft of appropriate size is chosen. The valve end of the graft is sutured to the aortic anulus with double-armed, pledgeted 2–0 Ethibond sutures, with the pledgets on the outside of the anulus.

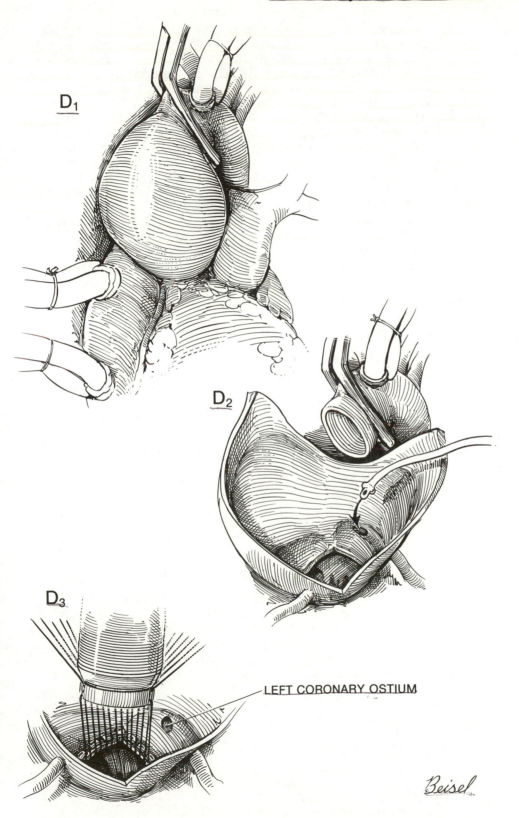

D₁

D₂

D₃

LEFT CORONARY OSTIUM

Beisel

E.—After repairing the valve, the ostia of the coronary arteries are visualized, and openings are made in the graft opposite the right and left coronary ostia using a sterile, battery-powered cautery unit.* Use of this cautery prevents fraying of the Dacron edges. The coronary arteries are sutured circumferentially with 4–0 Prolene to the openings made in the graft. Bites in the aortic tissue are taken approximately 2–3 mm away from the coronary orifice.

F.—The distal end of the graft is sutured to the aorta, and an external strip of Dacron felt is used to support mattress sutures of continuous 3–0 Prolene. An alternative approach is to suture the distal end of the prosthesis into the aorta inside the aneurysm, as shown in Fig 20–1A$_2$. Rewarming of the patient is begun at the beginning of this anastomosis. A needle vent for de-airing is placed in the most anterior portion of the graft, and the left ventricular apex is de-aired with a syringe and needle prior to the removal of the cross-clamp. The anastomoses are inspected for bleeding and reinforced with pledgeted sutures as necessary. Then the residual aorta is wrapped around the distal graft to aid in obtaining hemostasis.

---

* Concept Cautery: Concept, Inc.

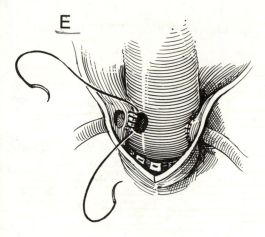

E

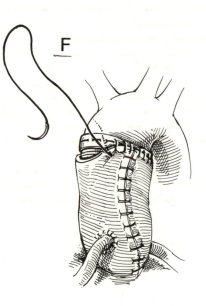

F

Beisel

REPAIR OF ACUTE DISSECTIONS OF THE ASCENDING AORTA EXCLUDING MARFAN'S SYNDROME

All acute dissections of the ascending aorta should be treated by immediate surgical intervention, before severe aortic regurgitation or rupture into either the heart or the pericardium occurs. We believe that in ascending aortic dissection with aortic valve incompetency that is not associated with Marfan's syndrome, the aortic valve in most cases can be preserved with resuspension sutures.

Fig 22–2, A.—Femoral artery cannulation is preferred in the acute setting of aortic dissection. At the same time, if the patient's condition is extremely unstable in the operating room, a venous cannula can be inserted into the common femoral vein for femoral vein–to–femoral artery cardiopulmonary bypass support while a median sternotomy is being performed. Although less desirable, systemic cannulation can also be achieved through the transverse arch, utilizing a partial side-biting vascular clamp and identifying intima to be certain the cannula is in the true lumen. On completion of the venous cannulation, cardiopulmonary bypass is begun. The heart is protected by systemic cooling, by using cold 4°C Ringer's lactate solution in the pericardial sac and by direct perfusion of the coronary ostia with cold cardioplegia solution. If the aortic valve can be preserved, the intima, media, and adventitia are reapproximated with double-armed, pledgeted 4–0 Prolene sutures with external supporting pledgets on either side of the commissures, as shown.

B.—The outer and inner layers of the dissection are reconstructed using outer, middle, and inner rings of Teflon felt. If the aortic layers appear to be strong, only the outer and inner rings of Teflon felt are used. A double-armed, parallel mattress suture of 3–0 Prolene is used to secure the Teflon rings to the walls of the aorta. This coaptation process obliterates the false lumen and holds the friable layers securely.

C.—A preclotted woven Dacron graft of appropriate size is selected. The tube graft is anastomosed to the proximal and distal portions of the aorta with a simple double-armed, running suture of 3–0 Prolene. De-airing is accomplished as previously described prior to aortic cross-clamp removal.

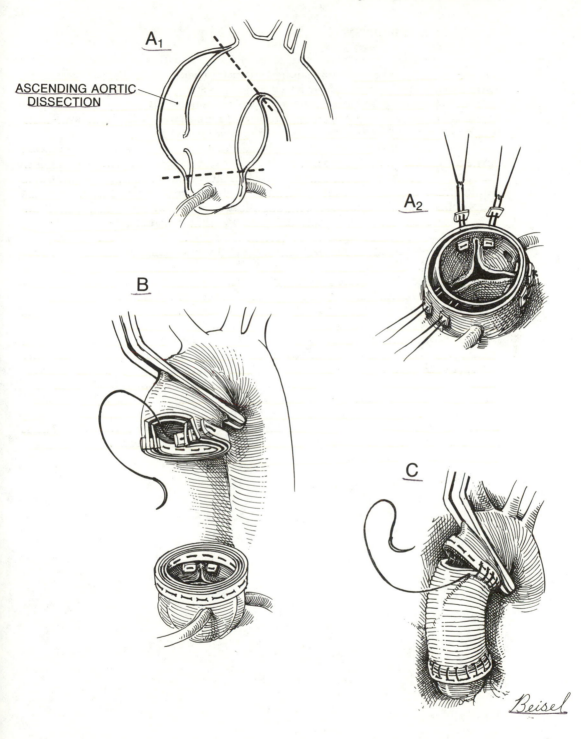

A₁

ASCENDING AORTIC
DISSECTION

A₂

B

C

Beisel

AORTIC ARCH ANEURYSM

An aneurysm of the aortic arch is usually a continuation of an aneurysm of the ascending aorta. It may be complicated by insufficiency of the aortic valve, which would require replacement of the aortic valve. Resection of a combined aneurysm of the ascending aorta and the aortic arch can be done on cardiopulmonary bypass using either separate cerebral perfusion or profound hypothermia. Profound hypothermia appears to be a safe technique for cerebral protection; it is less cumbersome and avoids the problems associated with separate cerebral perfusion such as cerebral swelling and hemorrhagic infarction. The technique requires reducing the core temperature to 15°C and maintaining this temperature before occluding the blood flow to the head. Packing the head in ice bags is also helpful. After clamping the brachiocephalic vessel, cardiopulmonary perfusion is reduced to 100–200 ml/min. When the aneurysm has been replaced with the graft, rewarming is begun, and the temperature raised 1°C every two to three minutes. The technique requires the availability of donor platelets and blood components to avoid excessive postoperative bleeding.

Fig 22–3, A.—Cardiopulmonary bypass is instituted with cannulation of the superior and inferior venae cavae, and cannulation of the common femoral artery. Exposure of the ascending aorta, the transverse aortic arch, and the brachiocephalic vessels is obtained while the patient is being cooled to a core temperature of 15°C. Once this optimal temperature is reached, the patient is placed in the Trendelenburg position, and the innominate, left carotid, and left subclavian arteries are individually cross-clamped. The aneurysm is incised longitudinally, and further cardiac protection is provided by direct infusion of cold potassium cardioplegia solution into the coronary ostia. A woven preclotted Dacron tube of appropriate size is anastomosed to the descending thoracic aorta within the aortic lumen, using a double-armed running suture of 4–0 Prolene, as shown. The suture line is checked for leaks by increasing the bypass flow to distend the anastomosis.

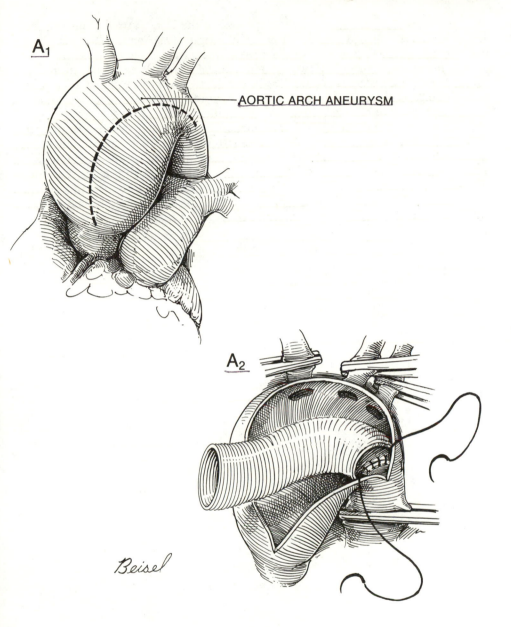

AORTIC ARCH ANEURYSM

Beisel

B.—An oval opening is made in the side of the Dacron graft. This is anastomosed within the opened aorta to the common origin of the innominate, left carotid, and left subclavian vessels in a single anastomosis. Again, the anastomosis is performed using a single running layer of 4–0 Prolene suture. When the anastomosis is complete, the graft is cross-clamped, air is eliminated from the graft, and the clamps on the brachiocephalic vessels are removed. At this point, rewarming is begun, and cardiopulmonary bypass flow rates are gradually increased to 2.4 L/min/m².

C.—During rewarming, the proximal anastomosis is performed from within the opened aorta, as described for the distal anastomosis, using a single double-armed running suture of 4–0 Prolene. Then the proximal portion of the ascending aortic graft is de-aired with a needle; the left ventricle is de-aired with needle aspiration of the left ventricular apex; and, when rewarming is complete, the patient is weaned from bypass. The wall of the aneurysm is trimmed and sutured around the graft while protamine, platelets, and clotting factors are administered as necessary.

B

C

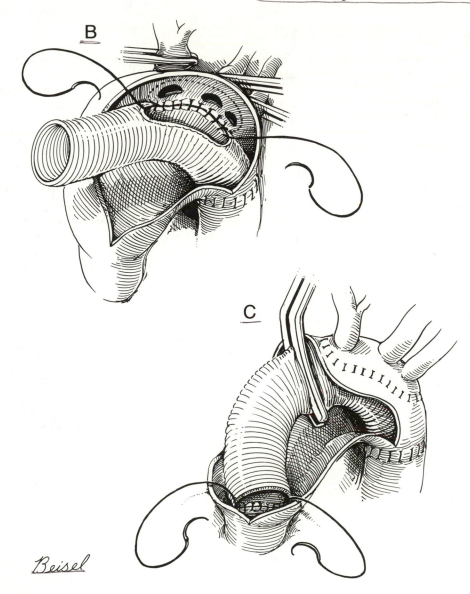

Beisel

ANEURYSMS AND DISSECTIONS OF THE DESCENDING AORTA

Aneurysms and dissections of the descending thoracic aorta are repaired by graft replacement through a left fifth intercostal space thoracotomy. The area of the left subclavian artery is dissected for proximal control of the aorta. An appropriate-sized Dacron tube graft is selected and preclotted. We prefer to use a simple temporary shunt to bypass the descending thoracic aorta and to provide blood flow below the distal aortic cross-clamp for organ perfusion. This eliminates the need for systemic heparin as well as for partial femoral vein-to-femoral artery bypass with a blood pump. Therefore, we use the cationic surfactant tridodecylmethylammonium chloride-coated (TDMAC) shunt,* which was developed by Gott.

Fig 22–4, A.—A site on the aorta that is proximal to the left subclavian artery is chosen for insertion of the proximal end of the shunt. Two pursestring sutures of 3–0 Tevdek are placed in the proximal aorta, and the shunt is inserted into a stab wound made with a bistoury knife. The cannula is secured with keepers and ties. The proximal shunt can also be placed into the ascending aorta or within the apex of the left ventricle using a similar technique. The left common femoral artery is then cannulated with the distal end of the Gott shunt. The aneurysm is isolated between vascular clamps. Bleeding from intercostal orifices within the aneurysm is controlled with figure-of-8 sutures of 3–0 absorbable suture material. The preclotted Dacron prosthesis is then anastomosed to the proximal aorta, using a double-armed, running suture of 3–0 Prolene.

B.—The distal anastomosis is performed with a double-armed, 4–0 polypropylene suture sewn in simple running fashion, as described for the proximal anastomosis. Following placement of the graft, the distal vascular clamp is removed. This is followed by the slow removal of the proximal vascular clamp. The Gott shunt is removed, and the cannulation sites are repaired. For the repair of an acute dissection of the descending aorta, the outer and inner layers are interposed between Teflon felt rings and held with mattress sutures of 3–0 Prolene. This technique obliterates the dissected lumen and creates a strong sewing ring for anastomosis to the Dacron tube graft.

---

* Gott Shunt: Argyle Division, Sherwood Medical.

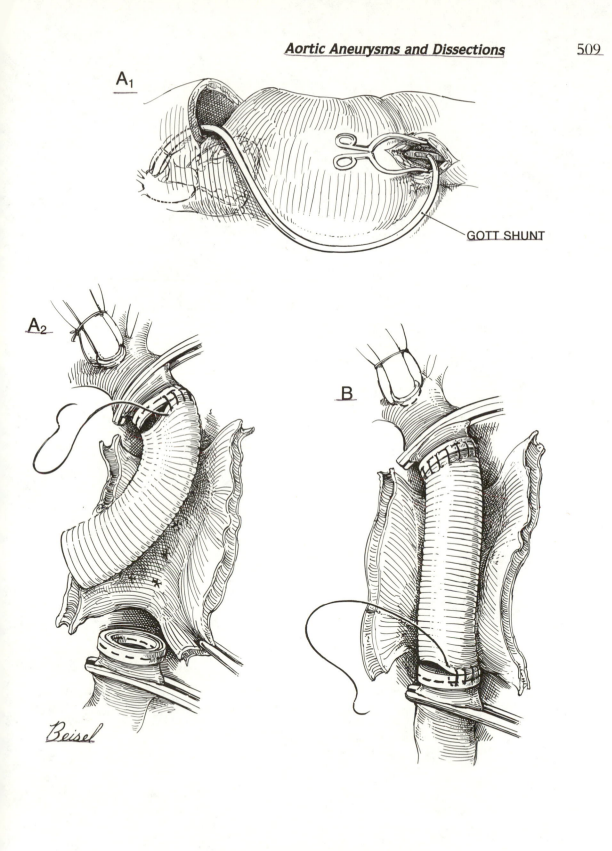

GOTT SHUNT

Beisel

CHAPTER 23

Decortication of the Heart

ONSTRICTIVE pericarditis can be confused with hepatic cirrhosis or various forms of myocardiopathy. Thus, cardiac catheterization is required to differentiate between myocardial and pericardial disease. Diagnostic pressure changes and hemodynamic patterns can be easily demonstrated during cardiac catheterization. Right atrial pressure is markedly elevated. There is an early rapid diastolic pressure elevation which plateaus throughout the remainder of diastole when measuring right ventricular pressure. In certain patients an accurate diagnosis can be obtained only by pericardial biopsy or myocardial biopsy.

The objective at operation is to remove as much as possible of the chronically inflamed, fibrotic, thickened and constricting pericardium, which limits diastolic ventricular filling. Usually, the scarred pericardium is densely adherent to the heart.

Fig 23–1, A.—A median sternotomy is employed. Adequate exposure of the left ventricle, great vessels, right ventricle, and right atrium is obtained. This exposure facilitates control of the lacerations of the thin-walled right ventricle and right atrium that can occur during removal of the fibrous peel. The incision also permits rapid institution of cardiopulmonary bypass if necessary to conduct a safe operation. Although cardiopulmonary bypass is infrequently used during pericardiectomy for constrictive pericarditis, its availability is a prime necessity.

B.—It is usually necessary to remove the epicardium of the heart if it has also become thickened and constricted. Special care must be taken to protect the coronary arteries during pericardiectomy, in particular the right coronary artery in the right atrioventricular groove. A knife is used to incise the pericardium to expose the heart anteriorly over the right ventricle. Cruciate incisions from this point then allow the development of three or four flaps of pericardium to be individually dissected from the heart. Great care is taken around the right atrium and the atrioventricular groove. The atrium is usually thin-walled, but small lacerations can be easily repaired with 4–0 pledgeted, double-armed polypropylene sutures. If the surgeon thinks that the pericardium and epicardium are too diffusely adherent to the region of the right coronary artery, a flap of scar tissue can be retained in the distribution of the right atrioventricular groove to avoid damage to the right coronary artery. Dissection is carried laterally over the left ventricle. The left ventricle should be freed beyond the phrenic nerve, leaving only a small pericardial patch posteriorly. The phrenic nerve and its vessels must be preserved as a pedicle. The right atrium is freed to the right phrenic nerve. Again, care must be taken to preserve the right phrenic nerve pedicle.

A

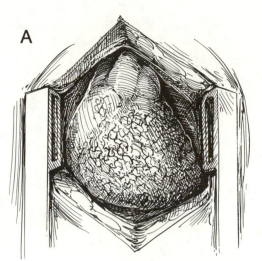

B

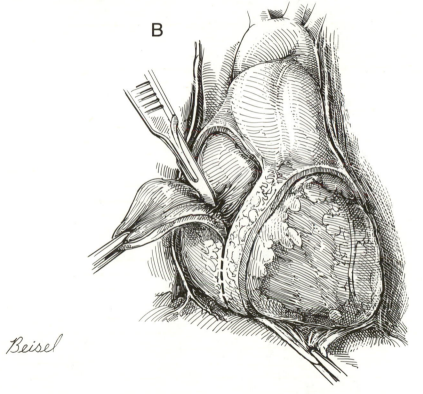

Beisel

CHAPTER 24

Transplantation of the Heart and Lungs

APREDICTABLE resurgence of interest in clinical heart transplantation is evolving in this country. Through the immense amount of scientific work that has been performed at Stanford University, cardiac transplantation today should be considered a reasonable and therapeutic treatment to extend life in selected individuals. A new immunosuppressive agent, cyclosporine, is a most promising adjunct to the success of transplantation. This drug has proven efficacy and appears superior to conventional immunosuppressive agents, when one compares the survival rates of patients who have received cyclosporine and low-dose steroid therapy to those of patients who have received maintenance therapy of azathioprine and high-dose steroids. This drug has also allowed the successful transplantation of the heart and lungs en bloc.

The donor heart is exposed through a median sternotomy. Following the dissection of the aorta, pulmonary artery, and vena cava, a sequence of steps takes place to ensure the rapid arrest and cooling of the donor heart. The major principle in heart procurement is to bring the heart rapidly from a beating, nonworking state to a cold, arrested state. This is accomplished by occluding the inflow tract (ligating the inferior and superior venae cavae), opening the left atrium to decompress the ventricle, rapidly cross-clamping the aorta, and, finally, injecting potassium cardioplegia solution into the aortic root to achieve cardiac arrest and rapid cooling. The heart is then excised by incising the left atrium circumferentially at the level of the pulmonary veins and severing the aorta and the pulmonary artery.

The donor heart is quickly placed into a basin of 4°C cold saline solution, and the left atrium and great vessels are prepared for transplantation. The left atrium is opened by connecting incisions through the pulmonary vein orifices. The circumference of the atrial remnant is trimmed to create a single left atrial remnant for anastomosis. The aorta and pulmonary artery are separated from each other. The remnant of the superior vena cava on the right atrium, which has been previously ligated, is secured with a figure-of-eight 4–0 Prolene suture. The inferior vena caval orifice is left open.

ORTHOTOPIC HEART TRANSPLANTATION

Fig 24–1, A.—The heart of the recipient is exposed via a median sternotomy, and cardiopulmonary bypass is established using two low-lying cannulas in the venae cavae and an arterial cannula in the ascending aorta. The patient is gradually cooled to 25°C on cardiopulmonary bypass. The vena caval tapes are tightened, and the aorta is cross-clamped well above the aortic valve. The recipient's heart is excised by cutting the atria just posterior to the atrioventricular groove and severing the great vessels distal to the aortic and pulmonary valves.

The first anastomosis, as shown in this figure, joins the left atrium of the donor to the left atrium of the recipient. This is accomplished with a 54-in.-long, double-armed 3–0 Prolene suture, started in the area of the atrial appendage and worked circumferentially until the entire suture line is completed. The atrial septa are brought together with full thickness bites of recipient septum to full-thickness bites of the donor atrium in the area of the donor septum. On completion of the left atrial anastomosis, a catheter is placed through the left atrial appendage of the donor heart, through the anastomosis which has just been completed into the left ventricle. Cold (4°C) saline solution is run through this catheter to achieve further myocardial preservation while the right atrial and aortic anastomoses are being performed. Also, the catheter can be used to decompress the left ventricle for a time after the aortic cross-clamp is removed.

B.—The artist's drawing shows the completed left atrial anastomosis and the proper way of opening the right atrium of the donor for anastomosis to the right atrium of the recipient. The incision is carried through the opened inferior vena caval remnant and is angled superiorly away from the junction of the superior vena cava and the right atrium of the donor. The incision is made in this way to avoid injury to the sinoatrial node.

C.—The right atrial anastomosis is performed with a double-armed, 54-in.-long 3–0 Prolene suture used in simple running fashion. The inferior margin of the donor right atrium is anastomosed with full-thickness bites through the atrial septal area of the left atrial anastomosis.

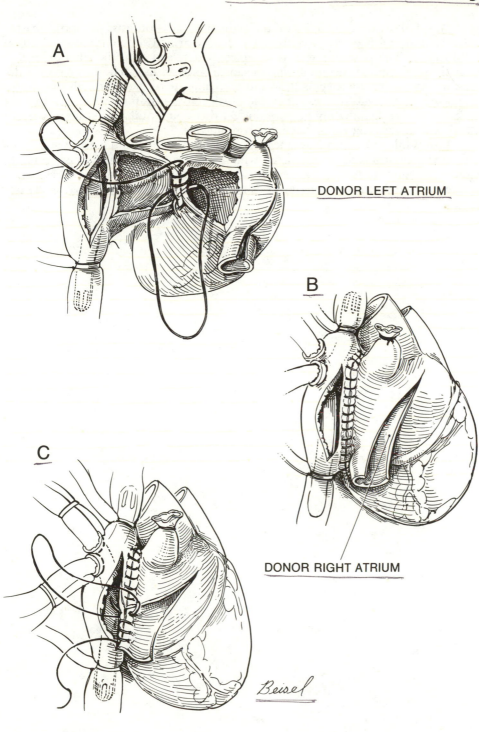

A

DONOR LEFT ATRIUM

B

DONOR RIGHT ATRIUM

C

Beisel

D.—Following completion of the right atrial anastomosis, the aortic anastomosis is accomplished with a continuous, double-armed simple running suture of 4–0 Prolene. The posterior wall is completed first, and then the anterior wall is sutured. Rewarming is begun during the aortic anastomosis. The aortic root is de-aired by decreasing the bypass flow and allowing air to vent through the almost completed aortic anastomosis, after the aortic cross-clamp is removed, and the patient is in the Trendelenburg position. At this point, full bypass flow is established, and rewarming of the patient is continued.

E.—While the patient's temperature is being warmed to normal, the pulmonary artery anastomosis is completed with a 4–0 Prolene double-armed, running suture technique similar to that performed for the aortic anastomosis. The heart is defibrillated, and after 20 minutes of support, cardiopulmonary bypass is discontinued.

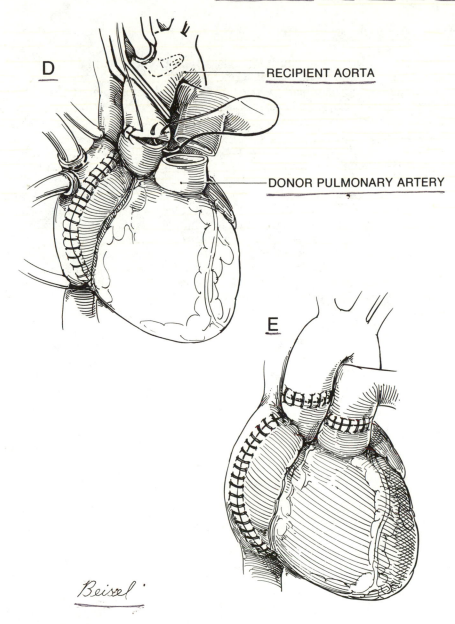

D

RECIPIENT AORTA

DONOR PULMONARY ARTERY

E

Beisel

HETEROTOPIC CARDIAC TRANSPLANTATION

Heterotopic, or auxiliary heart transplantation, has been championed by C. N. Barnard, M.D., and his colleagues in Capetown, Republic of South Africa. With their technique, the circulation of the patient is bypassed without interfering with the existing function of the patient's own heart. The basic concept of heterotopic heart transplantation has been critically analyzed at those institutions that perform primarily orthotopic heart transplantation, and the technique does have some merit, particularly when the patient requires immediate transplantation and the only available donor heart is too small for orthotopic heart transplantation. A major disadvantage, however, is the need for continuous anticoagulation therapy postoperatively.

The donor heart is removed by the same technique as described for orthotopic heart transplantation. The only modification necessary is the requirement for closure of the inferior vena cava and the provision for a suitable length of superior vena cava from the donor for anastomosis to the recipient superior vena cava.

Fig 24–2, A.—The recipient is placed on cardiopulmonary bypass, using the same technique as described for orthotopic heart transplantation. The left atrium is opened near the superior vena cava at the level of its junction with the right superior pulmonary vein. The incision is carried inferiorly to a level just below the entrance of the inferior vena cava into the right atrium. A side-to-side anastomosis is performed using a double-armed, simple running suture of 3–0 Prolene.

B.—The completed roof of the left atrial anastomosis is shown.

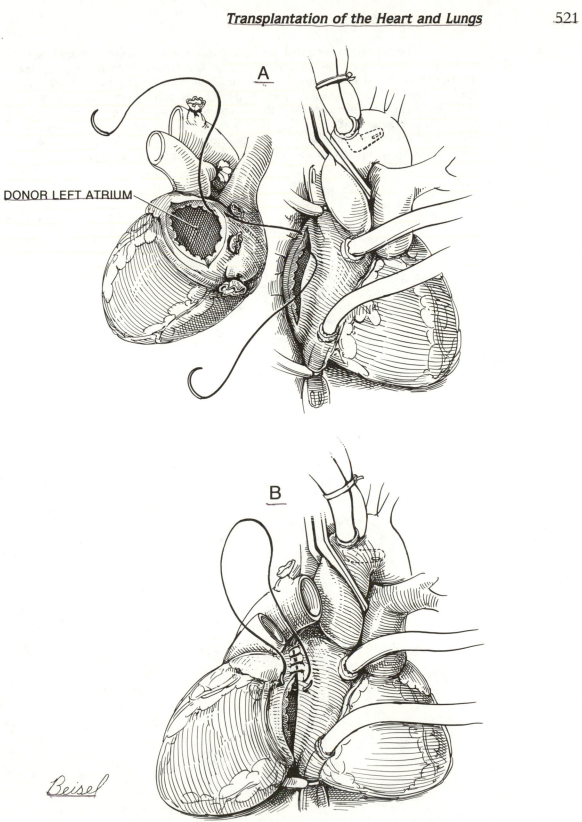

A

DONOR LEFT ATRIUM

B

Beisel

C.—The operation is carried out by anastomosing the donor's ascending aorta to the side of the recipient's ascending aorta. Next, the remnant of the donor's superior vena cava is anastomosed to the side of the recipient's superior vena cava. A third anastomosis is performed between the donor's pulmonary artery and the side of the recipient's main pulmonary artery, employing an appropriate-sized Dacron tube graft for length, if necessary. It is sometimes possible to avoid using graft material by preserving the donor's right pulmonary artery to the hilum of the lung and connecting it directly to the recipient's main pulmonary artery.

C

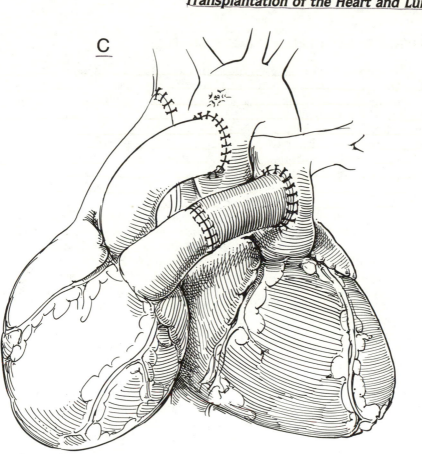

Beisel

COMBINED HEART AND LUNG TRANSPLANTATION

With the advent of cyclosporine immunosuppressive therapy, Bruce A. Reitz, M.D., and his associates at Stanford University conducted intense research in the field of combined heart and lung transplantation and devised a new life-saving procedure for a number of patients with a variety of devastating diseases. His improved operative technique for heart and lung transplantation includes saving the right atrium of the recipient to create a large atrial cuff to provide inflow to the heart and lung bloc, thereby eliminating the separate and time-consuming anastomosis of the vena cava. The three-anatomosis technique of heart and lung allograft implantation ensures preservation of the sinus node in the donor organ and the preservation of the recurrent laryngeal, vagus, and phrenic nerves.

Fig 24–3, A.—Cardiopulmonary bypass is established using the standard technique for orthotopic heart transplantation. Two venous cannulas and one high ascending aortic cannula are used for bypass. Resection of the anterior pericardium precedes the institution of cardiopulmonary bypass. The heart and lungs are removed. Care is taken not to injure the right and left phrenic nerves, the anterior vagus nerve on the esophagus, and the recurrent laryngeal nerve around the aortic arch. The heart and right and left lungs are removed separately to protect these important nerve structures adequately. In this situation, the heart is excised in a manner similar to that for removal for orthotopic heart transplantation. Pedicles of the right and left phrenic nerves are formed by incising the pericardium both anteriorly and posteriorly 2 cm away from the nerves and parallel to them. The pedicles must extend from the apex of the chest to the innervation of the diaphragm. In removing the heart and lungs en bloc, a portion of the pulmonary artery is left in situ near the recurrent laryngeal nerve to avoid injury to this nerve structure.

When the heart and lungs are removed separately, the heart is removed, and the pulmonary veins entering the left atrium are oversewn with running 4–0 Prolene sutures, while the pulmonary veins and pulmonary arteries are ligated individually and the stumps of tissue are left in place. In this technique, the bronchi are transected separately, and the stumps are clamped to prevent contamination. The trachea is transected just above the carina, and the small segment of distal trachea, with its bronchial stumps, is removed.

B.—The donor heart and lungs are brought onto the field, and the right lung is swung beneath the caval–right atrial remnant and the right phrenic nerve to lie in the right pleural space. The left lung is placed beneath the left phrenic nerve to lie in the left pleural space.

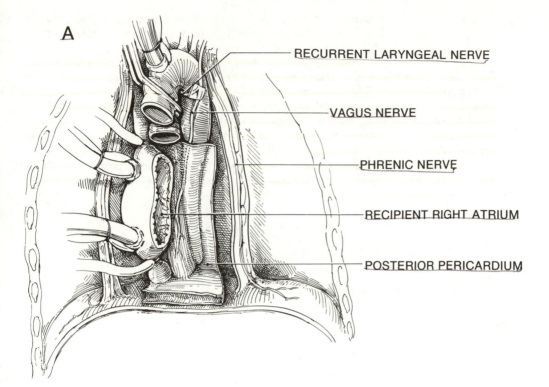

A

RECURRENT LARYNGEAL NERVE

VAGUS NERVE

PHRENIC NERVE

RECIPIENT RIGHT ATRIUM

POSTERIOR PERICARDIUM

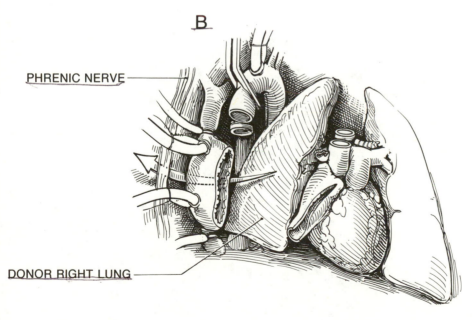

B

PHRENIC NERVE

DONOR RIGHT LUNG

C.—All anastomoses are carried out with double-armed 3–0 Prolene suture in simple running fashion. The first anastomosis to be performed is the tracheal anastomosis, as shown in this drawing.

D.—The second anastomosis to be performed is the right atrial anastomosis. An incision is made in the donor right atrium exactly as described for orthotopic heart transplantation. The incision is carried from the inferior vena cava toward an area anterior to the junction of the superior vena cava and the right atrium. The superior vena cava is ligated and oversewn as previously described for donor heart procurement. At the completion of this anastomosis, rewarming is begun and continued until the temperature reaches 37°C.

E.—While rewarming progresses the aortic anastomosis is performed. When this anastomosis is finished, the aorta is de-aired as the cross-clamp is removed.

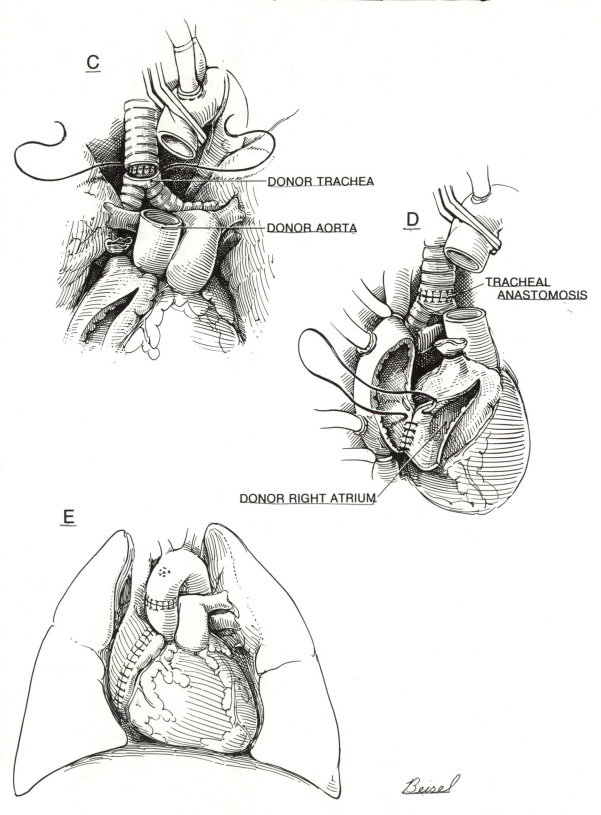

C

DONOR TRACHEA

DONOR AORTA

D

TRACHEAL
ANASTOMOSIS

DONOR RIGHT ATRIUM

E

Beisel

INDEX